INTRODUCTION TO
Nursing

THIRD EDITION

INTRODUCTION TO
Nursing

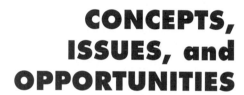

CONCEPTS, ISSUES, and OPPORTUNITIES

Janice B. Lindberg, RN, MA, PhD
Associate Professor of Nursing, Emerita and Former Associate Dean for Student Affairs
The University of Michigan School of Nursing, Ann Arbor, Michigan

Mary Love Hunter, RN, MS
Assistant Professor of Nursing
The University of Michigan School of Nursing, Ann Arbor, Michigan

Ann Z. Kruszewski, RN, MSN
Assistant Professor of Nursing
The University of Michigan School of Nursing, Ann Arbor, Michigan

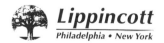
Lippincott
Philadelphia • New York

Acquisitions Editor: Susan Keneally
Assistant Editor: Stacy Jumper
Project Editor: Jahmae Harris
Production Manager: Helen Ewan
Production Coordinator: Mike Carcel
Design Coordinator: Doug Smock
Indexer: Nancy Newman

Edition 3

Library of Congress Cataloging in Publications Data

Lindberg, Janice B.
    Introduction to nursing : concepts, issues, and opportunities /
Janice B. Lindberg, Mary Love Hunter, Ann Z. Kruszewski. -- 3rd ed.
        p.   cm.
    Includes bibliographical references and index.
    ISBN 0-7817-9199-5 (alk. paper)
    1. Nursing.   I. Hunter, Mary Love.   II. Kruszewski, Ann Z.
III. Title.
    [DNLM: 1. Nursing.   WY 16 L742i 1998]
    RT41.L728   1998
    610.73--dc21
    DNLM/DLC
    for Library of Congress   97-35556
                                                              CIP

Care has been taken to confirm the accuracy of the information presented and to describe generally accepted practices. However, the authors, editors, and publisher are not responsible for errors or omissions or for any consequences from application of the information in this book and make no warranty, express or implied, with respect to the contents of the publication.

The authors, editors and publisher have exerted every effort to ensure that drug selection and dosage set forth in this text are in accordance with current recommendations and practice at the time of publication. However, in view of ongoing research, changes in government regulations, and the constant flow of information relating to drug therapy and drug reactions, the reader is urged to check the package insert for each drug for any change in indications and dosage and for added warnings and precautions. This is particularly important when the recommended agent is a new or infrequently employed drug.

Some drugs and medical devices presented in this publication have Food and Drug Administration (FDA) clearance for limited use in restricted research settings. It is the responsibility of the health care provider to ascertain the FDA status of each drug or device planned for use in their clinical practice.

9   8   7   6   5   4   3   2   1

Reviewers

Jean M. Dickes, RN, MS
Assistant Professor
Department of Nursing
Nebraska Methodist College of Nursing and Allied Health
Omaha, Nebraska

Norma J. Anderson, RN, BSN, MSN, EdD (candidate)
Assistant Professor
Nursing
Saint Anthony College of Nursing
Rockford, Illinois

Preface

The authors believe that an introductory text does not water down important professional ideas. Nursing is a caring science and how you learn and think about the important ideas in nursing is as important as how you learn to do any nursing activities. As a student you need to understand the concepts, issues and expectations of your profession. One reason you need to know this information early is to take action to shape your professional life in a way that is meaningful to you personally. The authors also expect you to be an active learner working to develop the basic skills needed for your profession. These basic skills include reading, writing, computer literacy, library search and interpersonal skills with peers and teachers as well as with clients.

Decisive changes in health care economics, delivery and staffing have occurred since the first revised edition of *Introduction to Nursing: Challenges, Issues and Opportunities.* The recent shifts to managed care and community based service are dramatic. While overall numbers of RNs have decreased in some settings, numbers of advanced practice nurses have increased in others. Although initial attempts at massive government reform of health care failed, health care reform continues both publicly and privately. Committed nurses of all educational levels, working with an increasingly sophisticated public, can accelerate substantive reform that maximizes community based health care and balances humane care with prudent economics. Additionally, advances in technology and electronic media are revolutionizing communications, health care and education in all settings. Access to information for both students and the general public has exploded. Amid these changes, the diversity of persons entering nursing continues. Today the community of nursing is both the local and the global community.

In this revision, all chapters have been updated. More active readers will recognize that our philosophical perspectives and critical thinking suggestions are intended to stimulate further individual exploration with colleagues and also through multiple media sources. Chapter 1, The Practice and Profession of Nursing, has been revised to introduce critical thinking, a concept that receives greater emphasis in Chapter 3, Nursing Today: The Health Science of Caring. Nurses need both critical thinking and leadership skills to supervise less prepared personnel and to assume advanced practice roles. Chapters 6, Health, and 7, Health Care Delivery, reflect recent changes in thought and practice. The concept of health is central to nursing science. Further, promoting, restoring, and maintaining health is vital to managed care. The relationship between clients' personal behaviors and health consequences grows more evident daily.

Chapter 9, Interpersonal Communication in Nursing, has been refocused to emphasize the communication skills that are used with both clients and colleagues. In Chapter 10, Learning and Teaching, greater emphasis has been placed on the nurse's role in furthering lifelong learning for both clients and self. The strategies for career development and lifelong learning have been expanded in Chapter 12, Opportunities and Challenges. Throughout the book, additional examples reflect the actual experiences of both practitioners and students.

A nursing student who had considerable international travel experience during her undergraduate education offered the following "Advice to students":

> Getting involved in nursing organizations and international nursing can be fun and rewarding but it is important to know how to manage your time and be careful not to overextend yourself. If you want to be involved, it is a good idea to talk to faculty, community leaders and other students about what opportunities are there. Make sure you keep your eyes and ears open for anything that might interest you. Use the resources at your school and in your community such as faculty members, University offices and international students. Do not be afraid to be creative or take initiative—write organizations for information, make contacts on the internet or get a group of students together who have the same interests as you have and work as a group. Keep a positive attitude! Sometimes it gets difficult to keep everything organized but stick with it because the rewards are worth it. To also help avoid burnout, get involved in activities that you truly enjoy. It is hard to motivate yourself if you do not really enjoy what you are doing. Most important, do not let anyone tell you that you are too young or inexperienced to be involved—you are a bright person with new ideas from which any organization could benefit!
>
> *Mary Pohanka (SN4)*

The authors believe that her advice captures the spirit with which this book was written. Whether you choose to be an armchair citizen of the global community or experience international travel personally, her advice could enrich your professional education.

Bon Voyage!

Janice B. Lindberg, RN, MA, PhD
Mary L. Hunter, RN, MS, CS
Ann Z. Kruszewski, RN, MSN

Acknowledgments

The authors gratefully express appreciation to certain individuals who offered special expertise:

Terry Allor, MPH, BS, faculty colleague, shared a lived experience in the Navajo culture.

Adem Arslani (SN_4 and computer consultant) contributed infectious enthusiasm about educational TV and potential internet resources for nursing students as well as innovative clinical suggestions for the use of videoconferencing technology.

Susan Boehm, RN, PhD, FAAN, faculty colleague and Associate Dean for Student Affairs at The University of Michigan School of Nursing, shared a research application of a computerized client/health professional communication.

Patricia Coleman-Burns, PhD, Director of the Office of Multicultural Affairs, The University of Michigan School of Nursing, reviewed and provided substantive suggestions on the cultural environment section as well as general wisdom and willingness to enlighten our cultural perspective.

Sandra Garr, RN, MSN, Assistant Professor of Nursing, The University of Michigan, shared her perspective on nursing's past.

Margaret Idour, long-time nurse educator and professional colleague, supplied an international perspective from New Zealand.

Michael Koteles, a former colleague now deceased, shared the lived experience of a person with AIDS so that nurses might know first-hand how they could demonstrate their caring.

Nina Lovern, BSN, RN, C, CDE, Patient Education Coordinator at Margaret R. Pardee Memorial Hospital, Hendersonville, North Carolina, reviewed the chapter Learning and Teaching.

Danyelle Lundy, offered an original and introspective poem written from an African American cultural perspective.

Bob Lupton, computer wizard and mentor extraordinaire, generously volunteered invaluable technical assistance.

Lillian M. Simms, RN, PhD, FAAN, Emerita and Associate Professor of Nursing, The University of Michigan, contributed her ideas about nursing's future.

Margaret R. Pardee Memorial Hospital, Hendersonville, North Carolina, through the sleuthing of Mary Ann Mooers, Director of Marketing and Public Relations, graciously provided photographs. Nina Lovern, Patient Education Coordinator and Peg Price, RN, MSA, CNAA, CHE, Chief Nurse Executive, also of Margaret R. Pardee Memorial Hospital, facilitated use of a Patient/Family Education Record that reflected the authors' philosophy of personalized care. Other photographs were furnished by The University of Michigan Hospital's Office of Planning and Marketing through the special assistance of Kristen Lidke Finn and also Randy Wendt.

Undergraduate students who have used the text offered student experiences that provide both credibility and remarkable insight. They are Jeffrey Adams, Nancy Bidlack, Andy Chan, Jennifer Jorrison, Lynn Michalski, Monica Patel. Mary Pohanka, Sonia Pritchard, Dave Svenson, and Katie Winnell.

Registered Nurses and R.N. students also contributed substantive examples, many that illustrated theory applications. They are Sharon Coyle, Ashling Farelly, Lisa Fulford, Pamela Giles, Betsy Hilton, Amy Hudson, Dorothy Morton, Kimberly Kenny-Sherlock, and Maricar Uy. Laura Knight, a Physical Therapy student, also contributed.

The authors have particularly appreciated the efforts and suggestions of the following persons: Acquisitions Editor, Susan Keneally; Assistant Editor, Stacy Jumper; and Project Editor, Jahmae Harris.

Once again, we offer a special thank-you to our families whose patience and lasting support have sustained us.

Contents

9
Interpersonal Communication in Nursing and Health Care *291*

10
Learning and Teaching *325*

11
Nursing Ethics and Legal Aspects *351*

PART FOUR

12
Opportunities and Challenges *395*

Part One

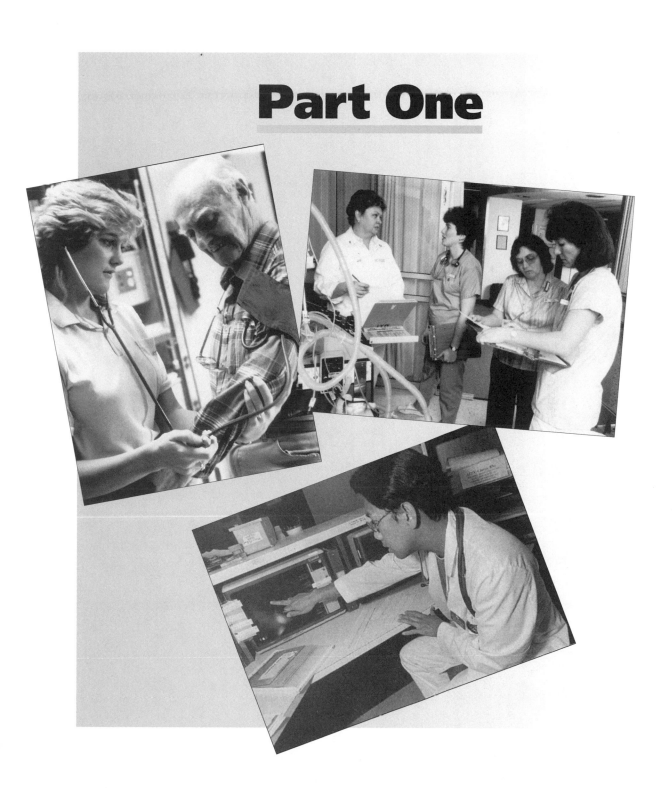

The Practice and Profession of Nursing

Key Words

Client	Health	Nursing process	Virtual reality
Critical thinking	Illness	Patient	Wellness
Environment	Leadership	Person	

Objectives

After completing this chapter, students will be able to:

Identify the expertise of the nursing profession.

Define critical thinking and leadership.

Identify common elements in several leaders' definitions of nursing.

Explain the concepts of caring and critical thinking in relation to nursing practice.

Identify the elements of person-centered nursing care.

Identify how caring relates to the concepts basic to nursing practice.

Can you tell which occupation meets the following criteria?

Is both new and old
Claims elements of art, science, and profession
Offers lifelong career opportunities without the requisite of changing fields
Serves society's health and well-being
Offers participation in life's major events
Offers interpersonal interaction in a high-technology world
Develops self-understanding
Provides immeasurable personal satisfaction

Confronts issues of humanism, ethics, legalities, and economics that shape
  public policy
Encourages entrepreneurs in the business of health
Offers wide diversity of career possibilities
Claims professional care as its area of expertise

Nursing certainly can be an answer to the preceding question. Advanced
practice nurses currently are a scarce human resource in society. Although professional nurses are generally admired by persons who have benefited directly from
their services, people who have not experienced nursing care directly often do
not understand nurses and their profession.

This text is an introduction to the nursing profession. Many ideas exist
about nursing. Common to many definitions of nursing is the idea of helping
persons. Throughout history, the potential for helping has been shaped by the
influences of society, by forces within the health care delivery system, and by
visions within nursing. Today, this helping potential takes many forms and is
bounded partly by the vision of nurses themselves and the dramatically changed
health care delivery system. Indeed, nursing today is both like and unlike
nursing of the past.

Nursing, which has always been the art of caring, is becoming known as the
health science of caring. In the past, it was nurses who most often were at the
bedside of ill persons. Although grateful patients acknowledged nurses' skill in
promoting, maintaining, and restoring health, nurses' unique expertise for health
received little emphasis.

Some of today's nurses remain at the bedside. The need for their expertise
in caring for ill persons continues. Traditionally, and in many ways, nursing
has emphasized its technical aspects. Currently, however, professional nursing
practice has room and need for greater creativity. Such innovation occurs at the
bedside and elsewhere. Nurses with advanced practice skills practice in both acute
care settings and out in the community. Today's nurses also enjoy practice opportunities as creative entrepreneurs, managers, administrators, teachers, and research scientists. Practice at different levels accommodates individual nurse interests, diverse ability levels, and varying career investments. Practice at any level
provides an important service to society and requires critical thinking.

Thinking is a primary skill for all scientific disciplines and professions. While
most of us may assume that nurses are thinking practitioners, one might suggest
that thinking has sometimes been underrated as a basic skill in our discipline.
Thinking is both a basic cognitive skill and a behavioral action. Meleis (1991),
a nursing leader, has written, "**Critical thinking** lies in the balance between
framework thinking and flexible viewing of a situation" (p. 123).

Framework thinking is thinking based on a generally accepted framework
of information or body of knowledge. Different sciences use different bodies
of knowledge on which to base their frameworks. Some life sciences, like
nursing, apply knowledge from several basic sciences in addition to developing
their own unique sciences. Knowledge of both basic and applied sciences is
organized in conceptual frameworks. Conceptual frameworks provide structures
for managing scientific or factual details, and for enabling persons to think

about information logically. Concepts also organize information to help us think both abstractly and concretely. The process of thinking in this logical and organized way involves deductive and inductive reasoning, the process of going from abstracts to specifics and vice-versa. This process is sometimes referred to as vertical thinking. Allowing oneself to think outside or beyond this vertical framework is sometimes called lateral thinking, flexibility or creativity. Critical thinking, as suggested by Meleis, combines both logical and creative thinking. Critical thinking is a professional skill that combines framework thinking and flexible viewing. Professional nurses use critical thinking in both clinical decision-making and professional leadership.

Leadership by nurses is needed for both nursing and health care. As Kelly (1991) said, leadership in many ways defies definition, but "in its simplest context, it is the ability to influence others, to lead, guide and direct" (p. 356). Nurses believe that they know many ways to lead their clients to better health, and many ways to guide the health care industry toward improved health care delivery. To extend these ideas beyond the nursing profession will require the persuasive demonstration of both critical thinking and leadership by large numbers of nurses.

The skills of critical thinking and leadership are not developed miraculously, nor are they developed without considerable effort on the part of learners and teachers. This text will assist you in developing critical thinking and leadership skills by giving you some of the means to empower yourself. First, you need the structure or framework for understanding nursing as science, art and profession. You need to understand the key words and ideas that form the structure or *metaparadigm* of nursing. The metaparadigm encompasses the broad concepts that prevail in the discipline, regardless of one's specific theoretical approach to the content of the science. You will need to be able to organize information to recognize patterns and to understand relationships. These skills require not only obtaining the information in the first place, but also taking time to reflect upon what the information means concretely and specifically, and also more generally or abstractly. Thinking abstractly is usually the more difficult skill to learn, because we may not have had obviously similar real life experiences on which to base our thinking. Further, some persons feel an initial resistance to reflection or abstract thinking, because many people come to nursing convinced that it should involve mostly learning and performing technical skills.

Upon reflection and with further investigation, nurses usually come to understand that critical thinking in nursing involves basic knowledge as well as the process of transferring and applying information to novel situations. An example of the latter is applying abstract or theoretical concepts to new clinical experiences which are the actual *doing* activities that may have attracted you to the profession in the first place. In classroom simulations, in tests, and in clinical situations, you will be asked not only to apply information and to analyze new situations, but also to synthesize or form new wholes from information of multiple sources. Clinical situations, because they involve unique persons and circumstances, are seldom routine. You will probably use case studies, and possibly **virtual reality,** to test hypothetically your diagnostic reasoning in the classroom. Virtual reality includes interactive audiovisual presentations via computer that enable a viewer to participate in realistic simulations of actual or imagined situations for entertainment or educational experience. Later, you will be expected to evaluate both your thinking and your application in clinical practice activities. Faculty will evaluate your thinking through your communications, both verbal and written, and also by your clinical performance. Beginning with this chapter, you will note that key terms and concepts are identified for you; you will be asked to apply these in many ways. The critical thinking questions that conclude each chapter give you the opportunity to begin individual exploration as the lifelong learner you are expected to become.

Now that we have described critical thinking in a formal way, a clinical example may help to clarify the concept.

Example: Note that as the nurse provides this example, she offers commentary on critical thinking as well.

Kerry who is 28 years old was hit from behind by a car after she stepped out of her car to check a flat tire. She sustained a fractured femur, pelvis and humerus (upper arm) and was now on our trauma step down unit. Her parents stayed with her continuously and were very anxious. Kerry was occasionally cheerful, but more often tearful and exhausted.

One evening I brought Kerry's pain medications and noticed immediately that she was pale and diaphoretic (perspiring heavily). My first concrete thought was to ask for her pain score. She said it was 3-4 on a scale of 10. I continued with concrete observations by taking her vital signs. Her blood pressure and respirations were within normal limits and her pulse oximetry (a measure of oxygenation) was a normal 98%. Her pulse, however, was bounding at 148 (normal = about 60-88). My next concrete observation was to check her urinary output. She did not have a catheter (continuous drainage through a tube). Moving into a more formal thinking mode, I wondered if she had been voiding (excreting) small amounts frequently indicating a full bladder. According to her chart, however, her output had been adequate over the past few days. I also checked her recent bowel movements. Long periods in bed can cause impactions (severe retention) that may alter vital signs. Again, her chart and her verbal report indicated normal output. This assessment took about five minutes.

I then considered what else might be happening. I knew that she could be bleeding internally or that she might have a pulmonary embolus (a blood flow blockage in the lung). In other words my reasoning was both deductive and inductive as I considered the pattern of the specific data and then formed a more abstract conclusion. My assessment, however, indicated a third possibility: as my thinking became more abstract, I checked her chart again for high pulse rates during the past several weeks she had been with us. I noted that frequently her pulse would reach the high 130s and often settled between 100 and 120. Although tachycardiac (abnormally fast), these rates were less alarming. Her father, sensing something was wrong, became increasingly agitated, needing reassurance and asking if I was going to call the doctor. I assured him that I would call the doctor when I had complete data that would help us make decisions.

The third possibility I was considering was extreme anxiety. I had known Kerry to be anxious before. Because her vital signs were normal except for the pulse, pallor and diaphoresis, I was fairly certain that this was a good possibility. I considered how vulnerable Kerry felt after being hit so unexpectedly and having her life disrupted. She was now both in

(continued)

pain and worrying about future surgery. In the past, these periods of anxiety seemed to come on her suddenly and without any apparent stimulus. When I asked Kerry what I could do for her now, she replied that she would like her usual evening Valium medication a little bit early. Although this request strengthened my opinion, I told Kerry that I must confer with the physician first, because Valium might obscure other problems. When considering this third possibility I had started with the abstract concept of anxiety and worked deductively to determine the specifics. The physician asked me the same questions I had asked myself. We discussed the fact that Kerry had experienced other tachycardic episodes and that she had been healthy prior to her injury. We decided that I would hold the Valium, check her during the next hour and then call the doctor back. This was a collaborative conversation that occurred easily because I had organized the data from a physiological framework.

Kerry's pulse did not change during that hour, and she continued to ask for her Valium. I talked calmly with her, frequently changing the cool cloth for her forehead and generally reassuring her. Kerry's father paced anxiously while I concluded that additional abstract thinking was needed. I told myself, Patience! Think Maslow, think Erik Erickson, think Helen Erickson and Jean Watson (see Chapters 3 and 4). I reminded myself of how vulnerable both Kerry and her parents felt. Their safety and security needs were unmet; they were struggling with whom they could trust and often they felt abandoned and helpless. They clearly saw their hold on control as weak. My thinking at this point was more abstract and within the frameworks of several theorists. In addition, I kept my concrete physiologic framework in mind, should Kerry show further signs of bleeding or embolus.

At the end of the hour I went through my concrete assessment again, found no changes except for a slight decrease in Kerry's pulse and so called the physician. The Dr. said to give her the Valium but to watch her closely. Again we were able to collaborate and conclude that no further expensive tests i.e., blood work or x-rays, were needed. This conclusion provided the added benefit of being cost effective.

Kerry was asleep within moments after I gave the Valium—sooner than it could have worked. She recognized, however, that relief had come. My observation of acute anxiety was probably correct: her condition remained stable and her pulse rate decreased throughout the night. Before I left that shift, however, I described my thinking so that the next nurse would continue to assess Kerry holistically. In this way I demonstrated clinical leadership by providing the nurse with a framework for organizing her own data. I appreciate receiving similar information from the nurse preceding me, because collaboration is enhanced and efficiency improved.

After this episode, and as I continued to work with Kerry, I planned her care to avoid provoking anxiety episodes. Interventions related to this goal included altering the environment according to her mood, ensuring that visitors did not stay too long, encouraging her parents to get more rest, and washing her hair frequently. Washing her hair kept her looking attractive for her fiancé and gave her a sense of being cared for and valued.

Note the movement of my thinking from concrete to abstract at first, and then the use of both modes as we moved away from the immediate crisis. I used many of nursing's technical skills as well. Note too that after working with many theories, both from nursing and other fields, I no longer need to reference them each time. Just reminding myself of Maslow, for example, enables me to move away from my own fatigue and impatience, and use a theoretical foundation. The interventions, while relatively simple in themselves, are based on both creative and logical thinking about my client's needs and concerns. Since I engaged Kerry frequently in her own care, I also empowered her, and that helped increase her sense of control and self-esteem.

In this chapter, we present an overview of nursing, both from our own perspectives and from the writings of acknowledged nursing leaders. This chapter also discusses concepts essential to nursing as a science: nursing, person, environment, and health. Additional concepts related to the practice of nursing within the health care delivery system are defined: nursing process, communication, learning and teaching, nursing ethics, and legal aspects of practice. Critical thinking, as a way of both thinking and doing, lays a foundation for translating all these basic concepts to practice. The translation of these concepts to a high standard of excellence gives nurses practice in providing exemplary care that can be a leadership example for nursing and health care.

Before beginning a detailed discussion of the individual concepts, it is important to understand clearly how these concepts relate to nursing. However, we first need to have a firm understanding of nursing. Beginning nursing students may be saying to themselves, "But I know what nursing is. I learned that from my relative who is a nurse [or from books, television, volunteer work in hospitals, guidance counselors, and so forth]." When asked to define nursing, most beginning students respond that it involves helping people. Our own concept of nursing is similar: we believe that the essence of nursing is caring for persons. This is the approach to nursing that inspired this textbook. We hope to provide our readers with an appreciation of the philosophy that underlies this text similar to the appreciation reported by the student in the following example.

Upon entering this class, I had a very limited view of nursing, and no appreciation of its history, or its future for that matter. The biggest insight I gained in this course was about my personal view and how narrow it had been. I had this stereotype of the hospital or doctor's office nurse. I had no idea that home health care was such a growing area, nor did I realize the importance of advanced practice nurses, especially in light of health care reform. Nurses are employed in virtually every setting, and their roles are much broader than I realized. They work in schools, communities, homes, with families and individuals, and as educators, researchers, and practitioners. The whole emphasis on health promotion and prevention was also relatively new to me, because I assumed I would be working with sick people rather than teaching well people how to maintain health. Finally, while I had some idea that nurses used a holistic approach, I lacked full appreciation of the implications of such an approach. I now realize the necessity of assessing the psychosocial, developmental, spiritual, cultural and physical aspects of the individual, because all these components contribute to health and wellness. Related to this, I have a new appreciation for the meaning of client-centered care. (Jennifer Jorrison, SN3)

Person-Centered Nursing Care

Many professions exist in society. Among this wide array, nursing is viewed as one of the health professions. Although the term *profession* has many common meanings, some writers have tried to define it more strictly. True professions are generally defined as having a body of knowledge on which expert skills and

TABLE 1-1 *Professionals and Their Fields of Expertise*

Professional	Expertise
Lawyer	Law
Pastor or minister	Spirituality
Physician or doctor	Illness, disease
Psychologist	Mind, behavior
Social worker	Societal support systems
Nurse	Caring for persons

services are based. Other criteria related to professional status are discussed in detail in Chapter 2. Table 1-1 lists some of the groups that are considered professions and identifies their expertise.

The emergence of professional nursing is usually attributed to the influence of Florence Nightingale, who practiced in the last half of the 19th century. Thus, nursing as a profession is relatively young compared with other professions. Nursing is an emerging profession, working to fulfill the criteria that define a profession. What is the expertise that nursing claims? It is, as you will discover, caring for persons—caring for individuals, families, and persons in the aggregate, that is, distinct individuals in a community group.

Caring as a Basis for Nursing

Nurses constantly use the term caring: "I'm caring for seven patients today," "Mr. Jones needs complete care," "Ms. Smith doesn't require much care." The term *caring*, however, is used in this text with a specific meaning in mind. Caring involves more than just carrying out nursing procedures, such as bedmaking and treatments. True caring is based on an attitude of nurturing, of helping another person to grow. Mayeroff (1971), a philosopher who explored the nature of caring, stated, "To care for another person, in the most significant sense, is to help him grow and actualize himself" (p. 1). He continued, "In caring, I experience the other as having potentialities and the need to grow" (p. 6).

A nurse–theorist, Jean Watson (1979), described nursing as the science of caring. She contrasted care with cure: with cure activities, the end is treatment and elimination of disease, whereas with caring, one assists persons to grow toward their potential.

> Human care . . . consists of transpersonal human to human attempts to protect, enhance, and preserve humanity by helping a person find meaning in **illness,** suffering, pain, and existence; to help another gain self-knowledge, control, and self-healing wherein a sense of inner harmony is restored regardless of the external circumstances. (Watson, 1985, p. 54)

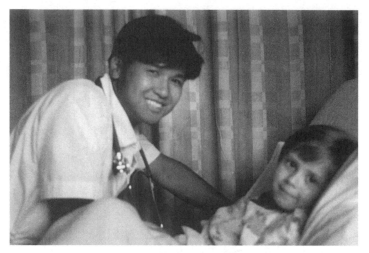

"Of all the nursing interventions that I do, it is basic caring that matters most."

Watson (1989) identified factors that are integral to the caring process, including:

❏ Cultivation of sensitivity to one's self and others
❏ Development of a helping—trusting, human caring relationship
❏ Promotion and acceptance of the expression of positive and negative feelings
❏ Provision for a supportive, protective, and corrective mental, physical, sociocultural, and spiritual environment
❏ Assistance with gratification of human needs (pp. 227–228)

Chapter 3 describes Watson's theory of caring in further detail.

Leininger, a nursing leader, believed that caring is essential to human development, growth, and survival. Leininger (1981, p. 13) described the following caring behaviors:

❏ Comfort
❏ Compassion
❏ Concern
❏ Coping behavior
❏ Empathy
❏ Enabling
❏ Facilitating
❏ Health consultative acts
❏ Health instructive acts
❏ Health maintenance acts
❏ Helping behavior
❏ Interest
❏ Involvement
❏ Love

❐ Nurturance
❐ Presence
❐ Protective behaviors
❐ Restorative behaviors
❐ Sharing
❐ Stimulating behaviors
❐ Stress alleviation
❐ "Succorance"
❐ Support
❐ Surveillance
❐ Tenderness
❐ Touching
❐ Trust

The expression of caring varies across cultures. The priority of a caring behavior, its form of expression, and the needs that the behavior satisfies may differ from culture to culture.

Caring nurses recognize that persons have strengths as well as needs, and that they possess worth and growth potential. Rather than seeing persons as helpless because they need care, caring nurses respect persons as autonomous. Caring nurses assist persons because of a desire to foster growth and independence. They want to enhance their clients' abilities to manage their own health needs as a result of the care received. As Mayeroff (1971) said, "To help another person grow . . . is to help that other person come to care for himself" (p. 10).

Definitions of Nursing

Thoughts on the caring nature of nursing are reflected in many nursing leaders' definitions of nursing. Table 1-2 summarizes definitions of nursing from Nightingale (1859), Henderson (1966), King (1981), Roy (1984), Orem (1984), and Martha Rogers (1970). The theme of helping or caring is inherent in each of their definitions. Likewise, other common themes in these writings are the nature of persons, environment, and health—the concepts on which this text is based.

Because nursing as a science and profession is experiencing evolutional growth of its own, we feel there is no single definition of nursing. You might develop a new definition of your own while reading this text. Whatever your definition, we hope that the element of caring for or nurturing persons is a motivation for your interest in nursing.

None of these thoughts on the definition of nursing is new. Nurses have always valued the idea of caring for persons; this idea attracts many nurses to the profession. Unfortunately, nurses sometimes lose sight of this goal in the reality of practice. For example, beginning students, at times, may find that they are so concerned about their own nursing skills that they forget to consider the anxieties of the person for whom they are caring. Even experienced nurses may become so overwhelmed by the complex technology involved in nursing care, or

TABLE 1-2 *Definitions of Nursing and Thoughts on Caring*

Definition	Thoughts on Caring	Related Nursing Concepts
Nightingale		
It is quite surprising . . . how many behave as if the scientific end were the only one in view or as if the sick body were but a reservoir for storing medicines into and the surgical disease only a curious case the sufferer has made for the attendant's special information (1859, p 70). What nursing has to do . . . is put the patient in the best condition for nature to act upon him (p 75). Nursing . . . ought to signify the proper use of fresh air, light, warmth, cleanliness, quiet, and the proper selection and administration of diet—all at the least expense of vital power to the patient (p 6).	The patient, rather than the disease process, should be the primary focus of health professionals.	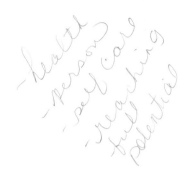
Henderson		
The unique function of the nurse is to assist the individual, sick or well, in the performance of those activities contributing to health or its recovery (or to peaceful death) that he would perform unaided if he had the necessary strength, will or knowledge. And to do this in such a way as to help him gain independence as rapidly as possible. This aspect of her work, this part of her function, she initiates and controls; of this she is master.	Caring is assisting persons in performance of activities they would accomplish independently given the necessary resources.	
King		
The focus of nursing is the care of human beings (1981, p 10). Nursing is defined as a process of action, reaction, and interaction whereby nurse and client share information about their perceptions in the nursing situation . . . leading to goal attainment (p 2). Nurses are concerned with human beings interacting with their environment in ways that lead to self-fulfillment and maintenance of health (p 3).	Caring for persons is the focus of nursing practice and is an interactive process.	Health is defined as dynamic life experiences of a human being which implies continuous adjustment to stressors in the internal and external environment through optimum use of one's resources to achieve maximum potential for daily living (p 5). Persons are open systems interacting with the environment (p 10).
Roy		
Nursing focuses on persons and how they maintain well-being and high-level functioning whether sick or well (1984,	The focus of nursing is persons and increasing their adaptive responses.	The person is an adaptive system (p 289). The environment is internal and external stimuli *(continued)*

TABLE 1-2 (Continued)

Definition	Thoughts on Caring	Related Nursing Concepts
Roy (continued)		
p 5). Nursing aims to increase persons' adaptive responses and to decrease ineffective responses. An adaptive response is behavior that maintains the integrity of the individual (p 37).		or all conditions, circumstances, and influences surrounding or affecting the development and behavior of persons and groups (p 28). Health is a state and a process of being and becoming an integrated and whole person (p 28).
Orem		
Nursing is deliberate action; a function of the practical intelligence of nurses . . . is action to bring about humanely desirable conditions in persons and their environments. Nursing is distinguished from other human services and other forms of care by the way in which it focuses on human beings, i.e., by its proper human object (1984, p 15). Nursing has as its special concern the individual's need for self-care action and the provision and management of it on a continuous basis in order to sustain life and health, recover from disease or injury, and cope with their effects (p 54).	Nursing's concern is persons and their self-care actions.	Health is used to describe living things when they are structurally and functionally whole or sound (p 173). The physical, psychological, interpersonal, and social aspects of health are inseparable in the individual (p 174). Each human being is a substantial or real unity whose parts are formed and attain perfection through differentiation of the whole during processes of development . . . (who moves) toward maturation and achievement of (his or her) human potential (pp 179–180)
Rogers		
Professional practice in nursing seeks to promote symphonic interaction between man and environment, to strengthen the coherence and integrity of the human field and to direct and redirect patterning of the human and environmental fields for realization and maximum health potential (M. E. Rogers, p. 122). Nursing exists to serve people (1970, p 122).	Caring involves promoting optimum human–environment interactions. Nursing's focus is human beings and their worth. *therapeutic touch*	Human beings are irreducible wholes that cannot be understood when reduced to their parts. Human beings and environment are energy fields that are integral with one another and are constantly evolving toward their higher potentials (M. E. Rogers, 1987, pp 141, 143).
Watson		
"Nursing in this context [science and discipline] may be defined as a human science of health–illness–healing experiences that are mediated by professional, personal, scientific, aesthetic, and ethical human transactions." (p 221)	"Nursing's social, moral, and scientific contributions to human kind and society lie in its commitment to human care ideals in theory, practice and research" (p 219)	

Both quotations from Watson, Jean (1989) Watson's Philosophy and theory of human caring in nursing. In Riehl-Sisca, J. (Ed.), *Conceptual Models for Nursing Practice* (3rd ed., pp. 219–236). Norwalk CT: Appleton & Lange.

by institutional demands, that they lose sight of the person who is the object of their activities. As one experienced nurse put it,

> "I had been teaching nursing for some time when I took a part time ICU [Intensive Care Unit] position. One day, early in my orientation, I was so caught up with the tubes, drugs and monitors that my preceptor finally had to say, 'your patient looks terribly uncomfortable.' I was embarrassed when I realized that she had slipped toward the bottom of the bed and was completely out of alignment."

Nursing texts frequently focus on concepts or techniques without considering how those techniques will relate to the persons who will benefit from them. For this reason, this text uses the term *"person-centered nursing"* as a reminder that caring for persons is the organizing focus for all aspects of nursing. Each of the concepts in the text is presented within this context. We have attempted to emphasize the person in each of our discussions, whether this means the nurse or the client.

Elements of Person-Centered Care

What is person-centered care? Carl Rogers provides many thoughts that can be applied to nursing. Rogers was a psychotherapist who challenged the traditional psychology focus on human behavior, particularly "abnormal" behavior. Rogers felt that, rather than emphasize what is wrong with a person, psychotherapists should concentrate on strengths to facilitate personal growth toward one's highest potential. He believed that all persons do not represent finished products but are, instead, in the process of "becoming"—that is, moving toward their potential. He also believed that persons move in a basically positive direction toward growth. Related to this belief is an appreciation of the value or worth of each person. Rogers stressed that facilitating optimal growth requires a strong interpersonal relationship between the therapist and the client. Through his experiences in psychotherapy, he came to believe "that it is the *client* who knows what hurts, what directions to go, what problems are crucial, what experiences have been deeply buried. It began to occur to me that . . . I would do better to rely upon the client for the direction of movement in the process"(C. R. Rogers, 1961, pp. 11–12). Thus, his "client-centered" approach to psychotherapy began.

Attributes of the therapist's use of a client-centered approach include the following:

❑ Trustworthiness
❑ Ability to communicate unambiguously (verbal behavior matches nonverbal behavior)
❑ A positive attitude toward the client built on a respect for the client's worth
❑ Ability to convey empathic understanding
❑ Acceptance of the client's feelings
❑ Ability to remain separate from the client (avoiding sympathy)
❑ Ability to allow the client to remain a separate person (avoiding taking over for the client)

❏ Acceptance of the client as a person in the process of becoming rather than as a fixed product or psychiatric diagnosis (C. R. Rogers, 1961, pp. 50–55)

Abraham Maslow, a psychologist who shared this humanistic view of persons, defined categories of basic needs ranging from the most fundamental (food, oxygen, shelter) to the highest level (self-actualization or the desire for self-fulfillment). Maslow's (1970) approach is also person centered because it focuses on assisting persons to meet basic needs, thereby freeing them to grow and achieve their potential.

Attributes of the Person-Centered Nurse

Many of the beliefs about nursing presented in this text evolved from the philosophies of Carl Rogers and Abraham Maslow. Because nursing is an interpersonal process, much of their work is applicable to our profession. We believe that nurses who give person-centered care will:

❏ Appreciate that each person is a unique product of heredity, environment, culture and spirituality. This means that we must interact with our clients on an individual basis, even though their health care needs may appear to be similar.
❏ Believe that persons strive for their highest potential. Nursing's function is to assist persons to achieve growth in relation to their health needs.
❏ Respect the worth of each individual. We appreciate each person's potential no matter how impoverished or ill he or she appears. We recognize that even the sickest or poorest of persons have strengths that can be mobilized to meet their needs and achieve their potential.
❏ Recognize our own humanity. Nurses are persons, too, with unique strengths and needs. To care effectively for others, nurses must have self-awareness to recognize both what they can offer another person and what their own personal limitations are.
❏ Be genuine. A nurse cannot be truly genuine without this self-awareness.
❏ Encourage the client to retain control. Nurses who are truly genuine and who are aware of and comfortable with their own feelings will be able to let clients be themselves. These nurses will not feel that they need to have authority over their clients, but instead will empower clients by engaging them in their own care (Patricia Coleman-Burns, personal communication, July 20, 1996). In other words, they will view clients as partners in the helping relationship. They will see the process of nursing as facilitating clients to meet their own needs. They will feel comfortable encouraging clients to express their needs freely and to set their own goals for nursing care.
❏ Recognize that persons have basic needs and are motivated to fulfill these needs. For this reason, a person's behavior is the result of his or her needs. This is an important idea, because it implies that each per-

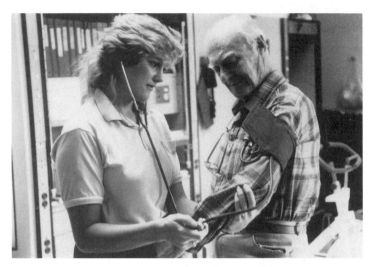

Person-centered care is nursing's unique contribution to the health professions.

son's behavior has meaning, no matter how different or "wrong" this behavior may appear.

❐ Realize all behavior has meaning. Nurses appreciate that a person's actions communicate messages about his or her feelings, beliefs, or physical functioning. The nurse respects the meaning of a person's behavior and avoids such labels as "wrong," "bad," or "weird," even though the behavioral manifestations may be perplexing or difficult.

Person-centered care can be given to any age group, from infancy through old age and from birth through death. This kind of caring is nursing's unique contribution to the health professions. What caring can mean to a client and how providing a caring experience can confirm your commitment to nursing are shared by a third-year student who wrote *On Becoming a Nurse*.

Example: It happens to all of us during our nursing education—an event, a moment so meaningful that you are profoundly changed. You are never the same again as a professional or a person. This is my moment. I want to share it with you, because I did not realize while it was happening to me that it was "my moment."

My level-3 clinical placement was with an instructor whose reputation preceded her. Words like "challenging opportunity" and "interesting teaching methods" were used to describe her. It was like describing a blind date as having a "good personality." I knew she would be tough, but I also knew that no one has ever had greater expectations of me than me.

The first day was a fiasco. She assigned me patient Betty Johnson, who was in hemodialysis and would not return to the floor until after preclinical time was over. Oh great! How was I supposed to do an interview and an assessment? And, of course, Ms. Johnson's daily chart and medical record had accompanied her to hemodialysis. The only information available to me was on the medication and nursing Kardexes.

I learned from the nursing Kardex that Ms. Johnson's medical diagnosis included gan-

(continued)

grene of the right lower extremity, with probable amputation, insulin-dependent diabetes mellitus, heart and renal disease, anemia, hypertension, uncompensated chronic metabolic acidosis, and two previous amputations. Oh, great again! This is my first "real" clinical experience. How am I supposed to take care of a person who is so sick? I needed to get more information about this patient, but how? I wanted to know more about her so I could give her the best possible care.

I decided to go to the patient's room to get a "sense" of who she was or what she was like. The room was empty except for a black overnight bag and a fuzzy pink sweater. There were no get-well cards or mementos to indicate family or friend support. This was strange since she had been admitted more than a week ago. I was becoming frustrated. I sighed and began to walk out of the room. Something bright in the corner caught my eye. It was her prosthetic limb. The flesh tone was dark, so I knew Ms. Johnson was a person of color. It was about the same size as my lower leg; we were probably the same height and weight. She must have a positive outlook despite her failing health, because the sock covering the foot part was bright red. I expected to see a very sick person with a good attitude.

Ms. Johnson was extremely ill indeed. She had a hypotensive crisis (extremely low blood pressure) in hemodialysis and was not feeling well at all. She was difficult to understand because she did not have teeth and was chewing a big wad of tobacco. She would not eat, even with assistance. Slowly, throughout the day, I was able to interview her and perform her physical assessment. My sense was that this patient needed one thing—to be cared for. I began by bathing her. She seemed to enjoy the bath; she would moan softly and sigh with pleasure. She said the warm water felt good. Then I decided to perform a full body therapeutic massage. The patient seemed to float. She repeated over and over how good it felt. She said "all of the people who come into this room either take something or hurt me, but you just give and make me feel good." I was embarrassed by her compliment, but I felt as though I had made a difference for her. I thought that what I did would help her to get well.

The next week I went back for my second assignment. I wanted to stop by to see how Betty was doing. I went to her room and she wasn't there. I found out that she had died two days before. I was shocked. I thought she would get better. I knew there would be a point in my career when I would have to deal with the death of a patient; I just didn't think it would be so soon. I cried. The only thought that helped me stop crying was that I knew I had made a difference for her. From this experience I learned that, of all the nursing interventions I perform, the basic caring ones are the ones that really matter. I promised myself that no matter how many technical tasks I had to perform throughout my workday, I would not forget to provide personal care.

I went home that night and shared my experience with my husband. I began to cry again and told him that I didn't know if I could be a good nurse, because I am emotionally affected by my patients. All he said was, "The day you stop being affected is the day you should stop being a nurse." I knew then that I had made the right decision to become a nurse. I will never forget that patient. I think of her fondly and I am grateful for the insights she gave me.

(*Michalski, L.* [written as an *SN3*]. *On becoming a nurse* [pp. 1–2]. *Unpublished manuscript.*)

The Person as a Recipient of Care: Patient Versus Client

Throughout this book, the word *person* is used when referring to anyone for whom nursing care is provided. Often, the word *client* also may be used and, occasionally, *patient.* There are some important distinctions to be made among these words, as indicated by their definitions.

The Patient

A **patient** is a person awaiting or under medical care and treatment, the recipient of any of various medical services. To be patient is to endure pains calmly and without complaint, to hold steadfast despite difficult circumstances.

These definitions of patient may help us realize that, although a person receiving health care and treatment may not behave in the manner described, that description represents what we, as health care providers, often expect. We wish our patients to be cooperative, to behave themselves, and generally to provide us with little trouble in this cumbersome business of getting them well. As you progress through the book, you may recognize that health care providers become distressed when their patients do not do as they are told. Keeping this idea in mind, we have attempted to underscore that the person receiving care is more healthy than ill, and more capable of strength than weakness. Persons who seek health care remain unique humans; although they share some characteristics with other persons, they nonetheless have their own individual thoughts, feelings, and ways of responding. That some persons may be patient during an illness is more characteristic of their individual personalities than of their roles as ill persons.

The Client

A **client** is a person who engages the professional advice or services of another; a person served by or utilizing the services of an agency. That is, a client contracts for services from another person who is qualified to provide those services. There is an assumption that the relationship is a negotiated partnership, and that clients are capable of taking the information provided and using it in some fashion. Should they decide it is useless, they generally feel free to take their business elsewhere. Although some persons approach health care with this sense of independence, most simply do as they are told, including going into the hospital when so directed. They may feel incapable of physically taking their business and moving elsewhere. That we, as health care providers, are well aware of this passive type of response is reflected in the name we have so frequently given these persons—*patients*—and the way in which we have often assumed control over so many facets of their lives.

You may not be aware that this inequitable relationship often exists between a person and the health services provider. We suggest that you accept the challenge to note this inequality as you explore the world of health care delivery. You are challenged, moreover, to look first at yourselves to become aware of the degree to which you share these attitudes, many of which are rooted in our history as a people and in our cultural value systems. Indeed, the receiver of health care services may be as likely to expect (and even want) control from the provider as the provider is likely to exert it.

It is our belief, however, that if nurses are to provide care that encourages each person to grow, we will view those who seek our services as unique beings. We will appreciate their worth, recognize their strengths, and offer a caring relationship in which they may truly be partners in this growth process. We would remind the reader, however, that our priority for persons as individuals does not preclude us from considering also persons in an aggregate, collective or community as clients.

Caring Related to the Concepts Basic to Nursing Practice

Concepts essential to nursing are nursing, person, environment, and health. In this section, we discuss caring as a framework for these essential concepts, and also the relationship of caring to additional concepts within the practice of nursing, namely nursing process, communication, learning–teaching, and ethics and legal aspects. The work of a variety of nursing leaders illustrates these concepts.

Caring gives priority to the needs of others in an unselfish way. Professional caring offers the knowledge and skills of the care-giver to the person needing assistance. According to Leininger (1991), care "refers to phenomena related to assisting, supportive, or enabling behavior toward or for another individual (or group) with evident or anticipated needs to ameliorate or improve a human condition or life" (p. 182). Professional nursing care is intervention to assist or enable another person to have a more healthful response to actual or potential health problems. Professional care based on critical thinking will be both scientifically sound and also personalized to individual situations. The public (nursing's clients) needs nurses and nursing to exercise leadership in demonstrating that such professional caring can be both humane and cost effective.

Nursing

The word nursing has its roots in the Latin term *nutricia,* which means to nurture or nourish. Nursing has been called the oldest of the arts and the youngest of the sciences. Art may be viewed as the systematic application of knowledge or skills. The art of nursing is the art of caring related to the health of persons, the "imaginative and creative use of knowledge in human service" (M. E. Rogers, 1987, p. 140). Nursing as an art has its origin in the caretaking activities of ancient humankind. Donahue (1985) wrote, "From the dawn of civilization, evidence prevails to support the premise that nurturing has been essential to the preservation of life. Survival of the human race, therefore, is inextricably intertwined with the development of nursing" (p. 2).

Science, conversely, is an organized body of knowledge covering general truths or the operation of general laws obtained and tested through research. Much of nursing's scientific and professional development, especially during the latter part of the 20th century, established nursing's credibility as a distinct scientific discipline and a profession separate from medicine. Particularly during the past two decades, nursing research has come of age, assisting the profession to identify a body of knowledge that is unique to nursing. Much of nursing's early theory development and research was modeled after biomedical sciences. Applying such an approach to the nursing of persons, however, has seemed foreign to many practitioners, students, and consumers. Although nurses appreciated the value of such a scientific method, this method did not fit nursing reality as many nurses knew it. A few nurse scholars, therefore, were drawn to theoretical approaches that were more like the humanistic, holistic approaches arising in psychology during the 1960s. With nursing's increasing scientific and professional maturity, more humanistic and culturally sensitive approaches are coming to the forefront of nursing science, just as caring, throughout history, has been at the forefront of nursing practice.

Leininger (1991), in conceptualizing her theory of culture care, stated, "I held this central tenet: care is the essence of nursing and the central dominant and unifying focus of nursing" (p. 35). Newman, Sime, and Corcoran-Perry (1991), in describing the focus of the discipline, wrote that "nursing is the study of caring in the human health experience" (p. 3). As Belknap (1991) suggested, "[We] are now beginning to understand that nursing's strength and power exists in nursing's ability to provide expert and compassionate professional care" (pp. 175–176).

These quotes suggest that care-giving and the study of caring reflect both the origins of the profession and discipline, and also nursing's focus for the future. Nursing dominates health care by the sheer number of its practitioners and the pervasiveness of their services. Nurses function around the clock, in all settings, and across the life span. Nursing care is the most needed service in any resident facility; nursing care is the reason for residency. Hence, **care facility** is the generic name for a place where nursing care is given. Similarly, intensive care, elder care, long-term care, and psychiatric care are synonymous with nursing care given to specific populations. Also, in such care settings, the care may appear nearly invisible to the untrained eye because it is expected, natural, and needed without question. Furthermore, because care is enabling and empowering rather than controlling, it may be underemphasized even when obvious.

Sometimes when caring is overshadowed by technologic interventions, nursing may seem to downplay its caring role. However, as Poulin (1987) has said,

> Ultimately the professionalism of nursing will be tested by the degree of its commitment to its caring function. It is a function which resides in every practitioner of nursing. It is a function that requires leadership on the part of each and every one of us. In essence it is the ethos of nursing. (p. 54)

As Leininger (1986) wrote,

> Indeed, what people want and need most from nurses has been and still remains quality humanized care. The dehumanizing effects of some mechanical technologies is becoming more evident, especially in people of different cultural values and life ways who fear mechanical care. (pp. 9–10)

Quality humanized care has different meanings for different individuals, and also different meanings for persons depending on whether they are care-givers or care recipients. Zane (1986) identified the 10 highest-ranked, nurse-identified caring behaviors:

(1) engaging in attentive listening
(2) comforting

(3) being honest
(4) having patience
(5) being responsible
(6) providing information so that the patient or client can make informed decisions *(legal & ethical)*
(7) touching
(8) expressing sensitivity
(9) showing respect
(10) calling the patient or client by name.

Additional caring behaviors identified with nursing include being competent and efficient. Some care recipients, if asked, may be able to clarify the specific nurse behaviors that exemplify caring to them personally.

Person

Because a **person** is the focus of nursing care, professional nurses need to be "person experts." Theories from biology, psychology, sociology, and philosophy have attempted to explain aspects of persons. Nurses need knowledge in all of these areas. Because persons are greater than the sum of their parts, we cannot learn about persons by viewing their components in isolation. The interactions of all the parts are what make persons unique. Nurses also need an unusually well-developed awareness of how all of the parts of an individual interact. Nursing theories attempt to explain these relationships. Nurse theorist Helen Erickson has established linkages among the concepts individually described by Maslow, E. Erickson, Engle, and others, for example:

1. The relationship between developmental tasks (Erickson) and basic need satisfaction (Maslow).
2. The relationships among satisfaction of basic needs (Maslow), object attachment and loss (Piaget, Bowlby, Engle), and developmental growth (E. Erickson).
3. The relationship between one's ability to mobilize coping resources (H. Erickson) and need satisfaction (Maslow).

Caring means that persons, the subjects of nursing care, are treated not as objects or impersonally, but always in a way that considers the essence of person. Caring is the opposite of mechanization and depersonalization. As Naisbitt and Aburdene (1990) remind us, "The most exciting breakthroughs of the twenty-first century will occur not because of technology but because of an expanding concept of what it means to be human" (p 16). The professional care of persons that nurses demonstrate is given unconditionally.

Caring is demonstrated also by service to persons that is sensitive to unique, cultural differences. "The cultural context and care values make a major difference in how care is expressed and how care takes on meanings to clients and especially families or cultures" (Leininger, 1991, p. 58). In our emphasis on person, however, we remember that individualism and "person-centeredness" is emphasized to a greater degree in North American culture than elsewhere in the world. Elsewhere, cultural care values related to person may include both family and community. This notion is well reflected in the recent text *Community as Partner: Theory and Practice in Nursing* (McFarlane & Anderson, 1996). Also, person–environment interaction may be a cultural value, as exemplified in the North American Indian culture in which harmony and reciprocity between people and environment are critical values. To care about various persons appropriately is to appreciate the concept of person in its various cultural contexts.

Caring is demonstrated further by service to persons that is sensitive to the individuality of gender differences, and also to sexual orientation. Just as cultural differences affect values, so do gender and sexual orientation. The caring nurse will appreciate these differences and avoid stereotypical generalizations that preclude individual care and that may be hurtful as well as inappropriate.

Environment

Nurses understand environment as more than the physical surroundings. **Environment** is both internal and external to the person's biopsychospiritual boundaries. The person needing nursing care is often in disharmony with his or her environments. Maintaining a healthful external environment was a caring environmental intervention of Nightingale's day. However, today, both internal and external environmental alteration as a caring behavior is certainly more technologic and sophisticated. On our shrinking planet, today's external environment is the world. Environment care therefore encompasses nurses' concern for pollution, radioactive hazards, toxic wastes, and other destructions of nature.

We also realize how the stress of an uncaring social environment affects health. Moccia (1986) suggested that "environment as social, political and economic structures"(p. 47) helps us to understand more fully today's health and illness situations. Williams (1991), in discussing why social activism is necessary, stated, "[A] society committed to democratic values must regard a health making environment as a basic human right" (p. 49). We know that joblessness and related poverty, inadequate insurance, decreased access to health care, and disrupted families all take their toll. Smith and Whitney (1991) labeled caring for the environment as the ecology of health. Whether through attention to the physical environment or attention to social, political, and economic structures, caring still manifests itself as interventions that are protective, supportive, or facilitative.

The concept of environment as milieu or cultural setting can also be related to the setting where nursing is practiced. Throughout the book, you will note both the increasing opportunities and trends for nursing care to be provided in less traditional settings.

Health

Health has been defined many ways; however, nursing leaders agree that nurses care for clients in the context of health. Although caring for our clients' health is assuming greater emphasis in nursing practice and science, the public and other health professionals have been slow to recognize this shift from illness care to health care. Nurses promote optimal functioning and biologic and psychosocial growth through health care. Through their care, nurses can enable their clients to be healthy (that is, to function at their optimum) even when elements of illness are present. With person-centered care, even the dying person who is functioning at his or her optimum may face death with a healthy sense of peace or well-being. If we remember that health is partly defined by our clients, then we will look for and maximize the strengths that mean health to our clients. As Davis (1990) suggested, "The most demanding and deeply human aspect of caring is the art of being fully present to another; it is both caring for and caring about" (p. 27).

From another perspective, health promotion is an anticipatory care intervention intended to enhance the **wellness** of persons at risk. Because health means different things to different people, caring about the health of the poor and underserved may mean social policy intervention, that is, political action to increase access to health care. Also, caring about the health of the elderly may mean advocacy for those who need basic care rather than heroic interventions.

> In a health-making society, all persons would have equal access to the resources needed for health, and individuals would not be exposed to health hazards beyond their personal control such as pollution, harmful biologic agents, intoxications of food and water, trauma, inducements for health-destructive personal behaviors, socioeconomic deprivations, and other health assaulting conditions. (Williams, 1991, p. 49)

Health Care Delivery

The illness care industry is often at odds with the health caring advocated by nurses. Society, however, needs caring nurses who are concerned about wellness and who are willing to work on influencing health care delivery so that it meets consumers' actual health needs. Improving quality of life is both a care process and care product about which nurses and their clients may agree, and which they may use as a goal for reform. Faced with cost cutting, professional nurses are challenged to demonstrate that high quality individualized nursing care can be delivered efficiently and effectively through innovative nursing processes in varying health care delivery systems.

Nursing Process

Nursing process may be a mysterious term to beginning students, yet it is nothing more than the problem-solving process involving critical thinking by which nurses meet a person's needs. The elaborations of nursing process fill entire textbooks. The problems, often referred to as "nursing diagnoses," currently are undergoing international standardization. Standardization, although logical in an age of globalization and computerization, is risky. To standardize is to risk overshadowing the caring that originally motivated a more scientific approach to improving nursing's problem solving. If standard diagnoses and standard care plans depersonalize rather than enhance individual care, much caring will have been lost in the name of scientific advancement. Therefore, caring nurses are challenged to use technologic advances to enhance and develop the caring traditions of nursing that are expressed through nursing process.

In a health care delivery system, client care needs may be an organizing focus for the delivery of care; that is, those persons who have common care needs are grouped together. Work assignments and staffing patterns may be built on the demand created by these client care needs, as demonstrated in certain patient care acuity models used for staffing. Because health care delivery is a big and serious business, both the care processes and care products need to demonstrate efficiency and effectiveness. Efficiency and effectiveness can be shown by decreased complications, decreased length of stay, and lower total cost per patient.

Communication

"The communication of a nurse–patient relationship that is therapeutic constitutes the essential caring in nursing" (Knowlden, 1990, p. 93). Nurses communicate their caring to clients directly through actions and words, and indirectly by advocating on behalf of their clients. Most of the caring behaviors identified earlier and by Zane (1986) are directly demonstrated through verbal or nonverbal nurse behavior. The behavior ranked highest by nurses—attentive listening—may be the behavior most likely to be compromised in the hustle and bustle of today's health care delivery.

Learning–Teaching

In the area of learning–teaching, caring meets needs as defined by the care recipient: the client. As health care delivery changes, clients need to learn many skills and behaviors related to maintaining and restoring health, and also to use the health care delivery system differently than in the past. Nurses can demonstrate caring by assuring that client learning needs are not ignored, and by innovating new ways to meet them. Caring puts the learner needs before teacher needs just as the nurse puts client needs before personal needs.

Ethics and Legal Aspects

Caring means balancing ethical rules and principles with the requirements, complexities, and exceptions created by individual circumstances. As Gilligan (1982) stated, "While an ethic of justice proceeds from the premise of equality—that everyone should be treated the same—an ethic of care rests on the premise of nonviolence—that no one should be hurt" (p. 174). Hurt can be both physical and mental, so caring is both physical and psychosocial. Not only will the caring nurse be competent personally, he or she will exercise caring judgment in delegating care activities to others. As more care workers are less or differently prepared than nurses, delegation and supervision become more demanding. The ethical and caring nurse is, however, nonjudgmental about client disease and health behavior. The caring nurse cares also about contributing to collective nursing knowledge and improving the nursing care standards of nurse colleagues.

In the following display, a beginning student shares her vivid memories of a dramatic, missed opportunity to demonstrate caring as a life ended. May her sensitivity and courage to share inspire your exploration of nursing as the caring science.

Example: An experience from my first clinical has remained with me more than any since—that of watching a "code" in the heart cath lab. The patient was a large man, lying naked on a narrow metal table, covered with only a sheet—dead. The lights were beaming down on him, the equipment was suspended overhead, monitors were everywhere. The table was completely surrounded with people—physicians, medical students, respiratory therapists, lab technicians, nurses. The first time they defibrillated him, he lurched up, his eyes popped open, his arms reached out, he bellowed. He fell back to the table, but the monitors did not indicate that his heart had restarted. The physicians yelled orders; the nurse administered drugs; everyone's attention was focused on the monitor—more defibrillation—no response. This went on for about 15 minutes, which seemed like an eternity. The patient's responses diminished to a slight fluttering of the hands as they dangled off the edge of the table. During this whole sequence, I was standing at the periphery of the room, with a clear view of the patient's head. I wanted more than anything to weave my hand in between the personnel and lay it on his forehead—it seemed to me he died such a stressful, lonely death. I still wish I would have been braver and acted on my impulse.
Sonia Prichard, (written as an *SN2*)

The authors contend that caring and critical thinking are themes that should pervade and guide any professional nurse's action in applying the concepts basic to nursing practice. The art of nursing, as defined earlier by Rogers, might be considered a precursor to what we now call critical thinking. Clearly the student above understood the framework of the situation, and yet in viewing it flexibly, saw a missed opportunity to intervene and demonstrate caring and leadership. If critical thinking lies in the balance between structured thinking and a more adaptable thinking, critical thinking by nurses is what many clients and their families would welcome in a time when technology and economics challenge humane health care delivery.

Because advances in technology and electronic media are revolutionizing communication, health care, and education in all settings, you will be expected to acquaint yourself with this new technology. If you do not have computer skills, you will need to acquire them. In this regard, more will be expected of you in some educational and practice settings than in others. Despite others' expectations, you should realize that computer skills in traditional and virtual library search, word processing, and communications are skills that will give you enormous personal and professional advantage throughout your nursing career.

KEY CONCEPTS

✔ Person-centered care focuses on the individual needs of clients and families, and is the expertise for which nurses are known.

Nursing definitions explain how different theorists conceptualize the ideas of nursing, person, environment and health that form the basis of professional nursing.

Critical thinking is a professional skill that combines the logical thinking of nursing science and the creative thinking needed for individual circumstances.

Caring is a framework for applying the basic concepts of nursing, person, environment, and health to the art, science, and profession of nursing.

Nursing uses the skills of nursing process, communication, learning and teaching, ethics and legal aspects, and leadership in the context of changing health care delivery and technology.

CRITICAL THINKING QUESTIONS

1. Examine your own thoughts about nursing and persons, and consider how the ideas presented in this chapter might affect you as you begin your nursing practice.

2. If you were to furnish and supply a nurse-run clinic, how would you equip it to demonstrate caring?

3. Interview three non-nurse acquaintances to determine their views about nursing as a profession. Using a critical thinking approach rather than merely a feeling response, analyze their views.

4. Do you already possess basic computer skills in library search, word processing, and communications? Do you use electronic mail, the internet, and the world wide web? If not, develop a plan for gaining these skills. Many libraries, college computer centers, individual peers, and faculty members can be of assistance.

5. Develop a personal strategy to keep informed about these chapter concepts as discussed in professional and lay literature and also in the multimedia.

REFERENCES

Belknap, R. A. (1991). Care: A significant paradigm shift and focus in nursing for the future. In D. A. Gaut & M. Leininger (Eds.), *Caring: The compassionate healer* (Publication No. 15-2401, pp. 173–180). New York: National League for Nursing.

Davis, A. J. (1990). Are there limits to caring?: Conflict between autonomy and beneficence. In M. M. Leininger (Ed.), *Ethical and moral dimensions of care* (pp. 25–32). Detroit: Wayne State University Press.

Donahue, M. P. (1985). *Nursing: The finest art—An illustrated history.* St. Louis, MO: C.V. Mosby.

Gilligan, C. (1982). *In a different voice: Psychological theory and women's development.* Cambridge, MA: Harvard University Press.

Henderson, V. (1966). *The nature of nursing.* New York: Macmillan.

King, I. M. (1981). *A theory for nursing: Systems, concepts, process.* New York: Wiley.

Knowlden, V. (1990). The virtue of caring in nursing. In M. M. Leininger (Ed.), *Ethical and moral dimensions of care* (pp. 89–94). Detroit: Wayne State University Press.

Leininger, M. M. (1991). The theory of culture care diversity and universality. In M. M. Leininger (Ed.), *Culture care diversity and universality: A theory of nursing* (Publication No. 15-2402, pp. 5–68). New York: National League for Nursing.

Leininger, M. M. (1986). Care facilitation and resistance factors in the culture of nursing. Topics in Clinical Nursing *8*(2), 1–12.

Leininger, M. M. (1981). The phenomenon of caring: Importance, research questions, and theoretical considerations. In M. M. Leininger (Ed.), *Caring: An essential human need* (pp. 3–15). Thorofare, NJ: Charles B. Slack.

Maslow, A. H. (1970). *Motivation and personality* (2nd ed.). New York: Harper & Row.

Mayeroff, M. (1971). *On caring.* New York: Harper & Row.

McFarlane, J.M., & Anderson, E.A. (1996). *Community as partner: theory and practice in nursing* (2nd ed.). Philadelphia: J. B. Lippincott.

Meleis, A.I. (1991). *Theoretical nursing: Development and progress* (2nd ed.). Philadelphia: J.B. Lippincott.

Moccia, P. (1986). *New approaches to theory development.* New York: National League for Nursing, Publication No. 15.

Naisbitt, J., & Aburdene, P. (1990). *Megatrends 2000.* New York: William Morrow.

Newman, M. A., Sime, A. M., & Corcoran-Perry, E. (1991). The focus of the discipline of nursing. *Advances in Nursing Science, 14,* 1–6.

Nightingale, F. (1859). *Notes on nursing: What it is and what it is not.* London: Harrison. (Facsimile ed., Philadelphia: J.B. Lippincott, 1966)

Orem, D. E. (1984). *Nursing: Concepts of practice* (3rd ed.). New York: McGraw-Hill.

Poulin, M. A. (1987). Leadership and the caring role. *Imprint, 34,* 51–54.

Rogers, C. R. (1961). *On becoming a person.* Boston: Houghton Mifflin.

Rogers, M. E. (1987). Rogers' science of unitary human beings. In R.R. Parse (Ed.), *Nursing science: Major paradigms, theories, and critiques* (pp. 139–146). Philadelphia: W.B. Saunders.

Rogers, M. E. (1970). *An introduction to the theoretical basis of nursing.* Philadelphia: F.A. Davis.

Roy, C. (1984). *Introduction to nursing: An adaptation model* (2nd ed.). Englewood Cliffs, NJ: Prentice-Hall.

Smith, M. N., & Whitney, G. M. (1991). Caring for the environment: The ecology of health. In P. L. Chinn (Ed.), *Anthology on caring* (Publication No. 15-2392, pp. 59–69). New York: National League for Nursing.

Watson, J. (1989). Watson's philosophy and theory of human caring in nursing. In Riehl-Sisca, J. (Ed.), *Conceptual models for nursing practice* (3rd ed., pp 219–236). Norwalk CT: Appleton and Lange.

Watson, J. (1985). *Nursing: Human science and human care—A theory of nursing.* Norwalk, CT: Appleton-Century-Crofts.

Watson, J. (1979). *Nursing: The philosophy and science of caring.* Boston: Little, Brown.

Williams, D. M. (1991). Health promotion, caring and nursing: Why social activism is necessary. In P. L. Chinn (Ed.), *Anthology on caring* (Publication No. 15-2392, pp. 7–58). New York: National League for Nursing.

Zane, R. W. (1986). The caring concept and nurse identified caring behaviors. *Topics in Clinical Nursing, 8,* 84–93.

Part Two

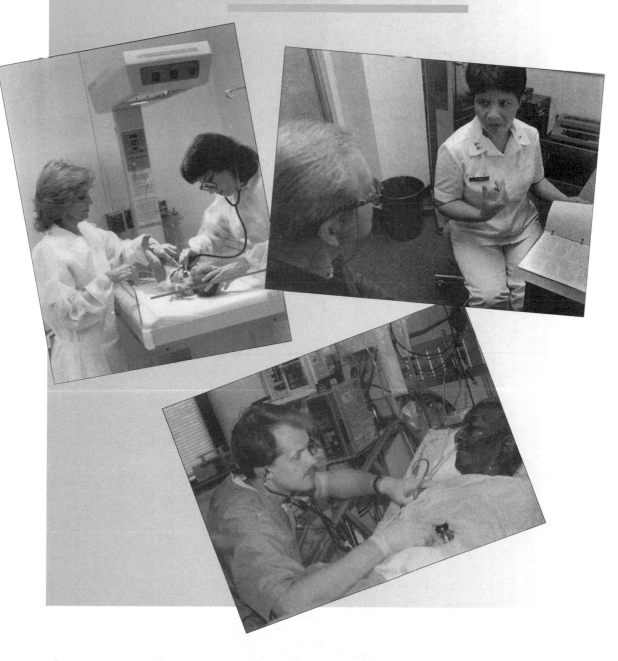

2

Nursing Through History: A Prelude to the Present and the Future

Key Words

| Accountability | Career | Professionalism | Science |
| Art | Certification | Professionalization | Standard |

Objectives

After completing this chapter, students will be able to:

Describe how social and philosophic systems have affected nursing through history.

Describe the highlights of nursing history.

Describe nursing's historical progress as art, science and profession.

Describe nursing's status in relation to each of the characteristics of professions.

History reveals deep-rooted philosophic traditions and social forces that have shaped nursing. The term nurse has been applied to persons with a wide range of skills and educational backgrounds. Additionally, history informs us that the caring tradition of nursing encompasses both art and science.

To *nurse* is to nourish or look after carefully—to promote growth, development, or other favorable conditions. To *doctor*, by contrast, is to diagnose, treat, and cure disease. Florence Nightingale (1859) used this common definition of nursing when she declared nursing to be both an art and a science, and differentiated nursing from medicine.

Throughout history, medicine and nursing have been closely associated. Not surprisingly, as the word *nurse* suggests, the nurse assumed the feminine caregiving role, tending to personal and comfort needs—especially for the ill and dependent patient.

A Philosophic Perspective

Hygeia of Greek mythology was the ancient goddess of health; nurses are described in Greek literature, although their gender is open for debate. Historical references to nursing parallel the beginning of Christianity.

Early values and beliefs created a philosophic base for the art and science that was to become the profession of nursing. Bevis (1989) described four philosophic periods of nursing history that have shaped the development of the profession and continue to influence nursing today; these elements of nursing's value system are asceticism, romanticism, pragmatism, and humanistic existentialism (p. 36). These labels, which reflect several philosophic influences on nursing's collective consciousness, provide a strategy for understanding nursing today.

Asceticism originated in the days of Plato. It arose from the idealism that projected an ultimate spiritual reality beyond physical reality. Asceticism was associated with a life of self-denial and devotion to duty and spiritual calling. Emphasis was on a service learned while doing. Learning was "training" rather than formal education. No wonder nursing originated as hard work, with employer exploitation and few monetary rewards. For many years, nurses themselves thought it was inappropriate to expect economic advantage from their calling. This belief, despite Nightingale's introduction of rudimentary nursing science and formal education, dominated nursing until well into the 20th century. The influences of this period are still evident, in that nurses are often expected to make charitable contributions to society and health care.

Romanticism developed from the emphasis on materialistic realism that grew out of the industrial revolution. Romanticism, the kind of escape from realism that created a fantasy experience, is reflected in the 19th-century music of Tchaikovsky and Schumann and the romantic canvases of the Victorian painters and the impressionists.

Nurses were romanticized in dress, paintings, and literature. Severe and plain religious garb gave way to elaborate uniforms and fussy caps, reflecting hospital school loyalty. Nightingale, rather than gaining wide recognition for her scientific and political acumen, was portrayed as "The Lady With the Lamp." If the Civil War dramatized the need for nurses, the late 19th and early 20th centuries romanticized their role. The romantic adventures of nurses in literature influenced young girls and women well into the mid-20th century. During this era of romanticism, nursing became medicine's loyal auxiliary. The lady-of-the-house role was assumed in hospitals, where students provided much of the domestic care. Even though graduate nurses were nursing supervisors, they reported to physicians and hospital administrative authorities. Bevis (1989) argued that the romantic era greatly influenced nursing education programs until past the mid-20th century. Nursing content was parallel to medical content: it focused more on diseases than on the recipients of care.

Throughout history, wars have reaffirmed the need for nurses. Not all wars, however, have had the same influence. World War I was a romantic war. World War II dramatically introduced a new era of realism that Bevis labeled *pragmatism.*

Pragmatism equated practical consequences with worth and truth. Bevis's philosophic interpretation of this era is particularly useful. Wartime casualties created an acute-care shortage. It was during this era that a group of health care workers, auxiliary to nurses, became prominent. Aides, technicians, and "practical" nurses gave much of the actual nursing care. The better-prepared nurses were needed to supervise and to instruct. Medical specialties dictated the most efficient care of hospital patients. Both health care delivery and nursing curricula were organized by disease. "The focus was on the problem, the disability, the disease, and the diagnosis, not on the person, his family, his needs, his wholeness, or his humanity" (Bevis, 1989, p. 39). Eventually, toward the end of this era, practical realities dominated. The need for intensive, rehabilitative, and ambulatory care units enabled nurses to return to their focus on care of client or human need. This transitional period signaled a forthcoming era of humanistic existentialism.

Humanism is a mode of thought in which human interests predominate. *Existentialism* is a modern philosophic view that accepts that reality exists in the mind of the person. Reality is unique to each person, and each person is a holistic being. The sum of a person is greater than the scientific study of the individual parts can reveal. Underlying this philosophy are choice for personal destiny and accountability. This value system elevates concern for others to a high priority for basic human reasons. The humanistic movement was popular in psychology as the "third wave" in the "me" era of the 1960s.

Current humanistic values in nursing shape the views of persons for whom nursing care is provided. These values also influence nurse–client interactions, nurse accountability, and professional autonomy. This dominant philosophic notion ushers in an exciting new era for the nursing profession. Humanistic nursing care can balance and complement the high technology of health care and provide cost-effective options in an era of rapid cost escalation.

Other Historical Highlights

During the late middle ages, religious orders of men and women began to nurse the sick. During the crusades to the Holy Land, knights served as nurses. These male military orders were called "Hospitalers." During this time, charitable secular orders of women also nursed.

The Reformation period ushered in a 300-year (1550–1850) dark period of nursing, when nursing conditions changed markedly. Male nurses nearly disappeared. Although religious orders of women (e.g., the Deaconesses, Sisters of Charity, and Sisters of Mercy) became prominent, women prisoners and prostitutes also were pressed into nursing service.

Florence Nightingale's era (1820–1910) marked the advent of modern nursing. Nightingale, a well-educated English woman, was born of wealthy and influential parents. She entered nursing at the age of 25.

> Called the founder of modern nursing, Nightingale was a strong-willed woman of quick intelligence who used her considerable knowledge of statistics, sanitation, logistics, administration, nutrition and public health not only to develop a new system of nursing education and health care, but also to improve the social welfare systems of the time. (Kelly, 1995, p. 24)

Florence Nightingale is credited with working miracles in the Crimean War and decreasing mortality in the Barrack Hospital in Turkey to 1%. Her greatest miracle, however, was the reform of nursing education. To some, Florence Nightingale was a saint; to others, she was a strong-willed eccentric. Regardless of varying views, she was a remarkable woman.

During the nursing reform, which began in mid-19th century England, three Nightingale Schools were established in the United States soon after the Civil War. During the Civil War, as in other wars, women left home and joined the work force. "Modern nursing," which originated during this Victorian era, prescribed women's roles as secondary to those of men, and nurses' roles as secondary to physicians'. However, despite their prominence in nursing during the Middle Ages, men were discriminated against during the post-Nightingale era.

Blacks and other ethnic minorities also suffered both discrimination and lack of recognition for their contributions. Documentation finally countered this lack of recognition. One classic documentation of black nurses' contributions was skillfully compiled by Mary Elizabeth Carnegie (1986), an outstanding African-American nurse–scholar. Multicultural ethnic groups within nursing have contributed essential knowledge and sensitivity regarding cultural differences. The Leininger book (1995) *Transcultural Nursing: Concepts, Theories, Research and Practices* and Spector's (1991) *Cultural Diversity in Health and Illness* present such knowledge.

Despite Nightingale's influence, early "training" for American nurses emphasized standard procedures, housekeeping tasks, and an ethic that was subservient to medicine. Although nursing has a wonderful heritage, it also carries historical baggage that influenced its art and deterred its scientific development from occurring earlier.

Nursing's more recent history in the 20th century also has influenced its development. The divergence between medicine and nursing, which has occurred since Florence Nightingale's death, provides such an example. This divergence also contributed to an understanding about nursing's development as art, science, and profession.

Development of Medicine and Nursing: A Comparison

At the turn of the 19th century, many similarities were evident between medical and nursing practice (e.g., similar knowledge and similar practitioners, such as the country doctor and the private duty nurse). Early in the 20th century, medicine made a purposeful assessment of its social responsibilities and its ability to meet them. This assessment resulted in a candid report on the condition of medical education in the United States (Flexner, 1910). Criticism abounded and targeted the students, faculty, clinical facilities, and libraries of the current medical establishment. Medicine and society took corrective action, and medicine skyrocketed to a position of professional prominence not held previously.

As a result of the Flexner report, medicine began to standardize its education programs in colleges and research universities. The Flexner report had specifically identified that society would be deprived of appropriate health care unless it was scientifically based and delivered. Medicine began to give considerable attention to accreditation and licensing issues. The Flexner report also emphasized that society would need to pay for the necessary improved and sophisticated education of physicians. Thus, an econometric model of reimbursement was created for medicine. Long formal education and clinical experience were rewarded by generous fees for service.

Nursing, conversely, remained charitable about the services it provided, and unassertive about its economic welfare. In 1923, the Goldmark Report (Goldmark, 1923) identified needs of nursing education and public health nursing. This report was the first of many studies by, about, and for nursing and its advancement. Despite repeated studies, a variety of programs proliferated in nursing that did not clearly or uniformly identify the kind of practitioners who were being prepared. In the 1970s, two reports about the scope of nursing practice created a great deal of reaction within and outside nursing. These reports were "Extending the Scope of Nursing Practice," from the Health, Education, and Welfare Secretary's Committee (1971), and "An Abstract for Action," from the National Commission for the Study of Nursing and Nursing Education (1970), chaired by Jerome Lysaught. The reports validated the divergence of medicine and nursing, and emphasized that nurses and nursing were not realizing their full potential. In 1980, Lysaught, describing the transformation of American medicine between 1900 and 1980 as a miracle, credited this fantastic change more to research than to technology itself.

Table 2-1 depicts a summary of the divergence between medical and nursing

TABLE 2-1 *Divergence Between Medical and Nursing Practice*

1900—Medical and Nursing Practice Similarities
Based on similar knowledge
Characteristic of the individual
Benevolent

1990—Medicine	1990—Nursing
Members educated largely in postgraduate university programs	Most members without baccalaureate education
Established scientific base	Developing scientific base
Established research effort	Developing research effort
Career commitment of members	Varying career commitment among members
Recognized professional autonomy and control of health care	Seeking professional autonomy and control of nursing
Recognized professional organization	Struggling professional organization and some unionization of members
Cost of services identified and collected privately or often reimbursed	Cost of services often not identified or reimbursed through third-party payers
Dominated by men	Dominated by women

practice in the 20th century. Clearly, the cornerstone of medical advance was education and research. This medical initiative was coupled with other scientific advances (e.g., the discovery of penicillin and technology for safer surgery). Medicine assumed a position of power to diagnose and to cure illness. Also, medicine built a cure system that was gratefully accepted by the public for decades. As the cure role grew for physicians, care and cure became increasingly dichotomized between physicians and nurses. Dock and Stewart (1938) had defined nursing as "not only the care of the sick, the aged, the helpless and the handicapped but the promotion of health vigor in those who are well especially the young growing creatures on whom the future of the race depends" (pp. 4–5). The concern for the care of the healthy was overshadowed, however, by rapid advances in the care of the ill. This situation further reinforced nursing's role as care of the sick. Nursing of the sick necessarily involves many physical care activities. Therefore, nursing often was seen as primarily concerned with physical tasks being done or as artful caring, rather than mental activity or science.

In her editorial in Nursing Science Quarterly (1989), Parse, a nurse–theorist, is even more explicit and detailed about the relationship between nursing art and nursing science as she envisions nursing in the future: "the set of fundamentals essential for fully practicing the art of nursing can be conceptualized as (follows):

- Know and use nursing frameworks and theories
- Be available to others
- Value the other as a human presence
- Respect differences in view
- Own what you believe and be accountable for your actions
- Move on to the new and untested
- Connect with others
- Take pride in self
- Like what you do
- Recognize the moments of joy in the struggles of living
- Appreciate mystery and be open to new discoveries
- Be competent in your chosen area
- Rest and begin anew

These fundamentals reflect values that emerge from nursing's unique knowledge base, that is, the extant frameworks and theories" (p. 111).

As the 20th century draws to a close, nursing and medicine share a resurgent interest in health, and nursing art is undergoing transformation. Regarding this transformation, note especially the attention to respecting differences in viewpoint, appreciating a mystery, and being open to new discoveries (referred to in Chapter 3 as diverse and divergent thinking and alternative hypotheses).

Nursing as an Art

Traditional nursing as **art** predominated in the first half of the 20th century when nursing was largely the care of the ill in the hospital and the care of mothers and children in the community. Nursing was primarily the art of caring, based on intuition and skill training rather than on science. Influenza, wars, and the Depression produced their share of ill and dependent persons who needed care. Thus, although the seeds of nursing science had been sown by Florence Nightingale nearly a half century earlier, social forces supported the growth of nursing as art and constrained its development as science.

Caring involves the ability to express oneself. Expression of self is, in turn, an element of art. The artistic or creative expression of self suggests the importance of developing unique aspects of personal ability. The intuitive nature of nursing has been identified and supported as the art of nursing; however, purposely developing the creative aspect of nursing has often been minimized.

Donahue (1985) wrote, "Nursing is not merely a technique but a process that incorporates the elements of soul, mind, and imagination. Its very essence lies in the creative imagination, the sensitive spirit, and the intelligent understanding that provide the very foundation for effective nursing care" (p. 10). The art of nursing was exemplified beautifully in Donahue's (1985,1996) classic volumes *Nursing: The Finest Art—An Illustrated History*. The book shows how individuals recognized as leading practitioners of the art of nursing have expressed themselves throughout history in the ministrations that gave them a prominent place in the annals of nursing.

Such creative nurses, too numerous to mention individually, include some names you may recognize:

- ❏ Florence Nightingale, the versatile genius who created modern nursing
- ❏ Lillian Wald, who pioneered public health/community nursing
- ❏ Mary Breckenridge, who founded the Frontier Nursing Service
- ❏ Virginia Henderson, who created a modern worldwide definition of nursing
- ❏ Martha Rogers, a contemporary catalyst for theory development

Other true artists of nursing toil with less recognition. However, they strive to use their unique personal attributes as they interact with clients of all ages in a variety of settings. In many ways, art is timeless—as represented by human creativity throughout the ages.

During the late 20th century, a renewed interest in art and creativity paralleled a growing interest in nursing as science and nurses as scholars. Scholarship, as Meleis (1991) reminded us, ". . . includes the creativity needed to consider ways to develop knowledge in a human science, ways that do not stifle the richness of its phenomena" (pp. 123–124). Certainly our nursing history has a heritage of creativity. Now, social and professional circumstances challenge us to rekindle that creativity to secure nursing's future and society's health. The future of nursing as art couples technologic and scientific advances with artistic creativity and critical thinking. Together, these advances will enhance the precious vitality of the interpersonal interaction that has been the essence of nursing.

From a slightly different perspective, art is also the reflection of feelings and perceptions. Because the core and essence of nursing is personal interaction, the art of nursing finds expression in many ways—including, for example, a nurse's sensitivity to and perception of a client's thoughts and feelings. Also included is the nurse's expression of thoughts and feelings to the client. That is, a nurse may express artistic sensitivity to a client's nonverbal behavior that indicates anxiety or pain. For example, a nurse could uniquely express unconditional positive regard for a person based on his or her worth as an individual. Although these behaviors can be learned scientifically, they also can be learned through experience and practiced intuitively as art. Nursing practice as both art and science offers the best of both worlds to society and also the widest range of practice expressions to nurses. Other references that speak specifically to nursing as art include Cohen (1991) and Chinn and Watson (1994).

Nursing as a Science

Florence Nightingale (1859) is often recognized as nursing's first scientist/theorist for her work *Notes on Nursing: What It Is and What It is Not.* She identified nursing as a scientific discipline separate from medicine. Perhaps her strongest action supporting this view was creating freestanding schools of nursing where nurses (rather than doctors) assumed responsibility for nursing education. Later Nightingale claimed that, with nursing, both a new art and a new science had been created. The early science of nursing was not a separate and recognized discipline like chemistry or psychology. Instead, it was a loosely defined body of scientific facts and principles underlying physician-prescribed nursing activities. For example, physicians taught nurses the knowledge of asepsis needed to perform the sterile technique of changing dressings and to assist with surgical procedures. In the early days, nurses often were taught the scientific applications necessary to perform their delegated duties safely, but were taught to do so without question.

A major breakthrough for the discipline of nursing came when nursing schools moved into university settings and nurses began to study the basic sciences and humanities on which nursing was thought to be based. This preparation served two major purposes. First, it gave nurses the educational foundation necessary to make the scientific applications themselves rather than to take them on faith. Second, it gave nurses basic college credit in scientific disciplines related to nursing, which, in turn, prepared nurses to earn advanced degrees in the biopsychosocial sciences; for example, nurses became psychologists, sociologists, anthropologists, and physiologists. Because a minimal number of programs within nursing existed to prepare scientists, theorists, and researchers, preparation in other fields was necessary. This preparation taught nurses the processes of science, including critical thinking and the theories of other scientific disciplines. Additionally, this advanced preparation enabled nurses to teach other nurses. Nurses also learned that within other scientific disciplines, especially biologic and physical sciences, specific laws and principles give direction for making predictions within the discipline.

When nursing did not have doctorate-prepared scientists within its own discipline, it also did not have the person power to develop and offer advanced nursing degrees. Only in recent years have nursing schools been able to recruit sufficient numbers of doctorate-prepared nurses to offer the nursing PhD in a large number

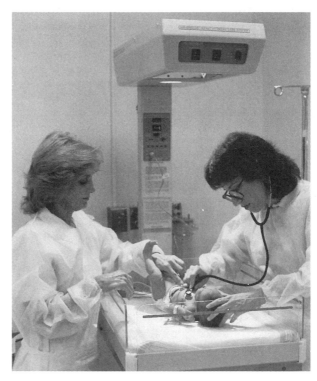

Nursing is both an art and a science.

of schools. Since the 1980s, the number of nursing schools offering the doctorate in nursing in the United States has jumped from a mere handful to over 50 (Baker, 1995). A recent, global, comparative study of nursing doctoral programs found more than 60 additional programs in 25 other countries. Doctorate-prepared nurses have the advanced research skills necessary to conduct independent scientific investigations and to contribute to nursing theory. Recent advances in technology have enabled that knowledge to be shared worldwide. Sigma Theta Tau International (STTI), for example, now has an electronic library, The Virginia Henderson International Nursing Library. The library houses the third edition STTI Nursing Research Classification System. "The Research Classification System is a representation of the language and structure of clinical nursing research knowledge" (Graves, 1996, p. 24). The system is a unique international resource that is both a registry of nurse researchers and a registry of nursing knowledge. One can search the resource for information related to any of the concepts basic to the metaparadigm of nursing, i.e., person, environment, health, and nurse. It is available on the internet as a subscription service.

Considering nursing's short scientific history and the 20th century divergence between medical and nursing practice, the past 45 years provide a startling contrast to earlier times. Selected highlights are summarized in Table 2-2.

TABLE 2-2 *Highlights of Nursing's Scientific History*

1950s	1960s	1970s	1980s
❏ Code of Ethics adopted by the American Nurses Association (1950)	❏ Postbaccalaureate programs in nursing specialty areas increase	❏ Nurse practitioners in expanded practice roles gain national visibility	❏ Master's and doctoral programs in nursing proliferate
❏ Nurses seek postbaccalaureate preparation in nursing; first graduate programs established for clinical nurse specialists	❏ Nurses establish National Clinical Specialty nursing groups	❏ Nurses' Coalition for Action in Politics formed	❏ Professional nursing journals increase remarkably (more than 80 by 1985)
❏ The professional journal *Nursing Research* is first published (1952)	❏ Nursing researchers pioneer clinical investigations	❏ American Nurses Association creates American Academy of Nursing to honor outstanding contributors to nursing	❏ By 1984, more than 20,000 nurses nationally "certified" in 17 specialty areas of practice
	❏ International Nursing Index categorizes worldwide nursing articles	❏ Nursing theorists come into national spotlight	❏ National Institutes of Health house a National Center for Nursing Research
			❏ Sigma Theta Tau, international honor society for outstanding baccalaureate-prepared nurses, numbers 75,000 members at mid-decade
			❏ Sigma Theta Tau launches 10-year plan, Focus on Scholarship, to increase the science of nursing and increase public awareness of research required

Nursing as a Profession

Most of us use the terms *profession* and *professional* rather casually. In some instances, we intend to convey the impression that a person is an expert; in other instances, we use the term *professional* politely, as a title of distinction. Accordingly, we describe someone as a professional athlete, musician, or engineer. We may ask someone "What is your profession?" when we mean "What work do you do?"

Professionalism is defined as professional character, spirit, or methods. Professionalism also encompasses teaching and activities found in various occupational groups whose members aspire to be professional. **Professionalization** is the process of acquiring or changing characteristics in the direction of a profession.

The debate about whether nursing is a profession has stirred and divided nursing throughout its history. With attention focusing on educational preparation for entry into professional nursing practice, professionalism in nursing remains a current and pressing issue. Because the issues related to professionalism present implications and challenges for every nurse and recipient of nursing care, the topic is important to practicing and aspiring nurses as well as to the public.

Historically, occupations traditionally accepted as professions have been medicine, law, and the ministry. Many other occupational groups now seek the status that has been assigned to these professions over time. Whether society views these aspiring occupations as professions is another matter.

You may or may not consider nursing to be a profession. At the very least, you are probably being confronted with a view of nursing that is somewhat different from what you expected. Often, as indicated earlier, beginning students regard nursing primarily as the mastery of many technical procedures. Indeed, such technical mastery is important, but it is only a part of the larger scheme of professional nursing practice. To clarify the notion of professional practice in nursing, it is helpful to reflect on the general criteria for all professions.

General Criteria for Professions

In general, all **professions** have the following characteristics:

❏ A body of knowledge on which skills and services are based
❏ An ability to deliver a unique service to other humans
❏ Education that is standardized and based in colleges and universities
❏ Control of standards for practice
❏ Responsibility and accountability of members for their own actions
❏ Career commitment by members
❏ Independent function (Schein & Kommers, 1972, pp. 7–14)

Let us consider each of these criteria for professions individually.

Body of Knowledge on Which Skills and Services Are Based

At one time in history, nursing skills and practice were based largely on intuitive knowledge. Today, as a practice discipline, nursing is called an applied **science.** If the person is the recipient of nursing, and each person is a biopsychosocial being interacting with his or her environment, then nursing applies concepts from many different basic sciences. Some nursing leaders have argued that nursing need not have a unique knowledge base. They believe nursing can be unique in its application of knowledge common to many disciplines. Other experts believe that nursing eventually will develop its own body of knowledge and its own theories.

Those who are particularly interested in nursing as science will be enriched by exploring further the work of nurse–philosophers, nurse–theorists, and nurse–researchers. The nature of knowledge development in many fields is changing from a deductive, reductionist, mechanistic, and quantitative view to an inductive, holistic, qualitative, and social view. This change may signal an era of science that is more supportive of the scientific agendas important to nursing. As Meleis

(1991) said, "It is a view that has shifted the focus from a causation to a more interpretive view" (p. 65). Meleis's book *Theoretical Nursing: Development and Progress* is an excellent resource for both a sophisticated scientific nursing perspective and extensive theoretical abstracts and bibliography.

Ability to Deliver a Unique Service to Other Humans

According to Henderson (1966), the unique function of the nurse is to assist a person in performing activities contributing to health and recovery, or a serene death, which the person would do for himself or herself if able. Furthermore, the nurse assists in a way that encourages independence. The current emphasis on nurses' promotion of self-care is consistent with Henderson's definition. In addition to a person-centered practice, the unique focus of nursing often is identified as health, not illness, which is the focus for medicine. Society validates its need for nursing by continuing to educate nurses. Currently, however, it is foolish to argue that all persons termed nurses provide the same unique service. Nursing's current statement of its social obligation is printed in Nursing's Social Policy Statement (ANA, 1995).

Standardized Education Based in Colleges and Universities

In 1859, Florence Nightingale advocated training schools that would be educational institutions supported by public funds. Although she thought the schools should be closely associated with hospitals, she also believed that they should be administered separately.

In 1909, Minnesota physician Richard Beard proposed and strongly defended university education for nurses. The first university school of nursing opened in Minnesota that year. A significant development in collegiate education for nurses occurred in the 1950s: Montag (1951) introduced associate degree (A.D.) programs to prepare nurse–technicians. The success of these programs, coupled with the general increase in numbers of community and junior colleges, resulted in a proliferation of A.D. programs. In 1974, the New York State Nurses' Association proposed that, by 1985, the baccalaureate degree would become the minimal educational preparation for entry into professional nursing practice. This proposal generated controversy among nurses, other health professionals, and hospital administrators, even though the suggestion of collegiate education was far from new.

In the past decade, from 1984/85 to 1993/94, the number of graduations from diploma programs decreased, from 11,892 to 7,119, to a level that was only one-third that number 20 years ago. During the same period, the number of graduations from Associate Degree programs increased from 45,208 to 58,839, while total graduations (including basic and registered nursing students) from baccalaureate nursing programs increased from 34,569 to 39,693. Statistics from the National League for Nursing (1995), the organization that accredits educational programs in nursing, document these trends.

The questions of how nurses should be prepared and titled have been ones of long-standing debate. During the registered nurse (RN) shortages of the late

1980s, many questions arose about how to prepare for and who will perform the basic tasks of nursing that had once been done by aides and licensed practical nurses. Whenever there are nurse shortages and/or pressing financial concerns, the creation of other lesser educated nonprofessional health care workers to fill in for professional nurses becomes an issue. An educational issue of the late 1990s, driven primarily by economic considerations, is **assistive personnel.** Assistive personnel are less expensive technical workers, minimally trained, doing activities formerly considered nursing. The NLN (1994) noted, however, that "the development of innovative flexible programs to allow assistive health care workers to join nurses' ranks is one example of how LPN/LVN education serves the profession and the health care needs of the nation" (p. 193).

Control of Standards for Practice

A **standard** is an authoritative statement or criterion by which the quality of practice can be judged. In the late 1950s, the American Nurses Association (ANA), nursing's professional organization, expressed formal concern for control of practice at a level above the legal minimum required for RN licensure. ANA first published *Standards for Organized Nursing Services* in 1965. These standards emphasized both systematic nursing plans providing for client participation and nursing actions to maximize health capabilities. The nursing practice standards assume individual nurse responsibility and accountability for meeting the standards.

ANA recognizes excellence in practice through a process called **certification.** According to the ANA (1980) social policy statement, "Certification of specialists in nursing practice is a judgment made by the profession, upon review of an array of evidence examined by a selected panel of nurses who are themselves specialists and who represent the area of specialization" (p. 24). Certification identifies persons who have obtained specialized knowledge, and affirms professional achievement. Certification also carries with it the endorsement of professional colleagues.

Responsibility and Accountability of Members for Their Own Actions

Accountability is responsibility for the services one provides or makes available. The concept of accountability is not new to nursing. Nurses are probably more concerned about accountability than many other professionals. Accountability has several dimensions, including legal, peer group, employer, and consumer accountability. Licensing boards can revoke licenses to practice for incompetence or certain violations of the law. Nurses are accountable to health care colleagues with whom they are professionally associated, as reflected in the increasing use of peer review within the clinical setting. Peer review may include evaluating the client's health record to compare actual practice with the ANA's nursing practice standards. Because nurses generally are not independent practitioners, they often are also accountable to hospitals or other employing agencies. Increasingly, nurses describe themselves as directly accountable to their clients. The concept of ac-

DISPLAY 2-1   **American Nurses Association Code for Nurses**

(handwritten margin notes)
- others
- cultural
- impact
- safety
- convey to another
- account for what you do!

1. The nurse provides services with respect for human dignity and the uniqueness of the client, unrestricted by considerations of social or economic status, personal attributes, or the nature of health problems.
2. The nurse safeguards the client's right to privacy by judiciously protecting information of a confidential nature.
3. The nurse acts to safeguard the client and the public when health care and safety are affected by the incompetent, unethical, or illegal practice of any person.
4. The nurse assumes responsibility and accountability for individual nursing judgments and actions. *(handwritten: coming forward w/ mistakes)*
5. The nurse maintains competence in nursing. *(handwritten: current)*
6. The nurse exercises informed judgment and uses individual competence and qualifications as criteria in seeking consultation, accepting responsibilities, and delegating nursing activities to others.
7. The nurse participates in activities that contribute to the ongoing development of the profession's body of knowledge.
8. The nurse participates in the profession's efforts to implement and improve standards of nursing.
9. The nurse participates in the profession's efforts to establish and maintain conditions of employment conducive to high quality nursing care.
10. The nurse participates in the profession's effort to protect the public from misinformation and misrepresentation and to maintain the integrity of nursing. *(handwritten: truth)*
11. The nurse collaborates with members of the health professions and other citizens in promoting community and national efforts to meet the health needs of the public.

(*From* Code for Nurses With Interpretive Statements (*p. 1*) by American Nurses Association, 1985, Kansas City, MO: Author.)

countability implies both that one is responsible for the consequences of actions chosen and also that one accepts the consequences of choosing not to act in particular situations.

Primary care is a mechanism whereby health care providers, including nurses, are accountable for the services rendered to specific clients. One usually thinks of accountability in this more narrow sense of specific care situations. In the broader sense, one is accountable for moving the profession toward professional goals. The individual is also accountable to himself or herself for achieving maximum potential.

CODE FOR NURSES

Another way professionals monitor conduct within their ranks is by formulating and enforcing a code of ethics. The Code for Professional Nurses was first outlined in the 1920s. It was adopted in 1950 and has been changed many times since

TABLE 2-3 *Characteristics of a Job Versus a Career*

Job	Career
A piece of work; may or may not be long-term employment	Life work; long-term commitment, long-term planning important, possibly involving a mentor
Variable initial training	Long training or education
Part-time or full-time	Usually full-time
Intermittent retraining possible	Lifelong learning necessary
Job selects person	Person selects career
Administrator evaluation primarily	Peer evaluation primarily

(ANA, 1985). This code not only guides members, but also serves as a proclamation to the public served by nursing (Display 2-1).

Career Commitment by Members

A **career** is what you do as your major life's work. It is sometimes described as the progress of a person through life. A career may be distinguished from a job, which is an individual piece of work done in the routine of one's trade or occupation. In earlier days, when women's life work was done primarily in the home, they had little opportunity for professional careers in the world of work outside the home. Today, most women work outside the home because of both economic necessity and a change in society's attitudes toward women's work. As women today consider employment, the choice between job and career is no longer made solely on the length of time one expects to remain in the work force. Most nurses who work probably do so for more than a quarter of a century, or one third of their lifetime.

The characteristics of jobs and careers listed in Table 2-3 may help distinguish between the two. The intent is not to imply that a career is inherently better than a job, nor is the contrast suggested as more than a guide.

Although the number of nurses being educated in college programs has recently increased, the impact of this number is deceptive. While most nurses maintain a current license to practice, 2,558,874 in 1996 (insert current# here), and fewer are leaving nursing voluntarily than is sometimes implied, restructuring of staffing in acute care settings has decreased the availability of traditional RN positions in many areas. Increasingly more nurses are employed in nontraditional community settings, and that trend is expected to continue.

Independent Function

During the first half of the 20th century, a view of nurses as handmaidens or assistants to physicians pervaded American thinking. The reason for this perception probably related more to deeply ingrained social values than to any inherent characteristics of nursing practice. State nursing practice laws generally do not prohibit nurses from behaving more independently in ways consistent with their knowledge and skills. At the same time, nurses are clearly restricted in diagnosing illness and in prescribing independently for its treatment. These two functions currently are the prerogative of medical practice.

As currently practiced, nursing has acknowledged independent and interdependent functions. Occasionally, nurses set up private practices outside a formal health care institution and practice independently. Society also receives great benefit from nursing's independent practice in the form of voluntary service or charity. Society often expects nurses to provide free advice and service in their neighborhoods and communities. It does not ask the same of law or medicine, in which most of the practitioners are men.

Additional Criteria

Two additional criteria of American professions identified by Lysaught (1980) are an active and cohesive professional organization and acknowledged social worth and contribution. In 1996, fewer than (one in ten licensed nurses) or 178,900, were members of ANA. Probably a comparable number belonged to other organizations such as specialty groups or honor societies. The membership of these combined organizations accounted for approximately one quarter of all RNs.

Professionalization is a dynamic process. Some people describe nursing as a semiprofession or an emerging profession. Others call it an aspiring profession. Just as humankind is viewed as being in the process of becoming, so might nursing be viewed. Thus, the terms *developing profession* and *aspiring profession* are useful, because they convey a possibility of striving to achieve a potential. As humans move from basic needs through growth needs, so nursing must move from occupational to professional criteria before achieving full professional status. Perhaps, then, nursing has reached early adulthood, not full maturity, as a profession.

Lessons of the Past

The following are three lessons of the past worth learning:

1. Issues and problems facing nursing today are neither as new as we sometimes like to think, nor do they need to be as immobilizing as some might suggest.
2. Just as yesterday's issues are today's history, today's issues will be tomorrow's history.
3. Today, as in the past, individual persons make things happen as they work alone and together for common causes. Ideas and actions begin with one person. Although society shapes the nursing profession, persons within nursing have determined and will determine much of what happens to nursing.

Historically, nurses were not always fully aware of their special contributions to health care. That is, they did not identify and articulate the essence of nursing.

Sometimes nurses minimized their abilities to develop trust between themselves and those they nursed, to identify the healthy aspects of the person, and to help individuals mobilize their own health qualities to achieve their personal potential. Nurses recognized that although people might have severe or even life-threatening physical problems, they were still unique individuals capable of growth. However, because nurses did not identify and articulate nursing's unique contribution completely, much of it was set aside as nursing entered an age of increased technology.

As technology flourished, much of nursing became "doing activities." Nurses and others measured their value by their skills in taking care of equipment. A unique nursing contribution was present in much of what nurses did, but it often seemed less important. It was not unusual for clients to describe their appreciation of nursing care and for the nurse to think or say, "But I didn't do anything!" Perhaps the nurse listened with trust and therapeutic purpose and helped the clients to recover control of their lives, to regain their sense of self-esteem, and to view their future with hope or a sense of well-being.

In the 1970s and 1980s, nursing made enormous leaps in practice, education, and research. The decisions to be made in the 1990s and the next millennium are understood better from a historical perspective. For the same reason that cultures find their roots important, nursing is experiencing a surge of interest in its roots. Today, a primary and specific purpose for considering history is to relate it both to the present and to the future. Many have written, explaining this well, including Aiken and Fagin (1992), Ashley (1976), Chaska (1990, 1983), Kalisch and Kalisch (1995), Kelly (1996, 1995), and Neil and Watts (1991).

Neil and Watts's (1991) edited work offers a recent feminist perspective of nursing. Their volume *Caring and Nursing: Explorations in Feminist Perspectives* explains in detail how various theories of feminism apply to nursing. For example, in that volume, MacPherson (1991) compared liberal, radical, and social feminist theories in "Looking at Caring and Nursing Through a Feminist Lens." As nurses turn the concept of caring toward themselves as persons, some nurses become concerned with what they consider to be the oppression of both women and nurses, and find that a feminist explanation for this oppression is helpful. Regardless of whether you subscribe to such a perspective personally, you will come to know that nursing's development as art, science and profession has been shaped by the fact that, to date, most practitioners have been women.

KEY CONCEPTS

✔Throughout history, nursing has been the art of giving care, centered on the individual needs of persons and families. Over time, the art has changed from intuitive to scientific.

✔Nursing is being recognized as an advancing science based on the recent development of its theory and research.

✔Nursing is developing the characteristics of recognized professions.

✔Recognized professions are characterized by unique knowledge and service, standardized collegiate education, independent function and control of practice, and accountability and career commitment.

CRITICAL THINKING QUESTIONS

1. How do you think nursing might have developed differently if:
   a. The majority of practitioners were men?
   b. The majority of nurses were baccalaureate prepared?
   c. All nurses accepted nursing as a career rather than as a job?

2. Using the criteria for professions given and your critical thinking abilities, how do you rate nursing on each criterion in comparison with other professions?

3. How might modern technology enhance or threaten nursing's:
   a. Development as a profession?
   b. Traditional values?

4. Using what you learned in this chapter, map a strategy for keeping current on issues that will affect nursing's professionalism.

5. How might you personally exert an influence on the professional status and perception of nursing?

6. Compare nursing with another art, science, or profession. How are they similar and how do they differ?

REFERENCES

Aiken, L.H. & Fagin, C.M. (1992). *Charting nursing's future: agenda for the 1990s*. Philadelphia: J.B. Lippincott.

American Nurses Association. (1995). *A social policy statement* (Publication No. NP-107) Washington, DC: American Nurses Publishing.

American Nurses Association. (1985). *Code for nurses with interpretive statements*. Kansas City, MO: Author.

American Nurses Association. (1980). *A social policy statement* (Publication No. NP-63 35M). Kansas City, MO: Author.

American Nurses Association. (1965). *Standards for organized nursing services*. New York: Author.

Ashley, J.A. (1976). *Hospitals, paternalism, and the role of the nurse*. New York: Teachers College Press.

Baker, C.M. (1995). Comparing nursing doctoral programs around the globe. *Reflections* 21(3), 2–3. Fall 1995.

Bevis, E.O. (1989). *Curriculum building in nursing: A process* (3rd ed., Publication No. 15-2278). New York: National League for Nursing.

Carnegie, M.E. (1986). *The path we tread: Blacks in nursing, 1854–1984*. Philadelphia: J.B. Lippincott.

Carnegie, M.E. (1995). *The path we tread: Blacks in nursing worldwide, 1954-1994.* (2nd ed., Publication No.14-2678). New York: NLN Press.

Chaska, N. (1990). *The nursing profession: Turning points.* St. Louis, MO: C.V. Mosby.

Chinn, P.L. & Watson, J. (1994). *Art and aesthetics in nursing* (Publication No. 14-2611). New York: NLN Press.

Cohen, J.A. (1991). Two portraits of caring: A comparison of the artists, Leininger and Watson. *Journal of Advanced Nursing, 16,* 899–909.

Dock, L.L., & Stewart, I.S. (1938). *A short history of nursing.* New York: G.P. Putnam's Sons.

Donahue, M.P. (1996) *Nursing: The finest art–An illustrated history* (2nd ed.). St. Louis, MO: C.V. Mosby.

Donahue, M.P. (1985) *Nursing: The finest art–An illustrated history.* St. Louis, MO: C.V. Mosby.

Flexner, A. (1910). *Medical education in the United States and Canada.* New York: Carnegie Foundation for Advancement of Teaching.

Goldmark, J. (1923). *Nursing and nursing education in the United States.* New York: Macmillan.

Graves, J. (1996). New classification system announced. *Reflections 22,* 24–28.

Health, Education, and Welfare Secretary's Committee to Study Extended Roles for Nurses. (1971). Extending the scope of nursing practice. *American Journal of Nursing, 71,* 2346–2351.

Henderson, V. (1966). *The nature of nursing.* New York: Macmillan.

Kalisch, P.A., & Kalisch, B.J. (1995). *The advance of American nursing* (3rd ed.). Philadelphia: J.B. Lippincott.

Kelly, L.Y. & Joel, L. (1996). *The nursing experience*: *Trends, challenges, transitions* (3rd ed.). New York: McGraw-Hill.

Kelly, L.Y. (1995). *Dimensions of professional nursing* (7th ed.). New York: McGraw-Hill

Leininger, M.M. (1995). *Transcultural Nursing: Concepts, theories, research and practices* (2nd ed.). New York: McGraw-Hill.

Lysaught, J. (1980, June). *Action on affirmation toward an unambiguous profession of nursing.* Paper presented at the biennial American Nurses' Association meeting, Houston, TX.

MacPherson, K.I. (1991). Looking at caring and nursing through a feminist lens. In R.M. Neil & R. Watts (Eds.), *Caring and nursing: Explorations in feminist perspectives* (Publication No. 14-2369, pp. 25–42). New York: National League for Nursing.

Meleis, A.I. (1991). *Theoretical nursing: Development and progress.* Philadelphia: J.B. Lippincott.

Montag, M. (1951). *The education of nursing technicians.* New York: G.P. Putnam's Sons.

National Commission for the Study of Nursing and Nursing Education. (1970). *An abstract for action.* New York: McGraw-Hill.

National League for Nursing. (1995). *Nursing Datasource: Vol 1, Trends in contemporary nursing education* (Publication No. 19-6649). New York: Author.

National League for Nursing. (1994). *Nursing Data Review 1994* (Publication No. 19-2639). New York: Author.

Neil, R.M., & Watts, R. (Eds.). (1991). *Caring and nursing: Explorations in feminist perspectives* (Publication No. 14-2369). New York: National League for Nursing.

Nightingale, F. (1859). *Notes on nursing: What it is and what it is not.* London: Harrison. (Facsimile ed., Philadelphia: J.B. Lippincott, 1966.).

Parse, R.R. (1989). Essentials for practicing the art of nursing. *Nursing Science Quarterly, 2(3),* 111.

Schein, E.H., & Kommers, D.W. (1972). *Professional education.* New York: McGraw-Hill.

Spector, R. (1991). *Cultural diversity in health and illness* (3rd ed.). Norwalk, CT: Appleton & Lange.

3

Nursing Today: The Health Science of Caring

To understand fully the career opportunities available in nursing, it is necessary to look at nursing from several perspectives. This chapter provides an introduction to the concept *nursing* that shapes nursing as art, science, and profession. The chapter offers a basic foundation for understanding the many intellectual and interpersonal nursing skills. It also provides a context for understanding the many technologic aspects of nursing that are necessarily a part of nursing education as well as professional nursing practice. *Professions* are applied sciences that must utilize theoretical knowledge to achieve practical ends, because one important characteristic of professions is their service to humankind.

The discussion of nursing as a theoretical science includes information that may be beyond the perceived need for some readers and insufficient for others. Likewise, some readers will not initially identify with the importance given to nursing research in an introductory text. However, the material included suggests a full range of nursing's potential scope.

As indicated in Chapter 2, people have always needed nursing care. As society evolved, attempts to meet nursing care requirements evolved, changing from familial and informal caregiving to caregiving based on formal education, state licensing, and national credentialing. Currently, society is accepting nurses practicing in expanded roles, as health care and health care delivery are changing rapidly. In 1987, the U.S. Department of Health and Human Services projected a deficiency of 600,000 nurses prepared at baccalaureate and higher levels by the year 2000 (Rosenfeld, 1987). This projected deficiency raised cries of both crisis and doom in the late 1980s. Now, the growing use of assistive personnel for nursing activities and the uncertainty of how health care reform will evolve make this an uncertain time for venturing predictions. Some who look to the future, however, foresee an era of golden opportunity previously unequaled for the profession of nursing.

Historically, when society recognizes a pressing, unmet, social need, as it does now for humanistic care, it may mobilize social forces to correct the situation. Thus, social need can create a window of opportunity to benefit both society and the professional group addressing that need.

The Nursing Concept Explored

Nursing is gaining professional and public recognition as the health science of caring. *Caring* is perhaps the one word or phenomenon most clearly associated with nursing over time. Caring involves having thought or regard for someone as a person, as well as giving watchful oversight or being an advocate for or assistant when an individual is unable to tend to personal needs. Caring is practiced: parent to child, lover to lover, well to ill, fortunate to less fortunate, or professional to client. Caring is the most intimate, tender, protective, and growth-producing of interpersonal interactions. However, caring and caring as science differ.

To call nursing the health science of caring is to value health and its promotion, to emphasize the science of nursing as well as the art, and to acknowledge that caring is a prime interpersonal interaction open to study. Caring is also an interpersonal interaction that transcends time, gender, and technology. In that spirit, nursing, the health science of caring, is a service basic to society. This service was born in the days of earliest humankind and has the potential to serve human needs as long as people inhabit the earth and the universe.

A century after Nightingale, Virginia Henderson (1966) wrote,

> The unique function of the nurse is to assist the individual, sick or well, in the performance of those activities contributing to *health* (emphasis added, p. 42) or its recovery (or to peaceful death) that he would perform unaided if he had the neces-

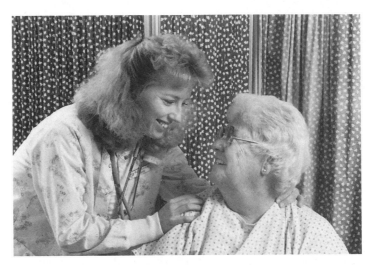

The science of caring is based on interpersonal interactions that are tender and protective and that value health and growth.

sary strength, will, or knowledge. And to do this in such a way as to help him gain independence as rapidly as possible. This aspect of her work, this part of her function, she initiates and controls; of this she is master. In addition she helps the patient to carry out the therapeutic plan as initiated by the physician (p. 15).

Henderson's emphasis on the nurse as ''she'' reflected an accepted reality, but one that overlooked a valuable human resource for society and nursing. In the 1980s, men's caring abilities finally received recognition and social approval. This recognition and approval may encourage men to choose nursing in greater numbers.

Another, more current, definition of nursing is from the Model Practice Act published in 1982 by the National Council of State Boards of Nursing. It states,

The ''Practice of Nursing'' means assisting individuals or groups to maintain or attain optimal *health* (emphasis added, p. 42) throughout the life process by assessing their *health* (emphasis added, p. 42) status, establishing a diagnosis, planning and implementing a strategy of care to accomplish defined goals, and evaluating responses to care and treatment (p. 2).

Also in the early 1980s, the American Nurses Association (ANA, 1980) issued a social policy statement with an emphasis on the importance of health. A few words from this statement took on the status of a national definition for nursing, namely, that nursing is ''the diagnosis and treatment of human responses to actual or potential health problems'' (p. 9). Notice that these last two definitions make no gender reference for nurse. These definitions suggest the need to clarify several terms to understand nursing as the health science of caring. The American Nurses Association reaffirmed its social commitment with a 1995 social policy publication.

Health is such an important concept for nursing that we have devoted an entire chapter to its elaboration. At this point, however, a few comments are enough to introduce the subject. Clearly, the definition of health is changing over time. Health is now considered to be a condition of the life cycle that is dynamic, adaptive, responsive to both internal and external stimuli, and influenced by the behaviors of the "person." Health has, as subconcepts, wellness and illness components. Wellness and illness often coexist in the same person.

All people have health needs—to promote, retain, or regain health, according to individual and varying potentials. These health needs exist across the life span in both well and ill persons. Any setting where nurses encounter persons with health needs is where nursing care can and should be delivered. For generations, and until just recently, the United States health care system has been primarily an illness-care system that has treated illness but has downplayed wellness promotion, health maintenance, and illness prevention.

That nursing is designated a health science is expanded on later. At this point, we can begin by saying that science is knowledge gained by systematic study. Science is also a particular branch of knowledge. An alternate and once popular definition of science—that is, knowledge as skill resulting from training—is no longer adequate. For example, what was once referred to as nurses' training is currently called nursing education and occurs with other higher education in colleges and universities. Nursing theory and the scientific knowledge gained by research help nursing gain recognition as the health science of caring.

Nursing Science

Nursing science is derived from scientific thinking about the discipline or field of nursing and the practice of the profession of nursing. As Torres (1990) states, "Basic to any professional discipline is the development of a body of knowledge that can be applied to its practice. Such knowledge is often expressed in terms of concepts and theories, especially in the area of behavioral or social sciences. Thus, nursing as a young, evolving profession is developing a body of knowledge in terms of the concepts and theories that support its practice" (p.1).

Before discussing nursing theory specifically, let us consider some more general ideas basic to scientific thinking. Two notions prominent among these general ideas are 1) critical thinking and 2) scientific method. One way to understand these notions is to talk about different kinds of thinking skills. Often we use such skills intuitively or without serious awareness of what kind of cognitive or thinking processes we are actually employing.

What is Critical Thinking?

Sometimes critical thinking is associated with logic or reasoning. Critical thinking is:

- ❐ Active
- ❐ Purposeful

❐ Disciplined and organized
❐ Expressed in reasoning or communication that influences beliefs and actions

It is also:

❐ Processing skills and abilities that involve both reasoning and creative thinking
❐ Open and reflective
❐ Reinforced by practice to become habit

Scientific method and nursing process (discussed in Chapter 8) are both ways to apply critical thinking.

Critical thinking is essentially both an activity of learning and the active processing of information. To process information, you must be able both to access it and to use it to some purpose. Critical thinking is a basic skill that is underdeveloped by the public education most students receive prior to entering nursing education programs.

This circumstance is unfortunate for many reasons:

❐ Critical thinking is expected of you in nursing education and practice.
❐ Confronting inadequate skills is uncomfortable.
❐ We often equate thinking and knowledge with information acquisition and memorization rather than with a level of understanding that is necessary for the critical thinking processes of applying, analyzing, synthesizing and evaluating information, regardless of its source.
❐ The half-life of information today argues for an education that focuses more on the process of developing thinking and learning skills than on facts alone.
❐ The amazing advances in the access of information through technology (i.e., electronic libraries and internet resources) make information much more available, detailed, current and flexibly organized than previously. These technological advances can free us to concentrate more on developing critical thinking skills that will empower us to adapt in personal and professional worlds of rapidly changing information and knowledge.
❐ You have the native intelligence and capacities necessary for developing critical thinking.

These capacities include:

❐ The ability to perceive in a number of dimensions, but especially to observe and to listen. Skills in these areas are seldom honed to their potential, because we are apt to fall into sloppy thinking habits of being lazy or inattentive.
❐ The capacity to explore and to be curious, to wonder and to be awed. Exposure to TV and other mass media may dull this capacity by encouraging passivity.
❐ The ability to deal with ambiguity. We often seek, however, to escape the unsettling discomfort that ambiguous situations can provoke.

The authors contend that critical thinking is a theme that should pervade and guide a nurse's actions in applying the concepts basic to nursing practice. The art of nursing, as defined earlier by Rogers, may be considered a precursor to what is today called critical thinking. Critical thinking is used to solve problems that you will often encounter in the everyday world of nursing practice, where nursing science is applied, as well as in the purely academic understanding of nursing theory. You will sometimes encounter problems that require more information or better techniques for handling information. These problems are often amenable to the logical and organized process of thinking that uses inductive or deductive reasoning and is called vertical thinking. Other times no new information is required, but to solve a problem you must, through a different way of thinking, rearrange information that is already available. This other way of thinking is sometimes called **lateral thinking** (deBono, 1970). It is also called flexibility, divergent thinking, or perhaps creative or innovative thinking. To be creative or innovative may seem to be more demanding than to allow yourself to be flexible and engage in divergent thinking.

Vertical thinking is probably the kind of thinking to which you are most accustomed, because most basic science courses have used this approach. Lectures often stress facts, principles, or expert opinion, i.e., general information which you are expected to apply in specific situations. This process is called **deductive reasoning**. In such lecture courses you may also have used what is called **inductive reasoning** to relate reality and past experience to principles or generalities that may be new to you. Vertical thinking through deductive and inductive reasoning is a way to reinforce concepts and facts, i.e., old knowledge. The counter side of such reinforcement is that it also tends to get our thinking mired in a "rut." Professional education both demands and offers more than "rut" thinking. It requires critical thinking that uses both logical (vertical) and flexible (lateral) thinking.

Consider the following contrasts of vertical and lateral thinking and summarize these skills: vertical thinking is intellectual ordering, while lateral thinking is intellectual searching. Vertical thinking is familiar and often conventional, conforming, convergent, accepted, and expected. Lateral thinking involves an attitude and a method of using information differently. Lateral thinking requires purposeful thought and practice, because the brain's memory system tends to create patterns and perpetuate them. According to deBono, vertical thinking is analytical, sequential, and correct. Lateral thinking is provocative, jumps by quantum leaps, and is not burdened by having to be correct. Provocative new ideas become correct only after testing and validation. "The most basic principle of lateral thinking is that any particular way of looking at things is only one from among many other possible ways" (deBono, 1970). Another principle involves challenging assumptions, i.e., asking *why?* Vertical thinking aims for a minimum solution to a problem, while lateral thinking increases chances of a maximum solution, but makes no promises. Vertical thinking and lateral thinking are complementary and not antagonistic thinking processes. Neither used exclusively is sufficient for our most productive or critical thinking.

A graphic representation may help you actually visualize these dynamic processes of vertical and lateral thinking (Fig. 3-1).

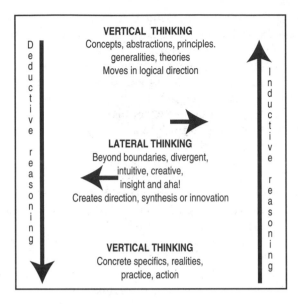

FIGURE 3-1 Vertical and lateral thinking.

Before turning to scientific method, with which you are probably somewhat familiar, consider actual ways you can develop critical thinking skills once you are open to the idea:

In keeping with the spirit of divergent thinking, this next section is purposely written in a highly personal and informal manner with the intent that you will actually think about how these suggestions might work for you. To understand nursing as science, it may be helpful *first* to realize that the skills nurse scientists, researchers and theorists use are the same skills that you will need in practice. Their development and application, though seemingly different, stems from the same foundation. Therefore, regardless of how you now think you intend to develop your personal nursing career, you can, early in your nursing education, acquire the skills that will enable and empower you to exercise many options beyond your present vision.

❏ First, acknowledge that these are skills you want to develop or hone more sharply.

❏ With the assistance of others, if necessary, assess your current cognitive skill level. Remember that the starting point of your skill development is less important than setting a goal.

❏ Focus on critical thinking as a *process* able to generate many useful *products*. Even complex products like nursing theory are outputs of the critical thinking process. Consider concepts, vertical and lateral thinking, and deductive and inductive reasoning to be tools to aid in the critical thinking process.

❏ Consider your life experiences, whatever they are, as a resource for critical thinking.

❏ Accept that original provocative ideas are a creation of cognitive thought, and therefore have some potential to be validated by testing. "Different" may or may not be better than "same old," but learn to suspend judgment.

❒ Bounce your ideas off other people. Remember that diversity in thinking begets excellence. Therefore, make it a purposeful habit to associate with others who are unlike yourself.

❒ Seek a mentor or patron who is wise and encouraging.

❒ Exercise your mind in fun ways so that the thinking habit becomes more pleasurable. You might also try reading for pleasure in an unfamiliar area, or learning bridge or chess.

You can develop your **vertical thinking** skills. Some ways to do this are to:

❒ Increase your repertoire of resource-searching strategies.

❒ Perfect your outlining skills.

❒ Limit highlighting of what you read to encourage a deeper understanding.

❒ Apply concepts to the real world as a self test, even when a faculty member does not require it.

❒ Use analogies to make vague and abstract ideas come alive. Concepts are based in facts and theories, but personalized and enriched through experience and practice.

You can also develop your **lateral thinking** skills. Some ways to do this are to:

❒ Practice reflective thinking, i.e., make time for personal contemplation and reflecting on the deeper meaning and significance of ideas. This is a skill that can be practiced while commuting, doing the household chores, or walking the dog.

❒ Share your divergent and reflective ideas with others for reactions, alternative views, and interpretations.

❒ Develop the habit of generating guesses or alternative hypotheses about ideas and problem solutions. Even if you do this silently only for yourself, practice improves competence.

❒ Put ideas into your mental creative thought processes and let them incubate or percolate.

❒ Keep a running list of divergent ideas on a yellow pad or in a computer file. Someday they may find an application.

❒ Break out of a group think mode. That is, come to class prepared with an open mind, interesting questions, and thoughts to share.

You can also practice other critical thinking skill development ideas:

❒ Hone computer word processing, electronic library, and information access skills. These skills will enhance your ease of capturing information and organizing ideas.

❒ Write!write!write! and expect to refine your writing through self-editing.

Remember, although computer-generated writing may look deceptively attractive, seldom is the first effort a finished product.

❏ Find an interest or activity connected to nursing that reflects your true creative self. Use your involvement in this activity to assist motivation, inspiration, and perseverance.

❏ Learn and practice APA style. Referencing according to the American Psychological Association style is both mental discipline for assuring future access to information as well as a way of documenting others' creativity in a scholarly fashion.

❏ Propose alternative ways of meeting course objectives; learn to negotiate as well as to challenge.

❏ Accept that divergent learning will feel different than rote memorization and regurgitation of facts.

❏ Learn and practice **critique.** Some persons equate critique with negative criticism, but critique is more accurately described as thoughtful and detailed response to intent of presentation, ideas, and communication. Consider critique a partner of reflective thinking.

In addition to depth, sophistication, and skill in vertical thinking, one of the characteristics that differentiates professional nurses (or nursing students) from other nursing personnel is their broader range of critical thinking skills. With practice you can function creatively by combining scientific principles with divergent intuitive thinking to achieve superlative results in the science and profession of nursing—including practice, research, and theory. Not surprisingly, one of the first and most satisfying discoveries of innovative professional nurses concerns the arena of practice. Although practice is partially defined by law and policies, there is much more opportunity for creative practice in nursing than most nurses realize. With health care reform, health care systems will require new ways to deliver nursing services. In "Critical thinking: taking the road less traveled," Stark (1995) suggests the importance of using intuition and following hunches as a way to be open to possibilities. Rubenfeld (1995) offers a detailed and interactive way for you to further hone your critical thinking skills, using problems and exercises. As Alfaro-LeFevre (1995) notes in *Critical Thinking in Nursing: a Practical Approach*, beyond clinical judgment and nursing research, other important areas for the application of critical thinking include moral and ethical reasoning, teaching others, teaching ourselves, and test taking (p. 70). Clearly, in both education and practice, you will have many opportunities to practice and use your critical thinking skills.

The Scientific Method

As Carl Sagan (1995) writes:

> Science is far from a perfect instrument of knowledge. It's just the best we have. In this respect, as in many others, it's like democracy. Science by itself cannot advocate courses of human action, but it can certainly illuminate the possible consequences of alternative courses of action.

The scientific way of thinking is at once imaginative and disciplined. This is central to its success. Science invites us to let the facts in, even when they don't conform to our preconceptions. It counsels us to carry alternative hypotheses in our heads and see which best fit the facts. It urges on us a delicate balance between no-holds barred openness to new ideas, however heretical, and the most rigorous skeptical scrutiny of every thing—new ideas and established wisdom. This kind of thinking is also an essential tool for a democracy in an age of change (p. 27).

The format of the scientific method is much the same whether used in physics, psychology, medicine, or nursing. The **scientific method** is the most advanced approach to acquiring knowledge, but it has limitations. It cannot answer ethical or value questions, nor can it overcome current inabilities to measure some of the concepts of interest to nurses. Furthermore, applying the scientific method in the real world of health care is much more difficult than in the confines of the laboratory. In nursing, the scientific method has been applied as **nursing process.** Nursing process can be used in conjunction with other critical thinking skills and nursing theory to solve practice problems.

The scientific method can also be purposefully used in both everyday and research situations to find an answer to a problem or perplexing question. The four steps of the scientific method are

1. Define the problem.
2. Collect data from observation and experimentation.
3. Devise and execute a solution.
4. Evaluate the solution.

Define the Problem

A basic but sometimes forgotten principle is that if you intend to solve or investigate a problem, you must know what the problem is. As described by de Bono (1970), a *problem* is the difference between the existing situation and a more ideal situation. Most problems are complex or multidimensional. Therefore, a general problem area may contain several related questions. Problems are often phrased in the form of what and how questions, although other words such as *who, when, where,* and *why* may also be appropriate. Questions asked this way, rather than in a way that anticipates a yes or no answer, lend themselves to exploring alternative solutions. Exploring alternative solutions is an important element of the scientific method.

Because beneath their individual differences people are alike in many ways, it is also possible to identify problems that apply to people collectively. This ability to generalize is the rationale for applying the scientific method to research, that is, being able to identify so-called researchable problems or problems that are of potential interest to large groups of people. For example, a general problem area of interest to both nurses and physicians may be how the risk of heart attack can be minimized for apparently healthy persons. Depending on the scientific and professional background and the hunches of the investigator, he or she might identify a variety of more specific problems (e.g., related to medication, diet, or exercise).

Collect Data from Observation and Experimentation

Experts in any scientific field are distinguished by their ability to use decision-making processes based on scientific principles. There is a large body of scientific knowledge about normal human functioning in biologic or physiologic, psychological or intrapersonal, and interpersonal areas. In health care, identifying problems of deviant function involves comparison with what a healthy or "normal" person should be able to do. The health care professional compares the information (data) received from the person to known standards or norms. Because persons are so complex, this task requires comparison with many normalcy standards. The definition of normal itself changes as scientific knowledge is added to a discipline—for example, information about what changes to expect in physiologic function with age. A full health history, physical examination, and laboratory tests, as well as an in-depth interview about how the person sees his or her current life situation, may yield valuable information to clarify the problem further. Such "experiments" as controlled tests of heart function may furnish additional information for comparison with normal expected values for persons of similar age, gender, and so forth.

For a particular situation, information (data), problems, and solutions may seem confusingly interwoven. Indeed, a certain amount of data collection precedes being able to even identify a general problem. Also, although we often diagram the scientific method in stepwise fashion, the process is less straightforward and more circular than usually imagined.

Devise and Execute a Solution

The solution or potential solution of a problem depends on the specific problem identified. Executing a solution is a process of selecting from among the alternatives those that seem likely to lead to a desired goal. Consider the problem and goal as two points, and imagine a number of paths linking them. Alternative courses of action provide paths or bridges between problems and goals. Considering alternative solutions forces choices among options. Problem statements that are too broad or too narrow can interfere with the discovery of alternative solutions. It is rare that a problem has only one solution. Some solutions, of course, will be more likely, less costly, and easier to execute than others. In research terms, alternative solutions are sometimes called scientific hunches or, more technically, hypotheses to be tested.

Evaluate the Solution

The scientific method does not guarantee the results of a problem-solving solution. Evaluation, although appearing to be a final step in the scientific method, is really a point in a circular process. Evaluation requires judging outcomes against specific criteria to determine the effectiveness of actions. Essentially, outcomes result from executing a problem solution. To be successful, an outcome must be a resolution, an alleviation, or a prevention of the original problem. This is both a reason for stating problems precisely and also evidence of the circularity of the process. Evaluation challenges the problem solver to move on to new problems or to readdress old ones.

Nursing Theory

What is Nursing Theory?

Now that we have explored some general ideas about scientific thinking, consider the scientific thinking called **nursing theory.**

Nursing theory is the systematic abstraction or formation of mental ideas about nursing practice reality. Its purpose is to describe, explain, predict, and control nursing action (caring) to achieve certain nursing practice outcomes. Theories interrelate concepts to provide new ways of looking at nursing care and improving nursing practice. Theories also assist in increasing the general body of knowledge within the discipline through the research implemented to validate (confirm) them (Torres, 1980).

Theories can be characterized according to their scope of focus. For example, a *grand theory* of nursing is broad, and encompasses supposedly everything a nurse needs to know. A *middle range theory,* on the other hand, is less broad and may, therefore, be pertinent to specific areas of nursing. Many other ways to describe theories are beyond the scope of these introductory remarks.

The Importance of Nursing Theory

Sciences develop and mature as the knowledge in the discipline increases and becomes unique, organized, and more complex. Nursing must create a distinct and unique theoretical science. The science must describe, explain, predict, and control the outcomes of nursing practice. Only then will nursing be fully recognized as a separate scientific discipline and a true profession.

Apart from the intellectual reasons for developing nursing theory, one might ask the logical question, "How does theory relate to nursing practice?" The basic answer is that practicing nursing from a theoretical perspective gives scientific credibility to practice. Theory provides a framework or paradigm to direct the action of practice. As Erickson, Tomlin, and Swain (1983) indicated,

> Basic needs can often be met in a very few actual minutes of care, assuming that a clear and purposive theory and paradigm [framework] are employed. If a substantial block of time *is* taken, it may in the long run preserve the nursing staff from even greater investments of time and energy extended over numerous future times. More strenuous efforts become necessary when complications occur that might otherwise have been avoided (p. 242).

An example contrasts two ways of looking at clinical situations, that is, with and without a theoretical perspective. Angry, anxious, frightened patients constantly call the nurse. The nurse can respond without theory and be exasperated, angry, disgusted, tired, bored, avoidant, and feel helpless. This response may lead to the nurse's complaining, scolding, or avoiding such patients. Or, the nurse can respond with theory and recognize patients' inability to maintain an image of the nurse when they cannot see him or her caring about them, be aware of the patients' feelings of insecurity in hospital settings, understand the grief process, and consciously plan theoretically-based nursing care for patients.

The purpose of both nursing theory and nursing research, an application of scientific method, is to suggest answers to puzzling questions from nursing practice. These puzzling questions are concerned with

- ❑ *Description*—Clarifying ideas, phenomena, experiences, or circumstances that are not well understood, for example, describing what pain really means to patients. This clarification is accomplished by presenting new information.
- ❑ *Exploration*—Exploring how ideas of interest are related, for example, what is the relationship between pain and patients' physical and psychological conditions?
- ❑ *Explanation*—Explaining, often within the context of an existing theory, the whys of events or occurrences, for example, why does pain occur more frequently and severely in persons whose physical and psychological resources are impoverished or reduced?
- ❑ *Prediction and control*—Knowing and foretelling correctly what will happen and also how to make it happen on command, and with some regularity, for example, in what specific ways can the nurse control the severity of pain for patients?

If nursing is the science of caring, then caring is a critical phenomenon of both theoretical and practical interest. Therefore, as nursing science develops, nurses will be better able to predict and control this caring phenomenon. Control will benefit individual patients, clients, and society in a unique way. Belief in nursing's extraordinary contribution to society has been the driving force that leads nurses to create nursing science and theories that are indeed singular to nursing. Scientific theories are built on concepts or general abstractions. The following are definitions of words we have used already and will be using in our discussion of theories:

- ❑ *Concept*—A mental image or classification of things and events in terms of similarities. In nursing, person, health, environment, and nursing itself are concepts of primary interest to theory and practice. Scientific concepts are the building blocks of theory and refer to the abstract notions that are related within a theory.
- ❑ *A conceptual framework or model*—A structure comprising concepts associated so that they form a whole, for example, a developmental model with concepts of infant, child, and adult.
- ❑ *Theory*—A group of concepts, definitions, and statements that presents an organized view of phenomena (e.g., caring) by specifying interrelationships among concepts with the intent of describing, explaining, predicting, or controlling these phenomena. A now well-recognized theory

that has moved from the realm of science to that of everyday life is Einstein's theory of relativity: E = mc squared.

Additional definitions related to theoretical ideas include the following: laws, for example, laws of physics, chemistry, or nature; and principles, for example, principles of sterile technique or thermodynamics. Perhaps nursing will have its own laws someday and its principles will be based less on traditions and more on research and theory.

Many theories in the same and in different scientific disciplines share similar notions or general concepts. Different sciences use the same or similar concepts in different ways. For example, the concept of human is used differently by those in the discipline of anatomy than by those in psychology. Anatomy is concerned with the human's body and the physical structure of its parts; in contrast, psychology is the science of human behavior and also is concerned with mental states and processes. Likewise, scientific nursing is built on common concepts, the most frequent of which are nursing, person, health, and environment. Except for nursing, all of these concepts are also pertinent to other disciplines. Theory within a science shows how the science uses concepts uniquely. Theory differentiates one science from others that are built on some of the same or similar concepts. Theory is important to nursing both to increase and to organize nursing's knowledge. Theory also helps establish nursing's credibility as a legitimate scientific branch of knowledge.

Some leaders within nursing have debated about the proper use of the terms *conceptual model* and *theory*. Conceptual models are more abstract and perhaps are a more accurate description for most of what are referred to as nursing theories. Others have referred to the works of some leaders as philosophies rather than theories. New professionals often experience frustration in dealing with abstract and philosophical ideas. Because conceptual models are so abstract, they can be mentally taxing. They may seem to have nothing to do with the real world of nursing care. True, they do not directly answer questions for practice and research. However, vague conceptual models and beginning efforts at nursing theories are the state of nursing science at present. Also, conceptual models and theories are more scientific than mere intuition. Theories and models provide many challenges. They also define the tasks yet to be accomplished by current and future nurse–scholars if nursing is to become a true science and full profession. The following are brief examples of how to use a conceptual model in practice, using illustrations from Orem's self-care theory and Erickson, Tomlin and Swain's Modeling and Role-Modeling.

Orem example: A student nurse was working with a six-year-old boy with fetal alcohol syndrome who was living with his foster family. The child had many developmental delays and was still wearing diapers. The foster mother stated that she had never considered toilet training because of the child's developmental difficulties. The nursing student, using Orem's self-care theory, assessed the boy's self-care agency [ability] and noted that he had adequate language skills to communicate toileting needs, could tell when he was wet or soiled, and was interested when other family members used the toilet. Noting that these are all signs of readiness for toilet training, the student successfully implemented a program to teach the child to use the toilet. By focusing on the child's self-care abilities, rather than his developmental delays, the student was able to teach a skill for which the child was ready.

Erickson, Tomlin and Swain example: A staff nurse in an intensive care unit noted that many patients with chronic lung disease were having difficulty weaning from the ventilator, even when they were physiologically stable and appeared ready to breathe independently. Using the concept of object attachment from the Erickson, Tomlin and Swain's Modeling and Role-Modeling theory, the nurse theorized that these patients were experiencing object loss when they were removed from the ventilator. She noted that the ventilator had been their link to survival and patients had developed an attachment to it. She developed a plan in which a staff nurse would become a substitute attachment object for the patients while they were being weaned from the ventilator. This nurse would stay with the patient, giving encouragement and support until the patient was breathing comfortably. This intervention was highly successful in reducing the number of patients who failed to wean from the ventilator.

Learning about theory is sometimes avoided, or theory is dismissed as unimportant. Aspiring nurses should recognize the Herculean efforts of a few especially valued nurse–scientists. These nurses take risks and blaze trails in nursing theory development. Some scholars have pioneered the way in nursing theory because of their dedication, conviction, and commitment. They value nursing as an important and distinct scientific discipline. They also value nursing as a practice profession that society needs. These nurse–scientists have boldly shared their conceptual and theoretical notions for which we can be thankful. Although it is not necessary that we all be theorists, it is necessary that we work together to push nursing forward and help it develop as both a mature science and profession.

Theoretical Foundations from Related Sciences

In the past, nursing has borrowed or used theories from other related sciences as the foundation for nursing. A major reason for this borrowing was the lack of well-developed nursing theories. Many problems arise when borrowing bits and pieces of theoretical foundations from related sciences. In this age of knowledge specialization, nurses cannot maintain the expertise across a wide range of disciplines that scientists within those fields have. This lack can lead to incomplete, inaccurate, or obsolete knowledge. It also leads to problems synthesizing information appropriately. Additionally, theoretical notions are meant to be used within the context of the specific theory and discipline for which they were designed. They may or may not be appropriate or compatible with other notions outside the theory. A theory that holds in nonnursing reality may not represent reality with the same accuracy in a nursing situation. The trick, of course, is to understand enough to make reasonable judgments and appropriate syntheses, which is one reason nurses need a liberal education.

Many kinds of theories from other disciplines have been applied to nursing with varying success, including, but not limited to, theories of stress, development, and learning. Borrowing will continue until nursing has its own unique and well-developed theories that are sufficient for not only describing outcomes but actually controlling results of our area of interest—nursing practice. Even then, some suggest, we will continue to adapt theories from other discrete disciplines, but will make unique linkages within a nursing context.

It is not surprising that nursing, the one concept unique to our discipline, is also the one concept that is least well developed in relation to the others we use. Nursing's interest in and application of any of the concepts it shares with other disciplines are different from those of the other disciplines, including medicine. For example, nurses' interest in anatomy, physiology, and pathophysiology is not to gather data for making medical diagnoses. Rather, nurses assess the functional disabilities and remaining strengths of persons to understand and to predict responses to altered health states. In turn, this understanding enables nurses to plan nursing care to enhance health.

Where disciplines overlap—for example, nursing and medicine or nursing and psychology—the overlap is significant because of common shared knowledge. What is often understood in other disciplines, but misunderstood in nursing, is that the area of no overlap between sciences is what becomes the content unique to a discipline. It is this area of no overlap, that is, the area unique to nursing, that will prove most fruitful in the development of nursing theory and science.

One Theory or Many?

In its present state, the developing science of nursing will need to approach theory building on many fronts. Multiple theories or conceptual frameworks will be pursued for many reasons—for example, the currently prominent conceptual frameworks require considerable development as theories to be truly useful in research and practice with any regular consistency; the scope of nursing is such that midlevel theories will be more realistic to construct and use; and the diversity of practice within clinical areas (which is one of nursing's most attractive features) supports theoretical diversity.

Remembering that nursing theories reflect both the private views of theorists and the world views of the times can be useful in understanding the direction of theory development over time. The subject matter common to all theories of nursing includes the concepts of nurse or nursing, human or person, health, and environment. Any combination of these concepts and others may be approached or developed in a variety of ways to create models that are primarily concerned with systems, human development, or interpersonal interaction.

Selected Contributors to Nursing's Theoretical Knowledge

This section presents a brief overview of selected contributors to nursing's theoretical knowledge.

There are many ways to organize a discussion of nursing theorists. For our purposes, we have chosen to first present some older and newer nursing philosophies, and Table 3-1 contrasts ''old'' and ''new'' world views that affect perceptions of concepts important to nursing as well as ways of knowing. Following this are grand and mid-range theories as identified in Table 3-2 and by Marriner-

Tomey (1994). As Fawcett (1993) stated, "The conceptual models of a discipline provide different perspectives or frames of reference for the phenomena identified by the metaparadigm of that discipline" (pp. 12–13). We have not included all of nursing's acknowledged theorists; at the end of the section, the reader is directed to the detailed works of these and other theorists and to works of nursing leaders who have thoughtfully critiqued nursing's experience with theory development.

In the last decade of the 20th century, the new world view has become more evident in nursing science. Three prominent theorists especially illustrate the shift from closed systems to open systems, and also from unidimensional to multidimensional views of person, environment, health, and nursing. They are Jean Watson (1940–), Madeleine M. Leininger (1925–), and Martha Rogers (1914–1994). These theorists, representing different levels of theories, present alternative ways for centering caring (which, according to the theories, is the essence of nursing) at the heart of both nursing science and practice. Increasingly, the works of these theorists are headlining conferences, dominating writing, and influencing curricula. Collectively, these works are theoretical and futuristic (e.g., Leininger, 1995a), yet practical. They portray a practice profession that is interactive, culturally and spiritually sensitive, and person centered, even when client is in a community. They typify nursing scholars' willingness to struggle with humanistic theoretical ideas that may have a great potential for nursing as it moves toward the 21st century.

In addition to presenting the essentials of the philosophical views and theories, we have, where appropriate, labeled particular perspectives on the theoretical concepts of nurse or nursing, human or person, health, and environment by highlighting the concept in **bold.** Note that Chapter 1 also cited some of these theorists' views in capsule form in Table 1-2.

TABLE 3-1 *World Views Old and New*

Old World View	New World View
Whole defined as sum of parts; people can be understood by studying parts (reductionism)	Whole defined as more than some of the parts (holism)
Knowing must be objective; only sensory data count (empiricism)	Many ways to know, including intuition, aesthetics, and so forth
Persons and environment are separate entities	Persons and environments are interconnected
Time and space are separate entities	Space-time is a unitary entity
Causation, linear processes, facts, and norms are the aim of discovery	Experiences, personal meanings, and mutual processes are the aim of discovery
Equilibrium (homeostasis) is the goal of living things	Growth and change (homeodynamics) are the goals of living things

TABLE 3-2 *Selected Contributors to Nursing's Theoretical Knowledge*

Philosophers		Theorists—Grand		Theorists—Middle Range
Nightingale	1820–1910	Watson[1]		Newman
Henderson	1897–1996	Rogers	1914–1994	Leininger
Benner[2]		King		Parse
		Orem		Erickson, Tomlin & Swain
		Roy		Pender

[1] Although Marriner-Tomey (1994) classifies Watson's work as philosophy, most scholars consider that her recent work meets the criteria for nursing theory.
[2] Dates are not given for living theorists.

Nursing Philosophies

FLORENCE NIGHTINGALE (1820–1910) *environment*

Nightingale's writings (1859) about nursing predated nursing's concern with either theories or concepts. Florence Nightingale was the first nurse to recognize the importance of environmental factors to health, believing that maintenance of a healthy environment is a primary concern of **nursing.** Her concept of nursing care focused heavily on modifying the physical environment. She clearly thought, as history has demonstrated, that hospitals of her time did not generally promote health. In the mid-1880s, little was known about principles of sanitation. Louis Pastuer's bacteriologic studies and Joseph Lister's research on antisepsis were in their early stages. Communicable diseases such as cholera and dysentery were the most common causes of death. Contaminated food and water and stale air contributed to the high incidence of bacteria-caused illness. Nightingale's writings show her interest in the concept of **environment,** with attention to the sub-concepts of ventilation, warmth, effluvia (smells), noise, and light. Nightingale believed that fresh air, pure water, sunlight, and attention to cleanliness were essential to the recovery of the sick (Nightingale, 1859, p. 14). Indeed, by using these sanitation principles, she was able to reduce the mortality rate of wounded soldiers in the Crimean War from an appalling 42% to just 2.2% (Kalisch & Kalisch, 1986, p. 51). She also discussed other environmental factors such as elimination of unnecessary noise, provision of appropriate environmental stimuli, quality of diet, and bedding. Nightingale's ideas relate closely to current scientific theories of adaptation, needs, and stress (Torres, 1980). Although current concepts of health and the environment are more complex than in Nightingale's time, most of her writing continues to be relevant for today's nurses. Long before others, Nightingale wrote of treating **persons** rather than disease. Nightingale believed that the human body had natural healing powers, and that the nurse's job was to put persons in the best possible condition for nature to act upon them (Nightingale, 1859, p. 75). She thought **health** was achieved by enabling natural processes to work. Given the general medical treatments at the time (bizarre herbs, heavy metals, fomentations), she was correct in her belief that the physician's care often did more harm than good.

VIRGINIA HENDERSON (1897–1996)

Virginia Henderson's classic book *The Nature of Nursing* (1966) provided a definition of **nursing** that was translated into many languages. It was also the definition of nursing accepted earlier by the International Council of Nurses (1961). This definition, along with a list of functional abilities she outlined for clients, provided a view of the scope of practice she thought nurses could initiate and control:

> The unique function of the nurse is to assist the individual, sick or well, in the performance of those activities contributing to health or its recovery (or peaceful death) so that he would perform unaided if he had the necessary strength, will or knowledge. And to do this in such a way as to help him gain independence as rapidly as possible (p. 15).

In Henderson's view, **health** was equated with the most independent functioning of which the person was capable. The activities, not unlike those performed by many nurses today, included the following:

- ❏ Breathe normally.
- ❏ Eat and drink adequately.
- ❏ Eliminate body wastes.
- ❏ Move and maintain desirable postures.
- ❏ Sleep and rest.
- ❏ Select suitable clothing—dress and undress.
- ❏ Maintain body temperature within normal range by adjusting clothing and modifying the environment.
- ❏ Keep the body clean and well-groomed and protect the integument.
- ❏ Avoid dangers in the environment and avoid injuring others.
- ❏ Communicate with others in expressing emotions, needs, fears, or opinions.
- ❏ Worship according to one's faith.
- ❏ Work in such a way that there is a sense of accomplishment.
- ❏ Play or participate in various forms of recreation.
- ❏ Learn, discover, or satisfy the curiosity that leads to normal development and health and the use of the available health facilities (pp. 16–17).

Henderson believed the **person** (patient/client) is a unique individual and that nursing as a profession makes a unique contribution to society. Henderson was concerned with nurses assisting clients in meeting their personal needs, and her ideas relate closely to Maslow's hierarchy of basic needs. She claimed to have been influenced by Claude Bernard, a physiologist, and Jean Broadhurst, a microbiologist. Within nursing, she cited as influential persons Ida Orlando (1961) and Ernestine Weidenbach. Generations of nurses began their basic study of nursing using the classic text *Textbook of Principles and Practice of Nursing,* written by Bertha Harmer and Virginia Henderson (1955). In 1991, Henderson revisited her earlier definition and updated its implications for practice, research, and education in the National League for Nursing (NLN) publication *Reflections After 25 Years, 1991.*

PATRICIA BENNER AND JUDITH WRUBEL

Patricia Benner (1984) is known also for her widely acclaimed book *From Novice to Expert: Excellence and Power in Clinical Nursing Practice*. Benner and Wrubel (1989) stated that their theoretical work, *The Primacy of Caring: Stress and Coping in Health and Illness*, presents "alternative approaches to health promotion, restoration, and even curing practices based upon the primacy of caring" (p. xi). It extends the ideas of Benner's earlier work. Both works take actual professional practice as their base.

The primacy of caring is a theory of practice and for practice based on lived experience of both patient and nurse. According to this theory, what gives life meaning and fuses persons' thoughts, feelings, and actions is connection with persons, events, and plans in a way that matters. Caring determines what is stress and coping, and creates the possibility of helping and being helped. Having a deep understanding of what the patients' lived experience means and being able to intervene in a way perceived as caring is what differentiates the expert nurse from the novice nurse. Caring is individualistic, that is, person centered. It is also relational to others and the environment, and therefore only occurs in and is describable in context. The theory, which views caring as the essence of nursing, reflects both phenomenologic and feminist philosophy.

Grand Theories

Although Marriner-Tomey (1994) classifies Watson's work as nursing philosophy, and Watson began her work as a philosopher, she is today more often grouped with the grand theorists.

JEAN WATSON (1940–)

Jean Watson's theoretical work *Nursing: The Philosophy and Science of Caring* (1979) presents a philosophic orientation that seeks to balance science and humanism. (See Chapter 1 for her definition of caring.) Watson (1988) identified the 10 primary carative factors that form a structure for studying and understanding **nursing** as the science of caring:

1. The formation of a humanistic–altruistic system of values
2. The instillation of faith–hope
3. The cultivation of sensitivity to one's self and to others
4. The development of a helping–trusting relationship
5. The promotion and acceptance of the expression of positive and negative feelings
6. The systematic use of the scientific problem-solving method for decision making
7. The promotion of interpersonal teaching–learning
8. The provision for a supportive, protective, and/or corrective mental, physical, sociocultural, and spiritual environment
9. Assistance with the gratification of human needs
10. The allowance for existential–phenomenological forces (p. 10)

Not surprisingly, Watson considers caring as the moral ideal of nursing.

Watson believes that, although medicine focuses on curing, **nursing** focuses on caring. She also believes that physicians can cure disease, but that without care the illness will continue. Thus, her model has spirituality as a critical element. Regarding what she called a phenomenological orientation to nursing, Watson (1979) went on to say the following:

- ❏ It concerns itself with the unique subjective and objective experiences of the **individual (or family or group).**
- ❏ It adopts a holistic, gestalt attitude toward the understanding of one's self and others.
- ❏ It holds the individuality of the person as its most important concern.
- ❏ It values people because they are inherently good and capable of development.
- ❏ It values the total person context or gestalt as a more important determinant of **health**–illness care than the patient's bacteria, organic pathogens, or disorders alone (pp. 208–209).

In 1985, Watson titled her work *Nursing: Human Science and Human Care—A Theory of Nursing*, indicating her clear intent regarding her work as theory. The philosophic foundations of her theory provide us with the basis for a number of theoretical perspectives and much food for thought. Sithichoke-Rattan (1989) applied Watson's perspective to nursing care of preterm infants and their parents. A more recent clinical example of Watson' theory applied is the following reported by a nurse manager:

> Rachel, aged 45 and a college teacher, suffers from life-long cataracts and glaucoma. These problems have required many surgeries and her vision is severely compromised. She wears heavy corrective lenses, and can see to read only by holding the printed material inches from her eyes. She confided in me, her nurse, that she offers her students extra points if they will type on the computer using 20 point font size.
>
> Vision is very precious, and while working with clients who come in for surgery, I have noted more acute anxiety than I have often seen even in persons facing cancer diagnoses. These patients find it extremely difficulty to wait even a day for the patch and shield to be removed from their surgical eye so that they can know what their vision will be. They probably listen more closely than most when we provide the home care post-operative teaching information, so fearful are they that something might happen to damage or infect their eye. Watson's carative factors, especially numbers 2,3, and 5 are most helpful when caring for these clients. A graphic drawing of Watson's transpersonal caring can demonstrate how the client and the nurse each are their own persons and function independently of each other. However, as nurse and client work together in a care situation, they become enmeshed as the nurse provides caring and the client receives it.
>
> Rachael was pronounced "difficult" by a nurse who had seen her for other surgeries. She warned me not to let Rachael "run the show". From this "data," I knew that control was critical to Rachael's basic need satisfaction, so I proceeded to let her do just that–"run the show". As I listened to her, I discovered that she could instill her own hope, that she had faith in God, and in the surgeon, and that she was proud of her adaptation to her decreased visual acuity. She was anxious

but stable in her belief that this surgery would help. Later, after surgery, she became alarmed at the pain, and since her eye was patched, she felt sure that something terrible was happening. Her comments suggested her belief that if we could stop the pain, we could stop any damage that the pain might cause. Although the pain itself was not likely to cause damage, it was preventing Rachael from being in harmony with her environment and the anxiety it caused could have affected the eye. It was first necessary to calm her, which I could do by thinking of the transpersonal caring model which calmed me as well. As Rachael became quieter, we were able to think rationally together and to develop a plan for pain management. As she left for home, her confidence and hope had returned.

MARTHA E. ROGERS (1914–1994)

Rogers's conceptual model of nursing was presented first in her 1970 book *An Introduction to the Theoretical Basis of Nursing*, and later (1989) as "Nursing: A Science of Unitary Human Beings" in J. P. Riehl-Sisca's *Conceptual Models for Nursing Practice*. In the spirit of Nightingale, she emphasized the knowledge base for nursing and also, in a more universal way, is concerned with the relationship of humans and their environment. Rogers is one of the first nurse–theorists to specify **humans or persons** as the major focus of nursing concern. Martha Rogers described person, that is unitary man (1970) and unitary human (1983) as synergistic: a whole greater and different than the sum of its parts. Rogers also first defined her unitary man as an energy field of four dimensions. The incorporation of the idea of space–time in her model shows the influence of Einstein. Later, she replaced "four-dimensional" with "multidimensional," and then "pandimensional" (M. E. Rogers, 1992, p. 29). Clearly, person as an energy field was conceptualized as more than visible physical being. According to Rogers, other characteristics of person are wholeness and the powers of perception and thought. "Abstraction and imagery, language and thought, sensation and emotion are fundamental attributes of man's humaneness" (Rogers, 1970, P. 67). These qualities take on importance as persons make choices about interaction with the environment and also convey to nurses their thoughts and emotions about changes in their health status. Rogers's distinctive theoretical characteristic of person, however, is the notion of person as energy field. This unique notion of person offers interesting appeal for high-technology and space-age health care. Initially, Martha Rogers viewed **environment,** also an energy field, as all the universe external to unitary man. In later writing, Rogers (1990) regarded person and environment as integral (belonging as a part of the whole) with each other (p. 7).

Nursing care is focused on participating with the person in the process of self-realization, strengthening of the human fields, and participation with repatterning. Although many students and practitioners initially have difficulty with the unusual terminology and mind-stretching ideas voiced by Rogers, her influence as a prototype of nurse–scholar remains strong. Other nurses including Newman (1979) and Parse (1992, 1981) have developed theories based on her conceptual model. With the increasing interest in space travel, parapsychology, and predicting the future, Rogers's ideas seem less foreign today than when they were first expressed. Her three revised principles of homeodynamics (1990) are as follows:

1. *Principle of resonancy*—Continuous change from lower to higher frequency wave patterns in human and environmental fields
2. *Principle of helicy*—Continuous innovative, unpredictable, increasing diversity of human and environmental field patterns
3. *Principle of integrality*—Continuous mutual human field and environmental field process (p. 8)

Not surprisingly, Rogers (1992) has written explicitly about "nursing science and the space age" (pp. 27–34).

DOROTHEA OREM (1914–)

Orem (1959) is credited with the first explicit use of the term *self-care* in nursing. Orem (1991) defined self-care as learned, goal-oriented activity of individuals. The impetus for such a model was the education of practical nurses. **Nursing** intervention was recognized as needed when persons had self-care limitations. Orem believes that self-care is a human requirement for both life maintenance and development toward optimal functioning. The persons who need the nurse's assistance with self-care are adults with health-related limitations, the young, the aged, the ill, and the disabled. Further, Orem believes that the self-care needs can be classified as universal (i.e., like Maslow's basic needs); developmental (i.e., a range of life events and developmental processes); and health deviation needs (i.e., relating to alterations in both human structure and function). "Functioning symbolically," as Orem suggested, might encompass both the psychological and spiritual elements of person-centered care. Her ideas (1991) about self-care include the following:

Self-care agency—Ability to meet requirements for care that regulates life processes and promotes health, development, and well-being (p. 65)
Therapeutic self-care demand—The measures of care required for persons to meet their self-care requisites (p. 65)
Self-care deficits—A relationship in which the self-care ability is less than that required to meet a known self-care demand; Persons who have self-care deficits have legitimate need for nursing care (p. 71)

A self-care theoretical approach is clearly person centered, consistent with the international definition of nursing, and places increased emphasis on the consumer of health care services. Orem's approach to nursing process delineates three steps: (1) diagnosing and prescribing or determining agency deficit; (2) designing and planning what she calls a system of nursing assistance; and (3) producing and managing the systems. A more recent book (1995) is *Nursing: Concepts of Practice* (5th ed.).

Orem (1980) defined a **person** as "a unity that can be viewed as functioning biologically, symbolically, and socially" (p. 120). In her model, persons who are healthy are able to care for themselves. Individual people have a need for nursing care when they are unable to care for themselves. The self-care agency also can be viewed as the person's self-care abilities with regard to the following six components of universal self-care:

1. Maintenance of sufficient intake of air, water, and food
2. Provision of care associated with elimination processes and excrements
3. Maintenance of a balance between activity and rest
4. Maintenance of a balance between solitude and social interaction
5. Prevention of hazards to life, functioning, and well-being
6. Promotion of normalcy (1995, pp. 440–455)

IMOGENE M. KING (1923–)

King's first book, *Toward a Theory for Nursing: General Concepts of Human Behavior* (1971), proposed a conceptual framework for nursing. A more recent book, *A Theory of Nursing: Systems, Concepts, Process* (1981), is a derivative of a systems approach. Her writings indicate how theoretical ideas develop over time. She offered an example of how inductive and deductive reasoning shape theory. Using **person** as a major concept, King included three dynamic interacting systems: (1) individuals; (2) groups; and (3) society. King's description of individual growth and development included thoughts of both Jean Piaget and Erik Erikson. She believes, as do other nurses today, that mutual goal setting by nurse and client is a condition of achievement of goals within the nursing process. King's underlying general assumption is as follows: "The focus of **nursing** is human beings interacting with their environment leading to a state of health for individuals which is an ability to function in social roles." (1981, p. 143). In 1992, she explicitly identified her theory as one of "goal attainment." In recent years, others (e.g., Frey and Sieloff, 1995) have advanced her theory through publication and as editors for international conferences and collaborations.

CALLISTA ROY (1939–)

Known as Sister Callista Roy in her earlier career, her adaptation model has undergone refinement and revision by the author since its first publication in 1970. She identifies the influence of other nurse–theorists including Martha Rogers and Dorothea Orem. Her later texts are *Introduction to Nursing: An Adaptation Model* (1984) and *The Roy Adaptation Model: The Definitive Statement* (1991).

The focus of **nursing** in Roy's model is on the individual as an adaptive system. The model also can be applied to family or community, and used in many settings. The adaptive behavior involves the whole person, who is seen as having great potential for self-actualization. The nature of human includes the biological level, with components such as anatomical parts which function physiologically. These anatomical parts function as a whole to contribute to the biological constancy of human. At the same time, humans have a psychological nature. The various biological systems, headed by the complex nervous system, together produce meaningful behavior. This behavior is organized in such a way that humans have constancy in their lives of perceiving, learning, and acting. Lastly, humans are social beings, and behavior is related to the behavior of others on groups levels such as family, community, and work groups (Roy, 1976, p. 11).

As an adaptive system, the individual is described as a whole comprised of parts that function as a unity for some purpose (Roy & Andrews, 1991, p. 11). Further, the **person** is conceptualized to have two internal subsystem mechanisms for coping with internal and external stimuli. One of these, the "regulator," works primarily through the autonomic nervous system. As Roy and Andrews (1991) described explicitly, the *regulator subsystem*

> responds automatically through neural, chemical and endocrine coping processes. Stimuli from the internal and external environment (through the senses) act as inputs to the nervous system and an automatic, unconscious response is produced. At the same time, inputs to the regulator subsystem have a role in the forming of perceptions (p 14).

The *cognator subsystem* "responds through four cognitive-emotive channels: perceptual/information processing, learning, judgment, and emotion" (Roy & Andrews, 1991, p. 14). The cognator assists with coping related not only to physiologic needs, but also to self-concept, role function, and interdependence—that is, the other adaptive "modes" of Roy's model.

Because Roy's nursing model is based on systems theory, it includes environment as an essential component. Roy defined the **environment** as all of the internal and external conditions, circumstances, and influences surrounding or affecting the development and behavior of persons or groups (Roy & Andrews, 1991, p. 18). Roy acknowledged both an internal and an external environment and classified environmental stimuli as follows:

> *Focal stimulus*—The internal or external stimulus most immediately confronting the person and the one to which the person must make an adaptive response; that is, the factor that precipitates the behavior.
> *Contextual stimuli*—All other stimuli present that contribute to the effect of the focal stimulus.
> *Residual stimuli*—Factors that may be affecting behavior, but the effects of which are unclear (1991, p. 8 & 9).

Changes in the environment provoke coping responses; behavior that promotes the integrity of the person is called an *adaptive response*. Nursing's goal is to promote adaptation (or a positive response to environmental change) by removing the focal stimulus or changing the contextual or residual stimuli. The activity of the two subsystem mechanisms is demonstrated by coping behavior in four specific "adaptive modes":

1. Physiologic need (e.g., elimination, nutrition)
2. Self-concept (sense of who we are)
3. Role function (socially expected behavior)
4. Interdependence (balance between independence and dependence in our relationships with others)

Roy (1984) defines adaptation as a positive response to the demands made on a person by the changing environment. Adaptive responses promote **health.** A person needs nursing care when his or her adaptive responses are ineffective.

The nurse intervenes through nursing process to promote adaptation in these four modes by modifying stimuli as needed. Roy is viewed as an outcome theorist whose approach is future oriented.

As these and other theoretical views of person are refined, they will undoubtedly influence both future nursing research and care delivery. Many aspiring professionals are strongly attracted to nursing because of the opportunity to work closely with persons in all aspects of their being: biologic, psychological, social, cultural, and spiritual.

Mid-range Theories

MARGARET NEWMAN

Margaret Newman was a student of Martha Rogers. She wrote *Theory Development in Nursing* (1979). A current theoretical work is *Health as Expanding Consciousness* (1994). Other writings of interest include a long futuristic poem, "Into the 21st Century" (1994). Given her mentor, it is not surprising that Margaret Newman's ideas are clearly futuristic and her concepts of theory are developed as energy process. **Persons** are viewed as belonging to and a part of "multiple systems levels in space" (Chinn & Kramer, 1995, p. 186). Although her theory is not yet widely applied, Margaret Newman is also widely known for and associated with the idea of **meta theory,** defined as theory about theory and how theory is developed.

M. M. LEININGER (1925–)

M. M. Leininger is a pioneer nurse anthropologist who created the concept of transcultural nursing. She wrote prolifically in this area and regarding human care theory. She was a leader in encouraging the incorporation of research-based cultural care content into nursing education programs, calling attention to the 21st Century as a *new age* presenting new multicultural challenges and requiring very different nursing practices (1995, p. 2). The definitive theoretical works of Leininger include the books *Transcultural Nursing: Concepts, Theories and Practices* (1978), and *Cultural Care Diversity and Universality: A Theory of Nursing* (1995b, 1991). Anthologies include *Caring: A Central Focus of Nursing and Health Care Services* (1980); *The Phenomenon of Caring: Importance, Research Questions and Theoretical Considerations* (1981); and *Historic and Epistemologic Dimensions of Care and Caring with Future Directions* (1990). After studying caring expressions in many different cultures, Leininger identified 20 caring behaviors. Leininger's model emphasizes the cultural expressions of care; that is, she believes that care can only be effective if it is culturally relevant. Caring behaviors identified by Leininger encompass, but are not limited to, comfort, facilitating, health instruction, protective and restorative behaviors, and support.

Leininger (1991) states that her theory of culture care is based on this central tenet: "[C]are is the essence of nursing and the central, dominant, and unifying focus of nursing" (p. 35). Leininger states further that cultures provide blueprints for living, including prescriptions for remaining healthy. Birth, illness, and death are experiences that are lived within a cultural frame of reference. To be meaningful, professional care must be congruent with the individual's cultural care values. **Health** is described as a state of well-being that is culturally defined, valued, and practiced. This state reflects the ability to perform daily activities in culturally patterned lifeways (p. 48). **Nurses** are concerned with how persons and groups experience health, the meanings they give to health, and how health is expressed. Nurses are also concerned with culturally defined meanings and patterns of care. With this knowledge, nurses are able to give culturally congruent care that is relevant and beneficial to their clients.

Leininger edited a chapter on her cultural care theory in Marriner-Tomey (1994) that defined **nursing** as:

> A learned humanistic art and science that focuses upon personalized (individual and group) care behaviors, functions, and processes directed toward promoting and maintaining health behaviors or recovery from illness, which have physical, psycho-cultural, and social significance or meaning for those being assisted generally by a professional nurse or one with similar role competencies (p. 430).

Leininger's culture care as defined has been extended beyond nursing to expand its applicability by persons other than nurses. Doing so, however, counters the theory as being exclusively within the realm of nursing.

R. R. PARSE

Parse's evolving theoretical work is published as *Illuminations: The Human Becoming Theory in Practice and Research* (1995). Much of its appeal seems to lie in its synthesis of concepts from human science, existential phenomenology, and the person–environment concept of Martha Rogers. Her acknowledgment of the person as controller of meaning and his health situation is in harmony with greater consumer responsibility in health care. Because her theory is abstract, extraordinary, and outside the realm of traditional nursing practice, its acceptance may be more limited than other theories seen as applicable within nursing process.

Perhaps Parse's greatest theoretical contribution to nursing theory may be a competing paradigm that has the potential to shift health care and nursing to a more humanistic and contemporary focus. In all sciences, paradigm (pattern) shifts precede scientific evolution and revolution. The world wide web provides access to a Parse Page at http://www.utoronto.ca/icps/index.html.

HELEN COOK ERICKSON (1936–)
EVELYN MALCOLM TOMLIN (1929–)
MARY ANN PRICE SWAIN (1941–)

The definitive work of these theorists is *Modeling and Role- Modeling: A Theory and Paradigm for Nursing* (1983). They acknowledged synthesizing the work of theorists from other fields, such as Erik Erikson, Abraham Maslow (1970), Hans Selye (1956), George Engel (1964), and Jean Piaget (1973).

Modeling is the process or means by which the nurse develops an image or understanding of the client's world from the client's frame of reference. Modeling is both art and science and involves the intake and analysis of information about the client and his or her world. Role modeling is the planning and implementation of nursing interventions uniquely for the client based on the client's model of the world.

Erickson, Tomlin and Swain (1983) believe that the role of the nurse "is to nurture biophysical, psychosocial, spiritual beings" (p. 2). **Person** is a unique being whose whole is greater than the sum of its parts. Three states are identified in their Adaptive Potential Assessment Model (APAM) that are similar to the three stages of Selye's General Adaptation Syndrome. However, instead of describing different adaptation responses, the APAM demonstrates the ability of the individual to mobilize coping resources. *Equilibrium* is an adaptive state in which persons have the potential to mobilize and use coping resources; *arousal* is a stress state in which a person is actively contending with stressors, using his or her resources; *impoverishment* is a stress state in which the person's coping resources are diminished or depleted. Persons can move among any of these states, depending on the coping resources available to them and the presence of new stressors. Persons may use energy from one subsystem to contend with stressors affecting another; for example, to cope with a stressful marriage, a person may tax the biophysical system and become vulnerable to physical illness. **Health** is viewed as physical, social, and mental well-being that is related to dynamic equilibrium among the various subsystems of the person. Helen Erickson's (Erickson et al., 1983) concepts of self-care incorporate ideas common to many nurse experts, including Orem, into her own special perspectives. Erickson's concept of self-care, when applied from her comprehensive framework or model for nursing, is equally useful with persons who are ill or well, and young or old, in whatever place they may be receiving or needing nursing care.

NOLA J. PENDER (1941–)

Pender's theory is the Health Promotion Model. Her books are titled *Health Promotion in Nursing Practice* (1996, 1987, 1982). In addition to being a theorist, Dr. Pender is a prominent nurse researcher who promoted the creation of the National Center for Nursing Research and provided research leadership in both Sigma Theta Tau and the American Nurses Association, as well as in academia. Her theory draws from social psychology and learning theory. In her model, cognitive-perceptual factors (e.g., perceived control of health) and various modifying demographic, situational, behavioral, biopsychosocial, and behavioral factors affect participation in health-promoting behavior. A health promotion model is both timely and especially reflective of nursing's scientific domain and Pender's commitment to health promotion, not disease prevention, as the hallmark for the next millennium. With health care reform looming on all fronts, and consumers taking more initiative for their health, this model seems destined to become more prominent.

Other Theorists

A section on nurse–theorists would be remiss without mention of other prominent nurses who have either developed their own theories or contributed significantly to our understanding of nursing theories over the years, and to whom the profession is indebted. We may not, however, have made specific reference to their theoretical works. Among these nurses recognized for their own theories are Dorothy E. Johnson, Myra E. Levine, Betty Neuman, Ida Orlando, Hildegard E. Peplau and Ernestine Weidenbach. Other nurses have provided careful compilation and critique of nursing theories. Among these nurses are Barbara Stevens

Barnum, Peggy L. Chinn, Jacqueline Fawcett, Julia B. George, Ann Marriner-Tomey, Afaf Meleis and L.H. Nicholl.

Sometimes theory within and beyond nursing is dismissed because either it is not readily apparent how it applies to practice, or it is not apparent that the theorist ever comes down from the ivory tower to confront the problems of the real world. The reader is directed to look for application to practice in the course of literature searches in current journals, books, and on the internet. Look also for books and articles about the theorists themselves written by their colleagues. *In Martha E. Rogers: Her Life and Her Work*, Malinski and Barrett (1995) write a tribute to the recently deceased theorist. They relate her vision and theory as it was developed and refined, along with glimpses of the real person. In "Nursing and the Next Millenium" Huch (1995), five theorists (King, Leininger, Parse, Peplau, and Rogers) provide a unique opportunity to read theorists' ideas as they chat among themselves at a nurse–theorist conference.

Now that we have explored critical thinking, scientific method, and nursing theory, we can focus on nursing research from a more informed perspective.

Relationship Among Theory, Research, and Practice

Both nursing science and nursing practice need theory and research. *To theorize* is to conjecture or construct the framework of a discipline or science. Theory systematically shows specific interrelationships for the purpose of describing, explaining, predicting, or controlling nursing practice.

Similarly, *to research* is to search into or to investigate thoroughly. Nursing practice and nursing research advance the discipline or science of nursing by shaping the theory. Conversely, the theory, knowledge, and research advance the quality of care and its delivery. As Chinn and Kramer (1995) wrote, ". . . practice contributes to and benefits from processes of creating conceptual meaning and deliberately applying the theories" (1995, p. 160).

Nursing research links **nursing theory** to practice in various ways. Sometimes theories give rise to hypotheses (hunches) that can be tested through research (experiments) in practice. Depending on whether the hunches are supported in the real world of practice, the theory is strengthened or weakened. A theory describes or explains a phenomenon, and research aims to test the description or explanation in either a simulated or natural setting. Research is a necessary intervening step to test possible applications to practice before implementing them full scale. Theories suggest general guidelines and possible outcomes. Research demonstrates how more specific guidelines actually fare in particular test situations. A theory predicts an outcome, and research attempts to demonstrate that prediction as true.

Sometimes notions generated from practice and tested through research become the concepts that, in turn, can build theories. The process of theory development requires many well-coordinated research studies over time.

Many realities cloud the theory–practice relationship. It is partly because nursing is a developing science and profession that the questions about these relationships persist. Theory, because it does not bring immediate answers to practice problems, is often considered impractical, if not useless. Also, the reflective thinking of theory is often at odds with the "doing" activities of nursing practice.

Many nurses, if they reflect thoughtfully on their practice activities, will recognize the kinds of observations that are important to theory—that is, how their patients respond to both health situations and nursing interventions. Concepts that come from practice are the mental images that become the building blocks of theory. This way of working inductively, that is, from specifics to generalities, provides a way to generate theory from practice (see the aggregation discussion in Chapter 8). Unfortunately, although trained to be careful observers, nurses often do not take the reflection and thinking time necessary to organize and synthesize their observations beyond individual care situations.

The term *grounded theory* has been used to identify a type of theory created inductively from systematic observation, analysis, and synthesis. In a famous study using this approach, Glaser and Strauss (1966) studied dying patients and related personnel in order to understand their shared reactions. The importance of their study was the light it shed on death as a reality that health care workers must accept.

Rather than create theory themselves, most nurses are concerned with how others' theories assist their practice. Because nurses desire to improve practice, and recognize that theory contributes to this end, they are tempted to make immediate application and expect immediate results. Reality demands considerable caution. A particular conceptual framework or nursing theory used for research will guide the nature of the problems and how they are studied. For example, using Orem's conceptual model, Denyes (1982) created a tool to measure adolescents' ability to care for themselves (Orem's self-care agency). The Roy Adaptation Model also has proved useful in guiding nursing research: Fawcett (1981) used the adaptive modes of the Roy Adaptation Model to classify survey data measuring fathers' responses to cesarean birth of their children.

In addition, several of the theoretical notions discussed earlier have been applied to a variety of practice situations. For example, Taylor (1991) used Orem's model to structure nursing diagnoses; Hanchett (1990) applied Roy, King, and M. E. Rogers to community as client; and Frey (1989) wrote of applying King's conceptual framework to the notions of social support and health.

In the past, nursing has borrowed many of its theories and its research methods from other disciplines. Furthermore, theory development and nursing research are often associated more closely with academic nursing than practice. Too often, the networking that could link theory, research, and practice does not exist. Perhaps nursing's conceptual frameworks will become well-developed theories unique to nursing. Ideally, increasing sophistication in research will yield better methods to measure results of holistic nursing interventions. Nursing needs to demonstrate how these interventions, derived from theories, make a difference in the health of persons and have economic value. With health care reform has come an emphasis on both collaborative practice and research. Brooten et al

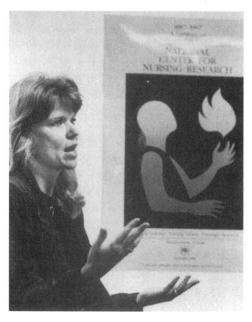

A nurse scientist talks about the art and science of nursing.

(1994) provide a good example of collaborative research, with a nurse as lead author and the research published in a respected medical journal. Within nursing, more nurses need to encourage and use research findings. In 1988, a new refereed journal—that is, one in which the articles are reviewed by peers in the nursing science community before publication—*Applied Nursing Research*, billed itself as "devoted to uniting the efforts of all professional nurses to advance nursing as a research-based profession." When the theory (research and theory)–practice relationships become clearer to all nurses, then theory will move from the realm of textbook discussion and academia into the center of professional nursing activity.

Nursing Research for Scientists and Practitioners

Nursing research is scientific study or investigation about nursing practice. Nursing research provides a purposeful way of seeking answers to questions about the specifics of nursing practice. Individual research studies do not prove or disprove scientific hunches. Multiple studies over time may provide strong evidence to support or refute educated scientific guesses about practice. Nursing research aims to answer both exploratory and complex questions. Exploratory questions concern the nature of nursing concepts (health, person, environment) or events (activities of daily living, such as sleeping). More complex questions ask about what will happen if specific nursing actions are practiced.

In this section, readers will find that research in nursing is based on the scientific method common to other scientific fields of study. Also, the various kinds of nursing research are introduced. Furthermore, readers will learn that although research is a relatively new activity for nurses, it is of rapidly increasing importance for nursing education, science development, and practice.

Many nursing journals can assist even the beginning practitioner to apply nursing research in the practice setting, as illustrated by examples from *Applied Nursing Research* and *Focus on Critical Care*. Kilpack, Boehm, Smith, and Mudge (1991) demonstrated in *Applied Nursing Research* that applying simple research interventions after a fall reduced the fall rate in an acute-care hospital. Falls, as a category of accidental death, are second only to motor vehicle accidents in the United States. After examining the relevant research, Schmitz (1991) in *Focus on Critical Care* concluded that "positioning can have a dramatic effect on oxygenation . . . (and) can result in improved clinical care for patients with pulmonary disease" (p. 64).

A decade ago, nursing research conferences were unusual. Today, they are commonplace in both schools of nursing and practice settings. ANA and Sigma Theta Tau International, the honor society in nursing, have become moving forces behind both nursing scholarship and research. However, nursing research concerns not only nursing scholars. Increasingly, nurses of all educational backgrounds and clinical specialties must see the political necessity of elevating nursing research to a priority of the profession. An important mandate regarding nursing research is clear: without an adequate research foundation, the unique knowledge of nursing science cannot be identified and developed. Because nursing is also a developing profession, it needs scientific research to further its growth as a profession. Without research, nursing will not maximize its scientific, professional, or social potential.

Development and enhancement of the profession of nursing is realized through knowledge acquisition. As Polit and Hungler (1985) wrote,

> The scientific approach is the most advanced method of acquiring knowledge that humans have developed. The scientific method incorporates several procedures and characteristics to create a system of obtaining knowledge that, though not infallible, is generally more reliable than alternative problem-solving approaches (p. 5).

Where Do Research Problems Come From?

A common question about nursing research is" Where do the problems investigated in research originate?" Nursing practice and nursing therapy generate problems for scientific investigation. As one head nurse in a busy acute-care hospital put it, "Reality, that is, practice, must drive both research and theory." To use these sources most effectively requires readiness to reflect on practice. Curious professionals also scour the nursing periodical literature to learn what others are thinking and doing. Perhaps the most important source of problems is less obvious: problems come also from the nurse–researcher's mind or imagination. The tendency is to minimize this source when we think of problems as coming from practice or theory. Problems do not materialize out of thin air. Whether they originate from theory or from practice, they are shaped in the mind of the practitioner–researcher.

Problems are the difference between the ideal and the real, and someone must

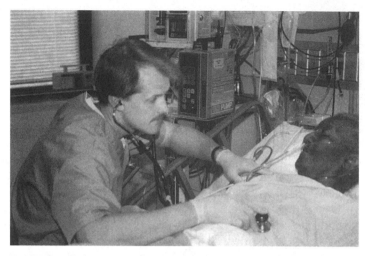

"Reality (practice) must drive both research and theory."

identify them as such. Dumas and Leonard (1963) made such an identification in a pioneering nursing study about the effect of nursing on postoperative vomiting. They envisioned as the ideal no postoperative vomiting for patients, but observed the reality to be frequent postoperative vomiting. In a controlled experiment, they intervened with some patients and found that the intervention decreased the incidence of postoperative vomiting. The study, based on Orlando's theory of interaction, illustrated that a research problem can be based on an abstract theory, made concrete for study, and yield results that can be generalized to a broad population for some practical application.

Since Dumas and Leonard's early clinical study, research has repeatedly demonstrated that nursing can make significant differences in both mortality and quality of life. Before a national health policy audience (the American Academy of Nursing meeting in Washington, DC), Fagin (1981) eloquently summarized many research examples of nursing effectiveness in her paper *Nursing's Pivotal Role in Achieving Competition in Health Care.* Unfortunately, such information often escapes widespread professional or public awareness. Lack of broad communication about significant nursing research results in a weak link in nursing's research chain.

Increasingly, and fortunately, individual nursing studies are finding their way into national journals. A landmark study demonstrating nursing's economic value was published in the *New England Journal of Medicine* by Brooten and colleagues in 1986. The study also made news in *The Wall Street Journal* and *The New York Times.* Nursing assessment and care by nurse specialists enabled premature infants to be discharged safely to home care, saving a single hospital hundreds of thousands of dollars yearly. Similar early discharge programs are being tried in other health care centers and with other populations—for example, elderly patients.

The particular problems chosen for nursing investigation will determine how the problems are best studied, and also will suggest the appropriate research methods to be used. Just as there is no one "best" theory of nursing, there is no one correct way to research all nursing problems. An important and ultimate aim of research in nursing is to enable clinical practitioners to improve care by being able to predict the patient outcomes of intervention (what will happen if . . . ?) and thereby develop prescriptions to achieve goals (how can I make . . . happen?).

Research Approaches

The variety of research approaches used in nursing parallels those used in other sciences. This section explores each of the following four research approaches. For detailed discussion of research methods, refer to Polit and Hungler's (1995) *Essentials of Nursing Research: Methods and Applications.*

Nonexperimental Research

Nonexperimental research is often labeled as ex post facto (after the fact) or descriptive. Descriptive theory and research in nursing also contribute important and necessary foundations for advanced research and theory development.

Experimental Research

Experimental nursing research, that is, true experiments with random selection of subjects to different kinds of care, is often difficult to carry out in real-life situations and in hospital settings. Nurses and health care administrators must weigh economic and ethical considerations in doing such experiments. Additionally, nurses must be able to control the experimental conditions. Because of these real difficulties, many past nursing studies have been studies about nurses rather than about nursing, or were nonexperimental. In recent years, the nursing profession has given the highest priority to studies, experimental or nonexperimental, that are central to clinical practice. Such studies clarify the effectiveness of specific nursing interventions, show the impact of nursing care on certain health problems and illnesses, or indicate the appropriate environment for effective nursing practice methods. Well-educated nurses are confident about how to study the phenomena that interest them.

Qualitative Research

A basic principle of research is that the nature of the problem will dictate the nature of the investigation needed to answer the research question. Much scientific research uses quantitative analysis, that is, the processing of numerical data for the purpose of describing phenomena and inferring relationships among them. With recent interest in humanistic nursing by such theorists as Watson and Leininger, it seems likely that use of qualitative research will increase in nursing. Qualitative approach organizes narrative or words to discover themes, and also relationships, among concepts in a nonnumerical way. Examples of such qualitative research strategies may have names such as human sciences research or phenomenologic approach.

An example of a qualitative study using a human science approach is Boodley's (1986) dissertation *A Nursing Study of the Experience of Having a Health Examination*. She sought to discover the meaning a person attaches to the health examination experience. Her rationale for this interest was quite simple:

> The health examination is probably the most frequent reason for a contact with the health-care system. Many basic expectations about how the health-care system functions and the person's role within it come from the experience of having a health examination. If nurses hope to understand more about the context for nursing practice, they must begin with an understanding of the meanings clients find in this common health-care experience (p. 5).

In a more recent study, Bauman (1994) used Parse's human becoming theory in an exploratory study of homeless mothers and children.

Interestingly, such a research focus is consistent with a more humanistic approach to "person" as a major theoretical concept. Swanson and Chenitz (1982) reminded us that the monumental scientific works of such scientists as Darwin and Einstein came not from counting how many, but from observing. Certainly, this gives us reason to be open to a variety of research approaches for nursing. Streubert & Carpenter (1995) offer a current viewpoint regarding advancing the humanistic perspective through qualitative research in nursing.

Historical Research

Another research method is historical research, which also may be called the literary or critical approach. This past-oriented research method seeks to illuminate a current question through an intensive study of existing material. In the historical approach, the researcher uses original or primary data whenever possible, gathered from actual historical documents. Philip A. Kalisch and Beatrice J. Kalisch investigated the image of nurses in the media. They used a clipping service to gather articles from newspapers to ascertain nurse image at a particular time. Their writings include "When Nurses Were National Heroines: Images of Nursing in American Film, 1942–1945" (1981) and "How the Public Sees Nurse–Midwives: 1978 News Coverage of Nurse–Midwifery in the Nation's Press" (1980).

In many ways, the image of the nurse has changed immensely since Nightingale's time. A place now exists in nursing for professionals who want to be researchers, and scientists who want to study health and people's adaptation to changes in their health. True, nurses have long been data collectors for physicians doing medical research. However, the emphasis here is on nurses doing nursing research. Nurses also work with physicians and other health care professionals to do collaborative research. Increasingly, government and private funding agencies are looking for evidence that health care professionals are working together to solve priority health care problems.

Nursing Research Comes of Age

Nursing is just coming into its own in terms of developing both its scientific base and its research visibility. You may have heard of the National Institutes of Health (NIH), which primarily is concerned with disease. It was not until 1986 that nursing found a home in the established research halls of NIH. This development occurred when a National Center for Nursing Research was created by congressional override of a presidential veto. To have key legislators speak to the value of nursing research was a major victory for nursing. In 1994, nursing research gained another recognition of its coming of age when the Center achieved full Institute status within NIH as the National Institute for Nursing Research. It seems only logical that nurses should have such a visible national institute; they are, after all, the largest group of health care professionals.

Ensuring funding for nursing research is an important beginning, and supports the work of nurse–scientists. The next step is to bring nursing research and nursing practice closer together so that nursing research becomes a reality for practitioners. Pioneering work in this area was done by Horsley, Crane, Crabtree, and Wood in the 1970s and reported as *Using Research to Improve Nursing Practice: A Guide* (1983). Horsley et al. emphasized the importance of working from a conceptual base and identifying particular clinical problems from which would come specific innovations that could be clinically evaluated. This model clearly followed the steps of the scientific method. Progress, however, comes slowly. In the mid-1980s, Butler (1987) investigated how innovations actually get used or ignored in nursing service organizations.

Nursing as an emerging science and profession clearly intends to monitor its continued research development, as evidenced by the recent ANA publication (1995), *Ethical Guidelines in the Conduct, Dissemination and Implementation of Nursing Research.* And we are reminded that national recognition is only a stepping stone to global recognition. Martha Rogers (1994a), one of nursing's most prominent and respected theorists, issued a clarion call for global nursing research, and encouraged us toward the"imaginative and creative promotion of well-being" of all people in a world undergoing rapid social change (1994b, p. 35).

While nursing is expanding its world view in theory and research, it is also honing its scientific discipline. As Newman (1994) wrote, "These two areas of theory and research–health and caring–emerged in the 80's as major emphases of the professional discipline that is nursing. But neither alone is sufficient to specify the focus of the discipline. But the two taken together, caring in the human health experience, specify a phenomenon of inquiry and a domain of service that nursing may call its own" (p. 55).

Although research may still seem mysterious, it is learnable and exciting to those who participate. Research progress in nursing has been slower than many nurses would like, but advances in the past decade have been dramatic. Nurses entering the profession should anticipate that they will encounter many research opportunities to enrich their careers. When nursing research becomes a usual and ordinary professional activity, rather than an extraordinary event, nursing will have come of age as a science.

KEY CONCEPTS

✓Critical thinking skills encompass inductive and deductive reasoning and flexible thinking abilities that can be developed with practice.

✓Scientific method is a problem-solving method that involves defining the problem, collecting data from observation and experimentation, devising and executing a solution, and evaluating the results.

✓From foundations in related sciences, nursing has developed unique philosophies and various theories using the concepts of nursing, person, health, and environment.

✓Nursing researches problems from clinical practice using various approaches in an effort to describe, explain, predict, and control outcomes of practice.

✓Nursing science uses theory and research to develop the scientific discipline that forms the basis of professional practice.

CRITICAL QUESTIONS

1. What priorities do you see for the development of nursing as a science in a) the immediate future; b) the next hundred years?

2. What strategies would you suggest for the discipline's success in addressing the priorities?

3. Considering one of the theorists featured (or another of your personal choice), reflect on what interests you most about this person and his or her theoretical contributions.

4. How would you explain the theorist selected above to a non-nurse peer who wants to know what the theory has to do with patient care?

5. Identify ways that interactive audiovisual presentations via computer (virtual reality) could be used to enhance nursing as science.

6. What extracurricular strategies might you personally use to become better informed about nursing as a science?

REFERENCES

Alfaro-LeFevre, R. (1995). *Critical thinking in nursing: A practical approach.* Philadelphia: W.B. Saunders.

American Nurses Association. (1995). *A social policy statement* (Publication No. NP-107). Washington, D.C.: Author.

American Nurses Association. (1995). *Ethical guidelines in the conduct, dissemination & implementation of nursing research* (Publication No. D-95). Washington, D.C.: Author.

American Nurses Association. (1980). *A social policy statement* (Publication No. NP-63 35M). Kansas City, MO: Author.

Bauman, S.L. (1994). No place of their own: An exploratory study. *Nursing Science Quarterly* 7(4), 162–169.

Benner, P.E., & Wrubel, J. (1989). *The primacy of caring: Stress and coping in health and illness.* Menlo Park, CA: Addison-Wesley.

Benner, P.E. (1984). *From novice to expert: Excellence and power in clinical nursing practice.* Menlo Park, CA: Addison-Wesley.

Boodley, C. (1986). *A nursing study of the experience of having a health examination.* Unpublished doctoral dissertation, The University of Michigan, Ann Arbor.

Brooten, D., Roncoli, M., Finkler, S., Arnold, L., Cohen, A., & Mennuti, M. (1994). A randomized clinical trial of early hospital discharge and nurse specialist home follow-up of women with unplanned cesarean birth. *Obstetrics and Gynecology 84,* 832–838.

Brooten, D., Kumar, S., Brown, L.P., Butts, P., Finkler, S.A., Bakewell-Sichs, S., & Gibbons, P. (1986). A randomized clinical trial of early hospital discharge and home follow-up of very-low birth-weight infants. *New England Journal of Medicine 315,* 934–939.

Butler, P.M. (1987). *Hospital embedding-diffusion mechanisms and nurses' knowledge of a diffused innovation.* Unpublished doctoral dissertation, University of Michigan, Ann Arbor.

Chinn, P.L. & Kramer, M.K. (1995). *Theory and nursing: a systematic approach.* St. Louis, MO: C.V. Mosby.

de Bono, E. (1970). *Lateral thinking: Creativity step by step.* New York: Harper & Row.

Denyes, M.J. (1982). Measurement of self-care agency in adolescents [abstract]. *Nursing Research, 31*(1), 63.

Dumas, R.G., & Leonard, R.C. (1963). The effect of nursing on the incidence of postoperative vomiting. *Nursing Research, 12*(1), 12–15.

Engel, G. (1964). Grief and grieving. *American Journal of Nursing, 64,* 93–98.

Erickson, H.C., Tomlin, E.M., & Swain, M.A. (1983). *Modeling and role modeling: A theory and paradigm for nursing.* Englewood Cliffs, NJ: Prentice-Hall.

Fagin, C. (1981, September). *Nursing's pivotal role in achieving competition in health care.* Paper presented at the American Academy of Nursing meeting, Washington, DC.

Fawcett, J. (1993). *Analysis and evaluation of nursing theories.* Philadelphia: F.A. Davis.

Fawcett, J. (1985). *Analysis and evaluation of conceptual models of nursing.* Philadelphia: F.A. Davis.

Fawcett, J. (1981). Assessing and understanding the cesarean father. In C.F. Kehoe (Ed.), *The caesarean experience: Theoretical and clinical perspectives for nurses* (pp. 143–156). New York: Appleton-Century-Crofts.

Frey, M.A. & Sieloff, C.L.,(Eds.). (1995). *Advancing King's framework and theory of nursing.* Thousand Oaks: Sage Publications.

Frey, M.A. (1989). Social support and health: A theoretical formulation derived from King's conceptual framework. *Nursing Science Quarterly, 2*(3), 138–148.

Glaser, B., & Strauss, A. (1966). *Awareness of dying.* Chicago: Aldine.

Hanchett, E.S. (1990). Nursing models and community as client. *Nursing Science Quarterly, 3*(2), 67–72.

Harmer, B., & Henderson, V. (1955). *Textbook of principles and practice of nursing* (5th ed.). New York: Macmillan.

Henderson, V. (1991). *Reflections after 25 years* (Publication No. 15-2236). New York: National League for Nursing.

Henderson, V. (1966). *The nature of nursing.* New York: Macmillan.

Horsley, J., Crane, J., Crabtree, M. K., & Wood, D. J. (1983). *Using research to improve nursing practice: A guide.* New York: Grune & Stratton.

Huch, M.H. (1995). Nursing and the next millennium. *Nursing Science Quarterly. 8*(1), 38–44.

International Council of Nurses. (1961). *ICN basic principles of nursing care*. London: Author.

Kalisch, P.A., & Kalisch, B.J. (1981). When nurses were national heroines: Images of nursing in American film, 1942–1945. *Nursing Forum, 20*, 15–61.

Kalisch, P.A., & Kalisch, B.J. (1980). How the public sees nurse–midwives: 1978 news coverage of nurse–midwifery in the nation's press. *Journal of Nurse–Midwifery, 25*, 31–39.

Kilpack, V., Boehm, J., Smith, N., & Mudge, B. (1991). Using research-based interventions to decrease patient falls. *Applied Nursing Research, 4*(2), 50–56.

King, I.M. (1992). King's theory of goal attainment. *Nursing Science Quarterly, 5*(1), 19–25.

King, I.M. (1981). *A theory for nursing: Systems, concepts, process*. New York: Wiley.

King, I.M. (1971). *Toward a theory of nursing: General concepts of human behavior*. New York: Wiley.

Leininger, M.M. (1995a). Teaching transcultural nursing to transform nursing for the 21st century [Editorial]. *Journal of Transcultural Nursing 6*:2

Leininger, M.M. (1995b). Culture care diversity and universality: A theory for nursing (2nd ed.). New York: McGraw-Hill.

Leininger, M.M. (Ed.) (1991). *Cultural care diversity and universality: A theory of nursing*. (Pub. No. 15-2402). New York: National League for Nursing.

Leininger, M. M. (1990). Historic and epistemologic dimensions of care and caring with future directions. In J. Stevenson & T. Tripp-Reimer (Eds.), *Knowledge about care and caring: State of the art and future developments* (pp. 19–31). Kansas City, MO: American Academy of Nursing.

Leininger, M.M. (1981). The phenomenon of caring: Importance, research questions, and theoretical considerations. In Leininger, M. M. (Ed.), *Caring: An essential human need* (pp. 3–15). Thorofare, NJ: Charles B. Slack.

Leininger, M.M. (1980). Caring: A central focus of nursing and health care services. *Nursing & Health Care, 3*, 135–43, 176.

Leininger, M.M. (1978). *Transcultural nursing: Concepts, theories and practices*. New York: Wiley.

Malinski, V.M. & Barret, E.A.M. (1994) *Martha E. Rogers: Her life and her work*. Philadelphia: F.A. Davis.

Marriner-Tomey, A. (1994) *Nursing theorists and their work* (3rd ed.). St. Louis: Mosby.

Maslow, A.H. (1970). *Motivation and Personality* (2nd ed.) New York: Harper & Row.

National Council of State Boards of Nursing. (1982). *The Model Practice Act*. Chicago Association.

Newman, M.A. (1994). "Into the 21st Century". *Nursing Science Quarterly, 7*(1), 44–46.

Newman, M.A. (1994). *Health as expanding consciousness* (2nd ed.). New York: NLN Press (Publication No. 14-2626).

Newman, M.A. (1979). *Theory development in nursing*. Philadelphia: F.A. Davis.

Nightingale, F. (1859). *Notes on nursing: What it is and what it is not* (1st ed.). London: Harrison. (Facsimile ed., Philadelphia: J.B. Lippincott, 1966).

Orem, D.E. (1995) *Nursing: Concepts of Practice* (5th ed.). St. Louis: Mosby

Orem, D E. (1991). *Nursing: Concepts of practice* (4th ed.). St. Louis, MO: Mosby–Year Book.

Orem, D.E. (1980). Nursing: Concepts of practice (2nd ed.). New York: McGraw-Hill.

Orem, D. E (1959). *Guides for developing curricula for the education of practical nurses*. Washington, DC: U.S. Government Printing Office.

Parse, R.R. (1995). *Illuminations: the human becoming theory in practice and research*. (Publication No. 15-2670) New York: NLN Press.

Parse, R. R. (1992). Human becoming: Parse's theory of nursing. *Nursing Science Quarterly,* 5(1), 35–42.

Parse, R. R. (1981). *Man-living-health: A theory of nursing.* New York: Wiley.

Pender, N.J. (1996). *Health promotion in nursing practice* (3rd ed.). Stamford, CT: Appleton & Lange.

Pender, N.J. (1987). *Health promotion in nursing practice* (2nd ed.). Norwalk, CT: Appleton-Century-Crofts.

Pender, N.J. (1982). *Health promotion in nursing practice.* Norwalk, CT: Appleton & Lange.

Piaget, J. (1973). *The psychology of intelligence.* Totowa, NJ: Littlefield, Adams.

Polit, D.F., & Hungler, B.P. (1995). *Essentials of nursing research: Methods and applications.* (3rd ed.). Philadelphia: J.B. Lippincott.

Polit, D.F., & Hungler, B.P. (1985) *Essential of Nusing Research: Methods and Applications.* Philadelphia, J.B. Lippincott.

Rogers, M.E. (1994a). Martha E. Rogers' clarion call for global nursing research. *Nursing Science Quarterly* 7(3), 100–101.

Rogers, M.E. (1994b) The science of unitary human beings: current perspectives. *Nursing Science Quarterly* 7(1) 33–35.

Rogers, M.E. (1992). Nursing science and the space age. *Nursing Science Quarterly,* 5(1), 27–34.

Rogers, M.E. (1990). Nursing: Science of unitary irreducible human beings—Update 1990. In E.A.M. Barrett (Ed.), *Visions of Rogers' science based nursing* (Publication No. 15-2285, pp. 5–11). New York: National League for Nursing.

Rogers, M. E. (1989). Nursing: A science of unitary human beings. In J. P. Riehl-Sisca (Ed.), *Conceptual models for nursing practice* (3rd ed., pp. 181–188). Norwalk, CT: Appleton-Lange.

Rogers, M.E. (1983). Science of unitary human beings: A paradigm for nursing. In E.W. Clements & F.B. Roberts (Eds.), *Family health: A theoretical approach to nursing care.* New York: Wiley.

Rogers, M.E. (1970). *An introduction to the theoretical basis of nursing.* Philadelphia: F.A. Davis.

Rosenfeld, P. (1987). Nursing education in crisis—A look at recruitment and retention. *Nursing and Health Care, 8,* 283–286.

Roy, C. (1984). *Introduction to nursing: An adaptation model* (2nd ed.). Englewood Cliffs, NJ: Prentice-Hall.

Roy, C. (1976). *Introduction to nursing: an adaptational model.* Englewood Cliffs, NJ: Prentice-Hall.

Roy, C. (1970). Adaptation: A conceptual framework for nursing. *Nursing Outlook, 18,* 42–45.

Roy, C., & Andrews, H.A. (Eds.). (1991). *The Roy Adaptation Model: The definitive statement.* Norwalk, CT: Appleton & Lange.

Rubenfeld, M.G. *Critical thinking in nursing: An interactive approach.* (1995). Philadelphia, J.B. Lippincott.

Sagan, C. (1995). *The demon-haunted world: science as a candle in the dark.* New York: Random House.

Schmitz, T.M. (1991). Fact or myth? Patients with pulmonary disease should be placed in semi-Fowler's position. *Focus on Critical Care, 18*(1), 58–64.

Selye, H. (1956). *The stress of life.* New York: McGraw-Hill.

Sithichoke-Rattan, N. (1989). A clinical application of Watson's theory. *Pediatric Nursing, 15,* 458–462.

Stark, J. (1995). Taking the road less traveled. *American Journal of Nursing 25,* 55.

Stevens, B.J. (1984). *Nursing theory: Analysis, application, evaluation.* Boston: Little, Brown.

Streubert, H.J., & Carpenter, D.R. (1995). *Qualitative research in nursing: Advancing the humanistic perspective.* Philadelphia: J.B. Lippincott.

Swanson, J.M., & Chenitz, W.C. (1982). Why qualitative research in nursing? *Nursing Outlook, 30,* 241–245.

Taylor, S.G. (1991). The structure of nursing diagnoses from Orem's theory. *Nursing Science Quarterly, 4*(1), 24–32.

Torres, G. (1980). The place of concepts and theories within nursing. In J.B. George, *Nursing theories: the base for professional nursing practice* (pp 1–10). Englewood Cliffs, NJ: Prentice-Hall.

Torres, G. (1990). The place of concepts and theories within nursing. In George, J.B. (Ed.), *Nursing theories: the base for professional nursing practice* (3rd ed., pp.1–12). Norwalk CT: Appleton & Lange.

Watson, J. (1988). Nursing: Human science and human care: a theory of nursing. New York: National League for Nursing (Publication No. 15-2278).

Watson, J. (1985). *Nursing: Human science and human care—A theory of nursing.* Norwalk, CT: Appleton-Century-Crofts.

Watson, J. (1979). *Nursing: The philosophy and science of caring.* Boston: Little, Brown.

4

Person

Key Words

Accommodation	Developmental task	Operation	System
Adaptation	Growth	Schema	Value
Assimilation	Holism	Self-concept	Value judgment
Body image	Maturation	Self-esteem	Variable
Closed system	Object permanence	Self-ideal	
Development	Open system	Structure	

Objectives

After completing this chapter, students will be able to:

State how the concept of holism applies to nursing.

Describe how the concept of system applies to nursing.

Relate the concept of the person's view of self to one's own self.

Describe several principles of growth and development.

Apply ideas from the theories of Maslow, Erikson, Piaget, and Carl Rogers to real-life situations.

Each person is a unique and complex human being comprising biologic, psychologic, and sociologic components. These components include unique characteristics as well as characteristics shared with other persons. As an open system, the components of the person are constantly interacting both internally and externally. Inherent in this interaction is a unifying element called the spirit. This component, although not necessarily religious in nature, may be viewed as such, and is the inspiring or animating principle that pervades thought, feeling, and action. Nurses view the person as a complete, holistic being who is greater than the sum of his or her parts, with a spirit that makes him or her unique from fellow creatures.

Each person in his or her uniqueness has the ability to grow and develop

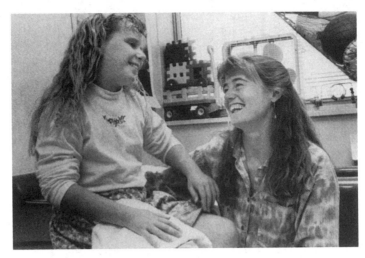

Nurses view each person as unique.

throughout the life span. Knowing this, nurses apply growth and development theories to the delivery of relevant and effective nursing care. In this chapter, we cite several classic theorists to provide background and resource material for understanding skills that nurses use in practice. We also include several examples from popular literature across the years to stimulate your analysis of growth and development and to encourage your professional application of the principles. For example, understanding how persons think assists health teaching. Being aware of psychosocial development provides nurses with guidelines for counseling. An appreciation of the physical growth patterns that occur in persons at different ages and stages helps nurses concentrate on pertinent areas when performing physical assessment. An appreciation of how these components of the person interact sets the tone for holistic care and demonstrates the unending potential of the human throughout life.

The subjects and theories introduced in this chapter are many. Students are expected to use the basic ideas presented to better understand aspects both common and unique to all persons. For a more thorough exploration, refer to the publications cited at the end of this chapter.

The Person as an Open System

Holism

The words *holistic* and *holism* are derived from the Greek word meaning whole. **Holism** is basically a theory in which the universe, and especially living nature, is seen in terms of interacting wholes that are more than the sum of their parts. Smuts (1926) indicated that holism is a theory that describes the parts of a person as dependent on each other and coordinated in a systematic fashion. According

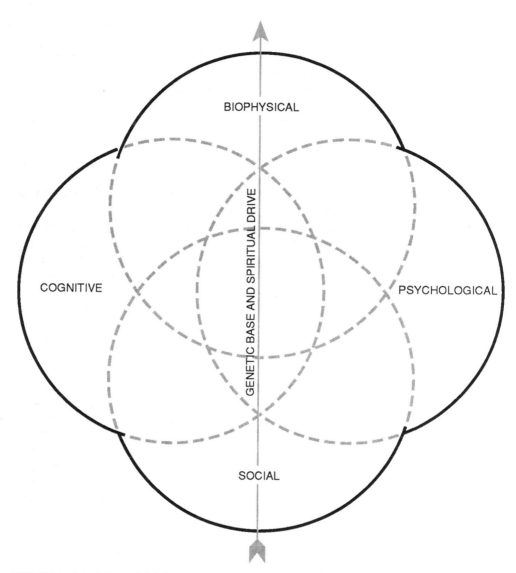

FIGURE 4-1   A holistic model. (Erickson, H., Tomlin, E., Swain, MA. [1983]. *Modeling and role-modeling: A theory and paradigm for nursing* [p 45]). Englewood Cliffs, NJ: Prentice-Hall.

to this theory, studying one part of a person indicates the need to consider how that part interrelates with all other parts of the person. An appreciation for the parts as a whole suggests the purpose and function of each individual part. The interrelationships also contribute to making the whole greater than the sum of its parts. This interrelation further increases the complexity of each of us as unique individuals. Figure 4-1 is a typical representation of the holistic person. Note the following three points reflected in the figure:

1. The subsystems represent interacting wholes that are greater than the sum of the parts.
2. The broken lines between the subsystems indicate the passage of energy among the subsystems.
3. Inherent throughout the whole are the genetic base and spiritual drive that make all persons unique.

General Systems Theory

The human is an open system. In discussing the meaning of system, Abbey (1978) stated that a **system** is "an organized unit with a set of components that mutually react. The system acts as a whole; the dysfunction of a part causes a system disturbance rather than the loss of a single function" (pp. 20–21). Systems are found everywhere. For example, a car is a mechanical system with many parts, all of which must function with reasonable precision for the car to move. A plant is a living system with interacting parts consisting of leaves, stems, roots, and many smaller structures. These parts function together to promote life and growth. These two systems—car and plant—have definite boundaries that are readily apparent.

Other systems within our social structure have less apparent boundaries. The public school system, as a social system, might exemplify this idea. Certainly each individual school has visible boundaries in the form of its building, teachers, students, books, and desks. However, each school district has its own school board, and each state has certain legislation relating to its particular school system. Financial support comes from a variety of sources. Philosophies of education, which may vary considerably across the United States, permeate each component of the system. In this large and unwieldy system, the interrelationships of the components are less evident. Consideration of each individual school and its parts in the system makes the functioning of the larger system more understandable. Thus we see that the public school system is made up of thousands of smaller systems that can be called subsystems. A subsystem has the same characteristics as a system, but is considered a part of the larger system as well.

General systems theory is a formalized means of describing the interplay of many systems. The idea of general systems theory was proposed by Ludwig von Bertalanffy in the 1950s. He wrote, "General systems theory then consists of the scientific exploration of 'wholes and wholeness' . . . the interdisciplinary nature of concepts, models, and principles applying to 'systems' provides a possible approach toward the unification of science." (von Bertalanffy, 1968, p. 30). Klir (1972) suggested the following definition: "General Systems Theory in the broadest sense refers to a collection of general concepts, principles, tools, problems, methods, and techniques associated with systems" (p. 1).

Open and Closed Systems

Systems are essentially of two types: open and closed. The distinguishing difference is the extent to which a system can exchange matter, energy, and information with its environment. The environment of the system has been defined by

Hall and Fagen (1968) as all factors that affect the system and also all factors that are affected by the system. The **open system** is one that can exchange matter, energy, and information with its environment; a **closed system** cannot. Because nearly all systems contain many subsystems, it is possible to have an open system that contains several closed subsystems. Systems that are essentially open include living, social, behavioral, and environmental systems. All of these systems contain closed subsystems.

As examples of open systems, persons constantly exchange matter, energy, and information with the environment. We hear, see, and process information received and then disseminate it to others. We adapt to the weather by changing clothes. We absorb energy from the sun, from food, and from other sources. As living systems, we are capable of self-regulation and growth.

Chemical reactions are examples of closed systems. Some compounds, when dissolved in water, dissociate. For example: lactic acid $\rightarrow H^+$ + lactate, carbonic acid $\rightarrow H^+$ + bicarbonate.

These systems will remain the same forever and will be unaffected by their environments unless new variables are added. Persons have closed systems within them: for instance, the chemical reaction in the preceding example occurs continuously within the body and helps to maintain an internal stability. Another example of a closed system is the withdrawal reflex that protects a person from painful stimuli. This reflex is an autonomic reaction within the system of the person in response to an outside stimulus.

Systems Theory Applied to the Person

The human contains many systems and subsystems that interrelate in an integrated fashion to become one total system. Each of the biologic, psychologic, social, spiritual, and genetic components that constitute this interaction could be considered a system having subsystems. For instance, the biologic system contains subsystems such as the neurologic, circulatory, and gastrointestinal systems, to name a few. The neurologic system, in turn, comprises the brain, the spinal cord, and the peripheral nerves throughout the body. Each of these parts is a subsystem in itself. The circulatory system consists of the heart and the blood vessels. These two systems interrelate as the brain sends messages to the heart that regulate its pumping. The heart, however, must pump to keep the brain functioning so that it can send signals. The psychological system contains subsystems that include thinking and feeling. Our feeling states also affect the autonomic nervous system, which signals the heart to beat faster or slower.

Systems such as those mentioned within the person are open when they exchange energy with other systems. Consider another example of this notion: the systems of the person constantly exchange energy not only among themselves, in the internal systems, but also with the outside environment.

Each system contains many variables. Polit and Hungler (1995) explain a **variable** as follows: "Within the context of research investigation, concepts are generally referred to as variables. A variable, as the name implies, is something that varies such as height, weight, body temperature, blood pressure, and preoper-

TABLE 4-1 *Selected Variables of the Person*

Biologic	*Psychological*	*Sociological*	*Spiritual*
Age	Attitudes	Basic needs	Beliefs
Genetic structure	Basic needs	Culture	Philosophy of life
Sex	Body image	Family	Religion
Race	Communication	Group membership	Values
Biologic rhythms	Coping mechanisms	Language	
Basic needs	Defense mechanisms	Life-style	
Growth	Feeling states	Relationships with others	
Acid−base balance	Level of develop-mental task resolution	Roles	
Circulation		Role prescriptions	
Digestion	Perception	School systems	
Electrolyte balance	Self-concept		
Immune response	Values		
Mobility	Cognition		
Reproduction	Consciousness		
Respiration	Knowledge		
Temperature regulation	Memory		
Physical health	Thought process		
Past illnesses			

ative anxiety levels'' (p. 22). Systems and variables are components of a larger whole. In many instances, both terms apply to the same object or event. Table 4-1 lists some of the variables that are part of the complex biopsychosocial system called the person.

Many of these variables, although associated primarily with the stated classification, also may be associated appropriately with another heading under certain circumstances. The concept of role, for example, is generally considered a sociologic variable. However, there are many psychologic components to this notion, and some might classify it with other psychologic variables.

Exchange of Energy Among the Subsystems of a Person

Systems have a certain amount of energy that can be exchanged within the subsystems and with the environment. If the person—a being greater than the whole of his or her combined parts—uses coping mechanisms that help achieve successful growth and development throughout his or her life, then each subsystem will retain its maximum potential health. However, if one component, such as the psychologic subsystem, becomes stressed, the person may be unable to cope effectively. At that point, energy may be drawn from another subsystem, which, in turn, may become less healthy.

To apply this idea to everyday situations, consider two kinds of examples:

those that represent a temporary breakdown in a system and those that reflect more far-reaching implications. Note the interactions of several subsystems in the brief but difficult common cold:

❒ A stuffed nose often causes a headache, difficult breathing, and unclear thinking.
❒ Constant nose blowing causes soreness to the skin of the nose.
❒ Muscles and joints often ache.
❒ One may act irritably, causing others to stay away.
❒ Often during a cold, persons have feelings of low self-esteem and inadequacy.

Mercifully, a cold is brief. Our natural recuperative powers quickly reassert themselves, and the brief unpleasantness is forgotten. The example, however, demonstrates the many effects of a "simple cold." Although it most specifically affects the upper respiratory system, it can also affect our general physical state and how we think, act, and respond to others. Energy is used to cope with the physical aspects, and we are often left drained psychologically and socially. Moreover, the cold is an event that may have been precipitated by other factors in our lives. For example, students who feel overburdened with course work and exams may be more susceptible to contracting a cold.

Sometimes persons with severe illnesses such as heart disease or cancer can point to events that they relate to their problems. One woman stated that her blood sugar had gone way up (900 mg/dl; norm = 90 to 110 mg/dl) when her son died. Furthermore, she indicated that it would not come down until she finally began to resolve her grief. This clinical example suggests that, in trying to cope with severe psychological stress, the woman drew on her physical energy as well. Others might not connect two events this closely, but nurses often note that clients develop illness 6 months to 1 year following a loss. For example, nurses often hear comments like the following: from a man who was hospitalized following a heart attack, "My wife died last summer and I haven't been right since"; or, from the man with a new diagnosis of bladder cancer, "My grandson was killed in a car accident last year." The man whose wife had died seemed to connect this with his heart attack. In other instances, nurses uncover the data while doing an assessment, or in another interaction. This was true of the man with bladder cancer. Research into the mind–body connection is ongoing, but the relationships are often noted. Consider how often we connect physical and psychological subsystems in our common language: we talk of aching or broken hearts, cold feet, a pain in the neck, eyes as the windows of the soul, and so forth. These examples suggest that one component of a person has an effect on the person as a whole.

In a Different Voice

Throughout the next several sections, we discuss certain aspects of human development using well-known authorities: Abraham Maslow, Erik Erikson, and Jean Piaget. Later, in Chapter 11, we discuss moral development using the work of

Lawrence Kohlberg (1987). Although the work of these authors has withstood the scrutiny of several generations of researchers, nonetheless, these male researchers developed their conclusions primarily from the study of males throughout the life cycle. Furthermore, they described the development of females (when considered at all) as a generalization from the conclusions drawn from the study of males. Even Piaget, whose own daughter is an early model in his work on cognitive development, described his observations through the male perspective.

In 1982, Carol Gilligan published her research in a book called *In a Different Voice*. She carefully reviewed and explored the work of the above-mentioned authorities and others as well. However, the essence of her work indicated that, with regard to psychosocial, cognitive, and moral development, males and females instinctively develop differently and offer different responses to ethical dilemmas, depending on their world view. Gilligan used Anton Chekhov's classic play "The Cherry Orchard" to demonstrate this belief. Lopahin, the young merchant, believes that we should "indeed be giants" because the Lord has given us immense forests, unbounded fields, and widest horizons. Madame Ranevskaya, however, states, "You feel the need for giants—they are good only in fairy tales, anywhere else they only frighten us." Gilligan, using this excerpt, noted, "Different judgments of the image of man as giant imply different ideas about human development, different ways of imagining the human condition, different notions of what is of value in life" (p. 5).

As Gilligan studied the issues of being male or female, she noted that masculinity is defined through separation (because separation from the mother is necessary for masculinity to develop), whereas femininity is defined through attachment (the identification with the mother is necessary for femininity to develop). Thus, she stated, "Since masculinity is defined through separation while femininity is defined through attachment, male gender identity is threatened by intimacy while female gender identity is threatened by separation. Thus males tend to have difficulty with relationships, while females tend to have problems with individuation" (p. 8). Gilligan did not discuss homosexuality or heterosexuality in her particular report, nor did she imply that these sexual identifications occur as a result of separation and attachment issues. Such conclusions would require further study.

Gilligan provided us with analysis based on research done by the aforementioned authorities. She indicated that, in moral development, males are generally more concerned with rules, debate, and logically drawn conclusions, whereas females are more concerned with relationships. She pointed out that although male researchers have often drawn similar conclusions, they have not changed their work (e.g., Erikson's chart of life-cycle changes remains the same). Moreover, male behavior has been regarded as the norm whereas female behavior has been regarded as a deviation from the norm, the conclusion generally being that something is wrong with the women (p. 14).

Although we will use the work of male authorities extensively in this book because we have often seen aspects demonstrated in both our male and female clients, more research is clearly necessary, using both male and female subjects and interpreters. In addition, discussions with students and colleagues suggest that, as the needed research is done, we may learn that differences are more generally people differences rather than gender differences. For example, we may learn, as suggested by the Modeling and Role-Modeling (Erickson, Tomlin, & Swain, 1983) theory for nursing, that we as persons respond according to our view or model of the world. This model is shaped by our past experiences and learning, our state of life, and our inherent qualities of genetic base and spiritual drive. As parents and teachers facilitate childhood development based more on inherent qualities and interests than on gender, we may see more person rather than gender identification. However, as in all things, balance is critical, and we also may see that males and females have differences other than physiologic ones. Genders bring their own strengths to the world: neither gender is a deviation from the norm; rather, both are necessary to the quality of life. For example, Ann Schaef (1990), in her book *Meditations for Women Who Do Too Much*, stated, "We have been taught to be afraid of our honesty. Yet it is the key to breaking down denial and the door to healing . . ."

Basic Needs of Persons

Maslow's Hierarchy of Needs

The extensive work of Abraham Maslow on the theory of motivation and the basic needs of persons has provided a framework through which nurses can understand both themselves and their clients. Maslow's basic belief was that each person wants to be the most self-actualized person possible. That is, the person wishes to reach the fullest potential and to become all he or she is capable of becoming.

This notion led Maslow to study how and why some persons become self-actualized and others do not. He stated (1970):

> If I had had to condense the thesis of this book [*Motivation and Personality*] into a single sentence, I would have said that, in *addition* to what the psychologies of the time had to say about human nature, man also had a higher nature and that this was instinctoid, i.e., part of his essence. And if I could have had a second sentence I would have stressed the profoundly holistic nature of human nature. . . ." (p. ix).

Although Maslow did not indicate it as such, inherent in the statement "higher nature . . . profoundly holistic" is an opportunity to recognize Gilligan's work. That is, both Maslow and Gilligan remind us that all humans have a higher nature and are profoundly holistic.

Maslow pointed out that if we are truly to understand persons, we must consider their highest aspirations: growth, self-actualization, the striving toward health, the quest for identity and autonomy, and the yearning for excellence. He believed (1970) that the "instinctoid nature of basic needs" constitutes a system of intrinsic human values that are not only wanted and desired by all humans, but also needed, in the sense that they are necessary to avoid illness and psychopa-

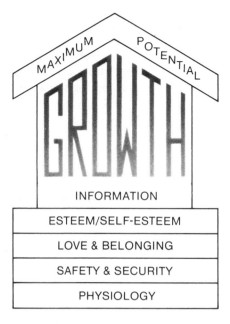

FIGURE 4-2 Maslow's hierarchy of needs. (Erickson, H., Tomlin, E., Swain, MA. [1983]. *Modeling and role-modeling: A theory and paradigm for nursing* [p 57]. Englewood Cliffs, NJ: Prentice-Hall.)

thology (p. xiii). This statement suggests the previous discussion on exchange of energy among the subsystems of the person.

Figure 4-2 is a representation of the hierarchy of human needs as identified by Maslow, beginning with the basic physiologic needs and progressing to the need for safety and security, the need for love and belonging, the need for self-esteem, and the need for self-actualization.

The following 12 ideas are extracted and adapted from Maslow (1970). Nurses may use these ideas to apply basic need theory to practice:

1. The basic needs are present in all of us all of the time, but if met, do not motivate our behavior.
2. Persons function from a state of deficit or a state of being. When a person experiences a deficit state (associated with unmet physiologic, safety and security, love and belonging, or self-esteem needs), one's behavior is motivated by those needs. When one is experiencing a being state, behavior is motivated by the growth needs that are self-actualization and the quest for knowledge, truth, and beauty.
3. The basic needs can be regarded as rights as well as needs.
4. As one group of needs is gratified, another of a higher order will appear.
5. Although all persons have the same basic needs, the means by which each person meets those needs will vary considerably.
6. The gratification of needs is not an absolute state. Rather, one level of needs may be gratified to a certain point and then another group will emerge.
7. The physiologic needs serve as channels for many other needs as well.

The person who thinks he or she is hungry may actually be seeking comfort or dependence rather than nutrition.

8. A conscious desire or motivated behavior may serve as a kind of channel through which other needs may express themselves. The person who seeks sexual encounters may be searching for a sense of belonging.

9. Although a person may be quite capable of meeting his or her basic needs and generally may be physically healthy, safe, loving, and self-actualized, stress may occur in this individual's life and cause a reappearance of a basic need, which the person will again strive to gratify.

10. Needs may be either conscious or unconscious.

11. The gratification of needs may be determined in some measure by one's cultural expression.

12. There are multiple motivations for and determinants of behavior. Thus, to say that a person would respond in any exact manner to this hierarchy of needs would be to oversimplify human nature.

If we accept the general premise that all humans strive for health and excellence, it makes sense for nurses to plan accordingly. This statement seems to be reasonable when we consider the many persons who certainly behave as if they were striving as suggested. We also encounter persons in a helpless–hopeless state and some whose behavior is antisocial or criminal. These persons may cause us to question the general premise. A further consideration of the basic needs may shed light on the meaning of certain behavior.

Physiologic Needs

A list of basic physiologic needs might include oxygen and gas exchange, fluids, food, elimination, rest, avoidance of pain, and sexual fulfillment. In translating these needs to our everyday existence, we remember instances when we were somewhat hungry, tired, or had a slight headache, and yet could continue with our usual activities. As the needs became greater, however, the urgency to gratify them became stronger. Usual activities were performed less effectively because the needs dominated our thoughts.

For most persons, it is a simple matter to obtain food or rest and to cope with a headache. Persons on strict diets, however, who often feel quite hungry, report that they have such a heightened awareness of food that they notice every picture of it, smell every aroma, and think and even dream constantly about it. As food is denied to a greater extent, all other wishes and desires may be lost, and the quest for food will dominate.

An extremely fatigued person, however, may find that the need for rest dominates even though he or she has not eaten recently. Generally, persons respond to basic needs according to a number of other variables. These may include lifestyle, cultural values, general health, and variables known by persons to be attainable. Other responses to hunger are also interesting. For example, consider the need to create, as expressed by the artist or the poet. These persons may avoid a steady-paying job and endure hunger so that they can continue to meet their self-actualization needs. The scholar may have the means by which to take care of his or her physiologic needs, but the scholar's work dominates this person's whole being. As long as life can be sustained, these persons may give little attention to gratification of the physiologic needs.

Consider the clinical example below:

One nurse told of an elderly man brought to the hospital by concerned neighbors. He obviously was starving, inadequately clothed, and confused. The neighbors said there had been no food or heat in the house and that the fuel tank was empty. The nurse assumed the man was poverty stricken. However, as she helped him to undress, she discovered wads of money in his pockets. Later, the authorities went to his home and found piles of money in drawers and canisters.

What prevented this man from using his money or accepting the assistance of neighbors is unclear. Consideration of the next level of needs may suggest ideas.

Safety and Security Needs

Safety and security needs might be listed as follows: security; stability; dependence; protection; freedom from fear, anxiety, and chaos; the need for structure, order, law, and limits; strength in the protector; and so forth (Maslow, 1970, p. 39).

Children frequently demonstrate these needs as they "test" their parents to determine whether limits will be set on their behavior. If children are permitted to throw temper tantrums, they may eventually feel unsafe; they may feel that adults will not stop them from behaving badly and thereby protect the children from themselves. Maslow believed that when safety and security needs are met in childhood they are less likely to surface in later years. However, when a severe stress occurs, an adult may feel unsafe. If the stress becomes overwhelming, and if safety is severely threatened—as may have been the case with the elderly man described above—the safety needs will dominate even the physiologic ones.

Nurses often see the safety of a relatively secure adult threatened when illness and hospitalization are experienced. At times, the safety need may be conscious and the person may express his or her fears. However, if the need is unconscious and fears are not expressed, we often see what is termed the "difficult client." This is the person who cannot participate well in his or her care. This individual may exhibit anger and hostility toward the nurses, yet call constantly with requests. Consideration of underlying factors associated with such behavior helps nurses to plan interventions to develop trust and meet safety needs.

Love and Belonging Needs

Needs for love and belonging include the following: affectionate relationships; a place in the family and in other social groups; the need for a spouse, sweetheart, lover, children, and friends; and the need for roots in a particular neighborhood

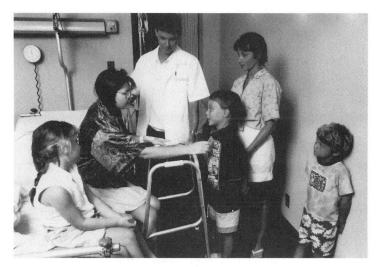

We empower our clients by engaging them in their own care.

or place. Maslow (1970) clearly pointed out that these needs include the need to give as well as to receive love, warmth, affection, and friendship. Persons who cannot meet these needs feel rejected, abandoned, and without roots. As they increasingly feel that no one cares about them, they develop a sense of helpless–hopelessness and diminished self-esteem (p. 43).

The sexual drive, a physiologic need, can be considered purely biologic in that context. Beyond that, however, sexual expression may be a channel through which love and belonging needs are met. Sexuality is usually considered an aspect of most intimate relationships. However, persons seeking gratification of love and belonging needs may engage in sexual activity that they sometimes regret. Their reason is that, at least for a little while, it helped them feel as if they belonged to someone.

Nurses often discover that persons whose love and belonging needs are met can respond readily to help and can mobilize their health resources with ease. They have a support system of family and friends in which they feel both a sense of belonging and a sense of security.

Esteem Needs

Esteem needs include a high evaluation of the self, self-respect, self-esteem, and the esteem of others. Maslow (1970) suggested that these needs can be divided into two subsets: those related to self-esteem (desire for strength, achievement, adequacy, mastery, competence, and independence) and those related to respect and esteem from others (reputation, prestige, status, fame, glory, dominance, recognition, attention, importance, dignity, and appreciation).

Those who can meet their needs for self-esteem will face the world with confidence and a sense of self-worth, capability, adequacy, and usefulness or purpose in the scheme of things. Those whose needs are thwarted will often demonstrate helplessness, inferiority, and weakness. They will be discouraged and nonassertive, demonstrating a diminished sense of the confidence they need to face their daily activities. Maslow (1970) also pointed out the danger that persons face if they gratify their esteem needs primarily from the opinions of others: to have the deserved respect of others is rewarding, but true esteem comes from within (pp. 45–46).

Self-Actualization Needs

The self-actualization need is the impulse to reach one's fullest potential, the need to become what one is capable of becoming, and the desire for self-fulfillment (Maslow, 1970, p. 46). Self-actualization needs emerge when the physiologic, safety, love, and esteem needs basically have been met.

Maslow (1970) described the self-actualized person as having a variety of characteristics, including spontaneity; the ability to center on problems rather than on self; an enjoyment of solitude and privacy; autonomy (independence from culture and environment); continued fresh appreciation for the basic goods of life; creativity; and the ability to develop deep and profound interpersonal relationships. Yet, these persons are not perfect. Maslow also described some of their shortcomings: they can be silly, wasteful, thoughtless, boring, stubborn, and irritating; they may be somewhat vain and have outbursts of temper (p. 175). Maslow also discussed two other higher levels of basic needs: the desire to know and understand, which is satisfied by acquiring knowledge through curiosity, learning, philosophizing, and experimenting; and the aesthetic need, the need for beauty and, specifically, for beauty in one's environment.

Erickson and colleagues (1983) described the self-actualization, knowing–understanding, and aesthetic needs as the growth needs. They indicated that persons who can generally meet their lower-level basic needs will begin to have a recurrence of these needs if they are thwarted in attempts to meet the growth needs. For example, professionals who perceive themselves as stagnant in the growth of their knowledge and development regarding their particular field may feel unsafe, inadequate, and without a group.

Spiritual Needs

Basic needs that flow from the biopsychosocial spheres of the person have been identified. Because persons also have been described as spiritual beings, it follows that needs are associated with the spiritual sphere. Although Maslow himself did not deal directly with this issue, some authors have attempted to describe the notion. Perhaps spiritual needs include the following: the need to believe in a Supreme Being or in a special order for the universe; the need to believe that one has a place in that Being or order and that life has meaning; and the need to feel hopeful about one's destiny.

We can speculate where spiritual needs might be placed on the hierarchy. Some might consider them a higher order of need, arising after others have been gratified. Others might suggest that they are present even before the physiologic needs described by Maslow. We might also consider that the spiritual needs are inherent in all the other needs, and therefore are inappropriately defined as a separate category. However we choose to look at this notion, we will want to be aware that most persons have a philosophy or a system of faith that directs their lives and serves as a refuge in times of need.

The Freedoms

Maslow (1970) indicated that, to meet any of the basic needs, certain conditions must exist. He listed those conditions as a series of freedoms. The freedoms include freedom to speak, to do what one wishes so long as it does not harm others, to express oneself, to seek justice, and to find fairness, honesty, and orderliness in the group (p. 47). Nurses will be more effective if they are aware of clients' basic needs and how the needs can be met by facilitating expression of thought and by protecting the freedoms.

Examples Using Maslow

In a course called Client-Centered Dimensions of Professional Nursing, registered nurse baccalaureate students worked on a term project in which they applied concepts from Maslow to clients from their own practice. Some of these examples were as follows:

Sam, aged three, had been beaten. The nurse states, ''In looking at Maslow's hierarchy of basic needs, Sam's physical needs were being met. He was fed, given water, warmth, and shelter. However, his safety and security needs were certainly in question. Had he been beaten before? Was he afraid to play loudly, or mess his pants, or leave his toys out for fear of being beaten? If these safety and security needs were not being met, then he would never move up the ladder of maximum potential. His sense of love and belonging and self-esteem would always be in question.'' Kimberly Kenny-Sherlock, RN

Lisa was twenty-six and badly burned in a fire. The nurse states, ''Lisa was very ill, and the doctors did not think she could survive. Lisa's parents went to her and asked if she wanted to continue treatment. Lisa told them she wanted to live. After I heard this, I realized that the only part of Lisa injured in the fire was her appearance, but what makes her the person she is was still fully intact. Lisa must have had a strong sense of self-esteem before the fire that enabled her to want to get her life back.'' Amy Hudson, RN

Jenna, in her late thirties, had lupus. The nurse states, ''The illness had physically consumed her energy and strength. She became dependent upon hospitalization for assistance to meet her basic needs. She was unable to focus on higher needs such as Maslow's self-actualization, as her energies were needed for survival.'' Lisa Fulford, RN

Marianne is elderly and lives in an extended care facility. Formerly homeless, she has no family. Tim, a kindly policeman who found her outside, cold and sick, now visits her regularly. Tim has become her father, son and friend. The nurse relays her concerns about Marianne's safety and security and love and belonging needs. She states, ''Marianne stares out the window at the diner across the road where Tim takes her. She constantly asks for Tim and has been known to leave the facility, dangerously crossing busy roads. When Tim arrives, she is like a child who is going out with her daddy. When he leaves, she returns to her depressed, zombie-like state. She eats better when Tim is with her, she looks to him as her source of protection, and while she feels abandoned and rejected when Tim is not there, when he is, her needs for love and belonging are gratified." Maricar Uy, RN

Jennifer is twenty-five and has come twice to the emergency department (ED) with a pseudo-seizure diagnosis. The nurse states, "Regarding Maslow's Basic Needs Theory, both of her visits to the ED revolved around her boyfriend not wanting to be with her. This unmet love and belonging need apparently led Jennifer to develop a psychological(ly) induced illness. Jennifer did not see life as worth living unless she was with her boyfriend." Dorothy Morton, R.N.

Person's Perception of Self

View of Self

As nurses work to help clients meet their basic needs, they learn how persons view themselves. Our **self-concept** is a collection of notions, feelings, and beliefs about ourselves with which we identify and through which we relate and communicate with others and interact with the environment. The ideas of self-concept are developed from many of the variables inherent in the biopsychosocial systems of the person (see Table 4-1). Persons generally have a self-ideal that might be considered the superego. The **self-ideal** refers to how we believe we ought to function and behave, given a personal value system and a set of personal standards. We develop this ideal with influences from family structure; cultural values; teachers; and our own talents, strengths, and goals for the future. Often we view ourselves as a reflection of how we believe that others see us. If others smile or nod, or if their eyes light up when they see us, our self-ideal is reinforced. Conversely, when we see anger or mocking, or if we are ignored, then we suffer. For some of us, these feelings may pass quickly, while others who are more sensitive may feel pleased or hurt for a long time. Thus we understand that a child's view of self is developed by the parents' response. Note that a child who has fallen quickly looks at mother to see whether he or she has been hurt. The child may cry if mother acts frightened or upset, but is less likely to when mother responds that all is well. The following example describes poignantly, in her own words, how a young woman felt during her adolescent years. Note how her inherent strengths overcome a negative view of herself as she strives to regain confidence and autonomy.

The Person In Me
Danyelle Lundy
Junior high wasn't one of the good experiences in my life.
I was going through puberty and I was not toughing it out like other preteens my age.
I wasn't happy with myself. I wasn't happy with myself because of other people's criticism about me being myself.
I can't remember and I don't think I'll ever recall why I deserved the treatment, but I always seemed to suffer some type of ridicule every single day.

They would talk about my clothing, my hair, my personality, my looks, my hygiene. They would even talk about my sexual preference, although I definitely preferred males.

I didn't let their words roll off my back. I took everything said very personal, everything said hurt. Soon my pride and self-confidence were shambles, but as stubborn as I was I didn't take the strong faith from my parents' as my own. Although my parents' support kept me from hurting myself later, my self-confidence would have to come from myself.

I had the hardest crushes on guys about this time. I had crushes on seemingly perfect and beautiful white boys, and I felt that the only solution to solve my problems of inadequacy was to have been born white.

Sometimes I felt so sad and hopeless. I found myself wishing to die.

Yet I would always hold back because I was afraid and uncertain of death. I didn't want to give up if things could change. I didn't want to lose my only hope and refuge, my dreams.

In my dreams, I could be anything.

In my dreams I would masquerade as a man. I would meet and befriend the man I unknowingly was destined to love. I would beat him at his own games and achieve higher than his goals. We would become close friends. I would become careless and he'd stumble upon the secret of my identity from where we would fall in love.

We would love as equals, even when my dreams led me to a time and place where equal relationships between lovers were unheard of.

These dreams seemed to be uplifting because they gave me the hope to feel better about myself and ignore the ridicule of others. I realized that being a different race other than the race *GOD* made me would not solve my problems. I learned in my heart that black is beautiful and *I* am beautiful. I realized that even if I wasn't black, *I* am beautiful.

The person in me is the person I am in my dreams; the daring, beautiful woman loved for who she is and for who she is behind the masquerade.

Danyelle

Body Image

An important aspect of self-concept is our sense of **self-esteem**—the personal judgment we make about our own self-worth. People may arrive at this perception by considering how they compare with their self-ideal and how often they attain personal goals. The ability to set and attain goals provides the person with a sense of control over his or her life, as well as a hopeful feeling about the future.

Another component of self-concept is **body image.** The body is the structural, functional, substantive, and visible part of the self. It is the packaging in which the self is enclosed and through which individuals interact with other persons and the environment. Our body image is how we view or think of that physical part of ourselves. Nurses often note that persons who are comfortable with their appearance generally have a high sense of self-esteem. Tolstoy (1904) said, "I am convinced that nothing has so marked an influence on the direction of a man's mind as his appearance, and not his appearance in itself so much as his conviction that it is attractive or unattractive."

When the view of the self does not correspond with what we actually see, self-esteem may decrease—as, for example, in persons who have had surgery, whether or not the surgical alteration is visible to others. Some theorists believe that *phantom pain,* which occurs in an absent body part such as an amputated limb, is the result of nerve activity. Others, however, suggest that the pain also may be associated with the alteration in one's body image or view of the physical self.

Some persons feel a disruption in their body image when they must wear glasses or a hearing aid. Others describe difficulty in communicating or in projecting themselves effectively when, in their view, their hair or clothes are not right. Daphne du Maurier (1957) described the feelings of her hero in *The Scapegoat* when he first notices the man who resembles him exactly:

> The resemblance made me slightly sick, reminding me of moments when, passing a shop window, I had suddenly seen my reflection, and the man in the mirror had been a grotesque caricature of what, conceitedly, I had believed myself to be. Such incidents left me chastened, sore, with ego deflated. . . . (p. 17).

Perhaps you can identify personally with the following example: One woman, after catching an unexpected glimpse of herself in a mirror, stated, "I wondered if I should accept what I saw and readjust my self-image, or if I should go on thinking of myself as before."

Inner Versus Outward Feelings

Our total self-concept consists not only of how we believe we appear, but also of the expectations we have of our behavior and achievements. Sometimes we are unsure of who that self is and how that person ought to be expressed. The expression *identity crisis* is common in our current Western culture; it refers to difficulty we sometimes have in grasping the meaning of our inner workings (thinking and feeling) or outward behavior. How we present ourselves to others may be vastly different from how we actually feel about ourselves.

Again we turn to du Maurier's (1957) hero as he talks of his struggle to understand his real self, as opposed to the self he presents to others. He appears to be a quiet, law-abiding professor, aged 38 years, but he wonders about the self, the man within.

> Who he was and whence he sprang, what urges and what longings he might possess, I could not tell. I was so used to denying him expression that his ways were unknown to me; but he might have had a mocking laugh, a casual heart, a swift-roused temper and a ribald tongue. . . . Perhaps, if I had not kept him locked within me, he might have laughed, roistered, fought and lied. Perhaps he suffered, perhaps he hated, perhaps he lived by cruelty alone. He might have murdered, stolen or spent himself in lost causes, loved humanity, embraced a faith that believed in the divinity of both God and Man. Whatever his nature, he always hovered beneath the insignificant facade of that pale self who now sat in the church. . . . The question was, how to unlock the door? What lever would set the other free? (pp. 14–15).

It is essential that nurses, as persons, understand themselves. As they become more comfortable with their own self-concept, they are better able to understand the strivings of their clients. As nurses become more aware of their own inner workings, they can more readily accept the inner workings of others as well as the facade persons present to the world. Such acceptance will enable nurses to find the uniqueness of each person and to use that uniqueness to facilitate growth.

Values

The particular value system a person espouses is another way in which he or she is unique and yet shares features in common with others. Our values help us to view ourselves in relation to others.

A **value** is a belief or a custom that frequently arises from cultural or ethnic backgrounds, from family tradition, from peer group ideas and practices, from political philosophies in one's country, and from educational and religious philosophies with which one identifies. Some values are unique to the individual; other values are more readily identified as arising from a particular group, philosophy, or culture.

Because we all form values and value systems, we also engage in a practice called **value judgment,** a personal decision about whether something is right or wrong. These decisions usually are affected by the society, culture, and period of history in which we live. We generally hold these decisions to be true and right and find support for them from others around us who agree and will support our claim to righteousness.

Because we are nurses as well as persons, we also have another set of values under which we operate. We are expected to provide care for others who often feel or believe differently from ourselves. The professional value system, as well as a personal one, often dictates that nurses must not abandon the person who has sought their care. Nurses can handle this situation in two different ways. First, nurses may decide to continue care. To maintain their own integrity, however, nurses may not become involved in the process, but merely support the person as that person carries out the plan himself or herself. The notion of empathy and techniques in problem solving discussed in succeeding chapters will be of use to the nurse involved in this kind of situation. Second, if values are seriously threatened, nurses may decide to find other nurses or agencies to assist the client.

Consider the example of a person who wishes to terminate his or her chemotherapy for cancer. The nurse may know, given certain statistics, that chemotherapy offers a chance for long-term survival, whereas termination may result in less than 1 year of life. The nurse may believe that stopping therapy is an inappropriate decision, but can remain objective and act as a listener so the person can explore his or her ideas. However, the nurse whose values are seriously threatened may want to engage another nurse, who is comfortable with the person's decision, to assist that person with planning and problem solving. Regardless of how we decide to handle a situation where our values are threatened, there is one overriding principle that prevails: we do not abandon our clients, but find proper help for them when we cannot offer it. This is as true with a value conflict as it is in any of the care we provide.

General Principles of Growth and Development

This section suggests an application of several growth and development theories to the delivery of effective nursing care. Growth and development are variables in the biopsychosocial functioning of the person. To provide background and resource material for understanding skills nurses use in practice, we wish to acquaint students with several prominent theorists. This knowledge increases our awareness of the total person concept. For example, knowledge about psychosocial development helps the nurse work with the teenager whose lagging physical development contributes to poor schoolwork. The most exciting reason for considering growth and development, however, is that it demonstrates the unending potential of the human throughout life.

The subject and theories of growth and development are far more lengthy than can be described in this section. We expect that students will use the ideas presented to understand aspects that are both common and unique to clients. For a more thorough examination of the subject, refer to the publications cited at the end of this chapter.

Growth

The term **growth** refers to an actual biologic or quantitative increase in physical size, that is, the enlargement of any body components by an increase in the number of cells. **Maturation** refers to the emergence of genetic potential for changes in form, structure, complexity, integration, organization, and function (Murray and Zentner, 1993, p. 175).

Some key ideas related to growth are as follows:

❏ Physical growth occurs at different rates among individuals.
❏ Growth of the body parts and systems of a person occurs at different rates; for example, a child may be within normal height and weight ranges at age 5 but have a less mature urinary elimination system that causes the child to wet the bed at night. During adolescence, a person's features may appear too large for the face, but will eventually be in proper proportion as the size of the head increases.
❏ A wide range of normal values exists for height, weight, muscle development, and physical abilities at all ages and stages of development. Charts that describe physical characteristics of different ages should be used only as guidelines.

Development

"**Development** is the patterned, orderly, lifelong changes in structure, thought, or behavior that evolve during maturation of physical and mental capacity, experiences, and learning and result in a new level of maturity and integration" (Murray & Zentner, 1993, p. 175). A **developmental task** is a growth responsibility that arises at a certain time in the course of development. If resolution of the task occurs, satisfaction and success with later tasks will probably result. Failure to resolve the tasks in a satisfactory manner leads to unhappiness, disapproval by society, and difficulty with later developmental tasks and functions (p. 175).

Three principles of development to consider are as follows:

1. Development that occurs in childhood provides a base for the rest of life.
2. Development proceeds in a predictable and sequential way throughout life.
3. The developing person acquires competency in four major areas across the life span:
   a. Physical: Gaining motor and neurologic capacities
   b. Cognitive: Learning how to perceive, think, and communicate thoughts and feelings
   c. Emotional: Developing awareness and acceptance of self as a unique individual, reacting to the environment, coping with stresses, assuming responsibility for personal behavior
   d. Social: Learning to interrelate first with the family, and later with different persons in many situations (Murray & Zentner, 1993, p. 176).

When performing a nursing assessment (see discussion of the nursing process, Chapter 8), it is especially useful to consider those aspects of development that are most pertinent to the client's age. For example, the 6-year-old child will be learning to write in school. Thus, an assessment of his or her fine motor development would be useful. The adolescent person who is struggling with identity and changes in body image may benefit from assessment and care planning related to secondary sex characteristics and the condition of the skin. Older adults experiencing changes in body structure will be helped if planning centers on their motor ability.

The following sections of this chapter describe the theories of Erik Erikson, a major theorist in psychosocial development, and Jean Piaget, a major theorist in cognitive development. These two men are well known and accepted in their fields. Their work provides nurses with a base for understanding the development of the psychologic and social components of the person. Again, however, we will consider Gilligan's (1982) comments as we read.

Psychosocial Development: Erikson

Erikson enumerated developmental tasks, as shown in Table 4-2. The following ideas from Erikson's (1963) classic work *Childhood and Society* can be used by nurses to apply concepts from psychosocial developmental theory to practice:

1. At each stage of development, a nuclear conflict arises (e.g., trust versus mistrust). Negative feelings (mistrust, shame, guilt, and so forth) as-

TABLE 4-2 *Developmental Tasks According to Erikson*

Age	Task	Favorable Outcome	Unfavorable Outcome
Birth–1 year	Basic trust versus mistrust	Lets mother out of sight without undue anxiety or rage	Senses an inner division; feels deprived or divided: feels abandoned
		Learns that mother has become an inner certainty and an outer predictability	Develops defense mechanisms, projection, and introjection against anticipated loss or disappointment Projection: "Attributing one's own thoughts or impulses to another person" (Stuart, 1995, p. 337) Introjection: "Intense type of identification in which a person incorporates qualities or values of another person or group into his own ego structure" (p. 337)
		Correlates inner remembrances and anticipation of sensation with outer sameness of experience; this leads to familiarity and prediction	
		Engages in constant testing of relationships both inside and outside	
		Begins not only to trust the outer provider but also to trust oneself and the capacity of one's own organs to cope with urges	
1–3 years	Autonomy versus shame and doubt	Develops a set of social modalities associated with holding on and letting go	Develops a set of social modalities associated with holding on and letting go.
		Benign expectations: Letting go (to let be); holding on (to have and to hold)	Hostile expectations: Letting go (letting loose of destructive forces); holding on (destructive or cruel restraining forces)
		Experiences definite wish to have a choice, begins to stand on own two feet, begins to develop a sense of self-control without loss of self-esteem; this can develop into a lasting sense of good will and pride	Shame: Becomes conscious of being upright and exposed; tries to get away with things unseen; could become defiant and shameless
			Doubt: Senses that one is dominated by the will of oth-

(continued)

TABLE 4-2 (Continued)

Age	Task	Favorable Outcome	Unfavorable Outcome
			ers; senses of loss of control and of foreign overcontrol; develops a lasting propensity for doubt and shame
		Develops basic faith in existence, autonomy fostered in childhood helps develop a sense of justice later in life	
4–5 years	Initiative versus guilt	Senses hope and new responsibility; a vigorous unfolding	Superego becomes cruel and uncompromising, causing repression in some persons (who become inhibited or impotent) and exhibitionism ("showing off") in others
		Learns quickly and avidly	
		Develops judgment; is active, energetic; develops direction; can undertake, plan, and attack a task	
		Cooperates, works with other children for a purpose, constructs and plans cooperatively	
		Establishes a moral sense that restricts the horizon of the permissible	Submerges rage, which causes self-righteousness; often psychosomatic disease is noted in the adult who fails to resolve this developmental task
6–11 years	Industry versus inferiority	Wins recognition by producing things, because this is the age of formal and systematic instruction, whether the school is the classroom, field, or jungle	
		Begins readiness to move beyond or outside the family	Remains unsure of status with peers and partners
		Begins to handle tools and develops skills with them	
		Applies self to skills and tasks	Feels unsure of skills and tools
		Directs attention and perseveres; goes beyond desire to plan and develops a sense of satisfaction in work completion	
		Senses a division of labor and differential opportunity	Restricts self and horizons to include only own work; becomes a conformist and thoughtless slave of the technology

(continued)

TABLE 4-2 (Continued)

Age	Task	Favorable Outcome	Unfavorable Outcome
		Senses the characteristics of the culture	Begins to feel the color of skin and background of parents and to feel judged by it
12–20 years	Identity versus role confusion	Questions continuity and sameness from past; searches for a new continuity and sameness	Confuses sex roles because of doubt regarding sexual identity
		Concerns self with appearance to others versus what one feels oneself to be	Overidentifies with heroes, cliques, and crowds (to the loss of individual identity) Behaves in a clannish and cruel manner to all those who are different (a defense against a sense of identity confusion)
		Develops a confidence that the inner sameness and continuity prepared in the past are matched by the sameness and continuity of one's meaning for others, as evidenced in the tangible promise of a career	
		Senses an ideology and a commitment to it; finds self in the stage between the morality learned by the child and the ethics developed by the adult	Becomes an easy prey to cruel totalitarian doctrines and ideology
20–40 years, early adulthood	Intimary versus isolation	Becomes eager and willing to fuse one's identity with others; ready for intimacy; has capacity to commit oneself to concrete affiliations and partnerships	Avoids intimate relationships and commitment for fear of ego loss; this leads to a deep sense of isolation and self-absorption
		Develops the ethical strength to abide by one's commitments.	Develops prejudice
		Welcomes situations that require self-abandonment: solidarity of close affiliations, sexual unions, close friendships, physical combat, and experiences of inspiration from teachers, institutions, and the recesses of the self	Fears others' encroachment on one's territory
41–60 years, middle adulthood	Generativity versus stagnation	Concerns self with establishing and guiding the next generation; mature persons need to be needed	Experiences a pervasive sense of stagnation and personal impoverishment; needs pseudo-intimacy
		Produces and creates	

(continued)

TABLE 4-2 (Continued)

Age	Task	Favorable Outcome	Unfavorable Outcome
		Believes in and has faith in the species, sees the child or the younger generation as a welcome trust	Indulges self; early invalidism, physical or psychological disorders become a vehicle of self-concern
61 years and on, late adulthood	Ego integrity versus despair	Sees self as the originator of others or a generator of products and ideas; in this person, the fruits of other stages of development gradually ripen: hope, willpower, purpose, competence, fidelity, love, care, and wisdom	Feels despair: time is too short to start over
		Senses an assurance that there is order and meaning in the sense of the world and of the spirit	
		Accepts one's own life cycle as the way it had to be	Does not accept one's only life cycle as the ultimate of life
		Experiences a sense of comradeship with the past	
		Defends the dignity of one's own life-style	
		Experiences a final consolation and emotional integration	Behaves with disgust, which hides despair and the fear of death
		Acceptance of death	

(From Erikson, E. H. (1963). Childhood and society (2nd ed., pp. 247–274). New York, W. W. Norton.)

sociated with each stage are the dynamic counterparts of the positive ones throughout life. Aspects of these counterparts are present in all of us at one time or another (p. 274).

2. Developmental levels are resolved, not achieved (p. 273).
3. At each stage of development, a ratio—preferably a favorable one—develops between the positive and negative senses of each nuclear conflict such that skills are formed throughout life for coping with stress. For example, trust is learned in infancy through satisfaction of basic needs (p. 274).
4. Stressors affect our lives, and new inner conflicts develop throughout the life span. Our ability to cope is closely associated with the ratio of resolution that has occurred during work on previous tasks (p. 274).
5. At each age, all the developmental tasks are present in us at some level (p. 271).

6. Each task exists from birth in some form before its critical time for resolution normally arrives (p. 271).

7. Theorists have suggested that the first two tasks (trust versus mistrust and autonomy versus shame and doubt) lay the groundwork for the person's future. Many conflicts that occur later in life may well reflect the ratio of resolution that has occurred in those early tasks. For example, Erikson believed that in society at large the resolution of basic trust is reflected in faith (religion, social action, or scientific pursuit). The resolution of autonomy is reflected in the principles of law and order (p. 274).

8. Evidence suggests that persons become physically and psychologically ill if the impact of stressors is overwhelming. This phenomenon is influenced by the achievement of coping skills through developmental task resolution (p. 274).

9. The strength acquired at any stage is tested by the necessity to transcend it in such a way that the individual can take chances in the next stage with what was most vulnerably precious in the last one. For example, as the child resolves autonomy versus shame and doubt, he or she can move on to the next task and not need to demand his or her own way unreasonably (p. 270).

10. Erikson believed these stages of development are present in all humans. The realization and demonstration of resolution may be reflected in the particular customs and styles of many different ethnic, cultural, and national groups. The essence of development, however, is the same for us all (pp. 271–272).

We continue to work on resolution of all the tasks throughout life. Erikson described the outcome potential of the favorable ratios of each stage of development. He called the words italicized in the following list the basic virtues. These basic virtues reemerge from generation to generation and constitute the spirit and relevance of human systems.

Basic trust versus mistrust: Drive and *hope*
Autonomy versus shame and doubt: Self-control and *willpower*
Initiative versus guilt: Direction and *purpose*
Industry versus inferiority: Method and *competence*
Identity versus role confusion: Devotion and *fidelity*
Intimacy versus isolation: Affiliation and *love*
Generativity versus stagnation: Production and *care*
Ego integrity versus despair: Renunciation and *wisdom* (p. 274)

Consider the following examples of a healthy child and an adult in different stages of Erikson's psychosocial development. Consider also, the examples offered by registered nurse baccalaureate students as they apply Erikson's ideas to their practice.

The theories of Maslow and Erikson blend well together. A person's ability to meet his or her basic needs is reflected by the degree to which the person has resolved the developmental tasks of trust and autonomy. When stress seriously affects one's sense of safety, adaptive coping can occur if the person has a sense of trust, self-control, direction, purpose, and competence. The ability to meet our basic needs on a daily basis is directly related to the number of skills we have developed through resolution of the developmental tasks.

Maslow emphasized that basic needs are satisfied not only by receiving but also by giving. Giving is essential to satisfaction. We provide a safe atmosphere and protect the safety needs of small children and others who are unable to do this for themselves. We wish to give as well as to receive love and friendship. Erikson pointed out the need to be trusted as well as to trust, to develop a sense of devotion and intimacy toward others, and to produce or care for the next generation. He maintained that the mature person needs to be needed and that the older adult develops wisdom that he or she wishes to pass on to the younger generation.

If, as persons ourselves, or as persons who are nurses, we consider our own development and ability to meet our basic needs, we can be more effective in helping others move toward the basic virtues and self-actualization.

Cognitive Development: Piaget

Piaget described cognitive development as a continuous progression from the spontaneous movements and reflexes of the newborn, to acquired habits of the infant, to the beginning of the development of intelligence that becomes apparent toward the end of the first year of life. Cognitive development is cumulative; understanding of new experiences evolves from what was learned during earlier ones. Piaget (1973) identified four major levels in the development of cognition or growth of thought.

Sensorimotor Level: Birth to 2 Years

The following describes the mechanism of progression toward the development of intelligence.

Assimilation

Reality data (i.e., input from the real world) are treated or modified such that they become incorporated into the structure of the person. Piaget used **structure** to describe how information is organized within the person to make a simple mental image or pattern of action. Although the necessary mental structures are genetically destined, these structures mature with age. The organizing activity of the person is as important as the relationships inherent in the external stimuli. This idea might be represented as follows: stimulus $\underset{\text{person}}{\longleftrightarrow}$ response.

The input stimulus is filtered through a person, who develops action-schemes or, at a higher level, the operations of thought, which, in turn, are modified and enriched when the person's behavioral repertoire increases to meet the demands of reality. **Assimilation,** then, is the process of taking novel information and making it fit a preconceived notion about objects or the world. Later, the child will be able to find new ways of looking at things.

Accommodation

Accommodation is the alteration of internal schemes to fit reality: reconciling new experiences or objects by revising the old plan to fit the new input. Singer and Revenson (1996) provided an example of this process in the infant. Initially, the child attempts to understand something new by using old solutions, that is, by assimilation. When this does not work, the youngster is forced to modify his or her existing view of the world to interpret the experience. The baby who attempts to drink milk from the rattle (assimilation) quickly learns that rattles make noise but do not yield milk. The rattle no longer substitutes for feeding (accommodation).

This dual process of assimilation–accommodation leads to **adaptation,** which is a continuing process of learning from the environment and learning to adjust to alterations in the environment. Adaptation allows the child to form a **schema,** a more complex mental image and action organization that a person uses to explain what he or she sees and hears (Singer & Revenson, 1996, pp. 15–17).

From birth to 2 years, the infant relies on his or her senses and his or her motor activity for information about the world. Reflex actions occur during this period. The infant recognizes these as successful actions, but has no knowledge about them. The infant's understanding of the world involves only perceptions and objects with which he or she has direct experience. As language appears, usually at about age 1 1/2 to 2 years, the development of symbolic or preconceptual thought begins. Toward the end of the sensorimotor phase, the child begins to understand the concept of **object permanence:** the child begins to realize that objects can exist apart from himself or herself. When the child cannot see an object, he or she begins to understand that it is still there. The child can accept the parent leaving his or her sight because the child knows the parent is near and will return.

Preoperational Level: Age 2 to 7 Years

The preoperational level is the period of curiosity, questioning, and investigation. Children become interested in their environment, but still interpret it according to their own viewpoint. This approach is called *egocentrism*. The child uses explanations of the world he or she knows and makes up others to answer his or her questions. An especially descriptive example of preoperational thinking found in literature is the following discussion between Scout (Jean Louise Finch) and Miss Maudie Atkinson in Harper Lee's (1960) novel *To Kill a Mockingbird*. Scout, age 6, is asking questions about Boo Radley, a reclusive man who lives in her neighborhood, and whom Scout has never seen:

"Miss Maudie," I said one evening, "do you think Boo Radley's still alive?"

"His name's Arthur and he's alive," she said. . . .

". . . Yessum. How do you know?" . . .

". . . What a morbid question. But I suppose it's a morbid subject. I know he's alive, Jean Louise, because I haven't seen him carried out yet."

"Maybe he died and they stuffed him up the chimney!" (p. 44)

In this conversation, both Scout and Miss Maudie deal with object permanence and preoperational thinking. Scout worries that if she cannot see the man, then he does not exist. However, if he has died they must have done something with him, because no one was seen carrying the man out. Thus, the solution—stuffing him up the chimney—satisfies her to some extent. Miss Maudie believes that if she has not seen him carried out, his death has not occurred. However, she is more concrete than Scout, and does not create a silly explanation to satisfy her curiosity. Still, we can make the observation that even adults may revert to earlier thinking when things become too confusing or overwhelming.

Consider the following display about three-year-old Luke:

Example 1: Three-year-old Luke has been working through autonomy versus shame and doubt. Luke was taking a boat ride with his parents. When his mother opened some packages of cheese for snacks, Luke said, in a perfect imitation of his day-care teacher's voice, "Now we do not throw the papers in the water; we take them back home and put them carefully in the trash can." In this way, Luke demonstrated his developing autonomy as he instructed his elders on the correct way of doing things. In another situation, Luke had a different experience. Billy had come to Luke's house and Luke was not happy because Billy took his toys and would not let Luke play with them. When Luke's mother took him to the bathroom, he was distressed and afraid to leave his toys. When he returned, he saw that Billy had usurped more of his toys, and he yelled, "I just went to the potty and you took my toys."

In this example, Luke demonstrates how children make connections using preoperational thinking (Piaget). Luke uses the bathroom and "Let's go" (Erikson), and in doing so, he loses control (Billy takes the toys). For a healthy child who has a supportive family, such an incident, rather than being a detriment, can help the child develop residual strengths. Luke's parents hugged him and explained that Billy was playing here for a while but would not take the toys home with him. Though minimally comforted at the moment, Luke realized later that Billy did not get to keep the toys. Thus, the part of his personhood that was connected to the toys was affirmed and he was again in control. Issues of control, however, may surface in adults who, as children, were overwhelmed by similar incidents and not given the support they needed.

Example 2: Growth and development in the adult has a similar appearance. Consider Claire, the director of a hospice agency. She is concerned about the development of standards of care (see Chapter 8) for hospices in the United States. She stated, "We have been on a journey with hospice. We began several years ago, and now are working toward putting the pieces together. Each piece is like a building block as we work to make the whole for hospice care everywhere." Claire is demonstrating generativity versus stagnation. She has begun her work and now is looking to the next generation. She hopes to prepare hospice care for the future.

*C*oncrete *Operations Level: Age 7 to 11 Years*

Piaget (cited in Singer & Revenson, 1996, p. 129) defined an **operation** as an interiorized action, or an action performed in the mind. Several qualities characterize the concrete operations level:

Reversibility—The direction of thought can be reversed mentally. When children learn addition, they can then learn subtraction. The child knows how to find the way to school and how to turn around and find the way home again.

Seriation—The child has the ability to arrange objects mentally according to a quantitative dimension such as size or weight.

Conservation—The person has the ability to see that objects or quantities remain the same despite a change in their physical appearance. The child understands such quantities as number; substance (mass); area; weight; and volume. He or she can understand that a quantity of liquid is the same whether it fills a short, fat container or a tall, thin one.

The child applies his or her concrete operations to objects that are physically present. As adults, we often use concrete operations when we first learn a new skill. We wish to be told how to proceed step by step. Later, we can think more broadly and develop our own process while continuing to follow the basic principles. Some people learn more quickly than others, depending on background, knowledge, skill, and general abilities.

*F*ormal *Operations Level: Age 11 to 16 Years*

The child can now consider objects that are not present and perform formal operations by considering the future and the abstract. As the child reaches adolescence, he or she can problem solve using more rational and scientific processes. The child's thinking is more flexible, and he or she can consider various ways to solve a problem or view an experience. The child can make relationships among several pieces of information and draw rational conclusions. Piaget (1973) hypothesized that we do not develop any new mental structures after the stage of formal operations. He believed that intellectual development from this point on consists of an increase in knowledge and depth of understanding.

An Example of Piaget's Theory
   Kathleen Norris (1996) in her book *The Cloister Walk,* describes a day in fourth grade when she suddenly had an "epiphany" (a new understanding of an old concept) about numbers. Always anxious about math, she was doing a problem on the blackboard and botched it badly. The teacher grabbed the chalk, fixed the problem, and announced that it was "as simple as two plus two is always four." Norris states, "And without thinking, I said, 'that can't be'. Suddenly I was sure that two plus two could not *possibly* always be four. And of course it isn't. In Boolean Algebra, two plus two can be zero, in base three, two plus two is eleven. I had stumbled onto set theory, a truth about numbers that I had no language for. As this was the early 1950's, my teacher had no language for it either, and she and the class had a good laugh over my ridiculous remark. I staggered away from my epiphany and

went back to my seat...Briefly, numbers had seemed much more exciting...but if two plus two was always four, then numbers were too literal, too boring...I wrote math off right then and there...

In a way though, this experience had a positive side, as the beginning of my formation as a poet. Whenever definitions were given as absolutes, as *always*, I would have that familiar tingle—*that can't be*—and soon learned that I could focus on the fuzzy boundaries, where definitions gave way to metaphors.''

In this anecdote, Norris shows us how the concrete thinking of childhood, two plus two equals four, can give way to formal thinking where operations become exploratory, creative, and yet logical. At first, because she had no language for the formal math, she used a preoperational approach—that is, making up something to describe the sudden insight she had had. However, now that mathematics has been more thoroughly developed, we know that she actually experienced a revelation, probably because of her budding creativity, that was the formal operations of cognitive ability as described by Piaget.

In following Norris' example, one nurse clinician and instructor states, ''when I was less experienced, I tended to put forth my opinions as correct and exact. However, as I gained in cognitive development, I learned to listen carefully to the ''ridiculous remarks'' of others. As I worked with new ways of thinking, I became more effective in explaining misconceptions, but I also learned to view concepts from a variety of perspectives, thus further growing in my own formal thinking operations.

A Woman's Perspective

Before beginning a discussion of nursing implications using the Erikson and Piaget theories of growth and development, a look at several other female writers may be helpful. Deborah Tannen (1990), for example, indicated throughout her book *You Just Don't Understand* that men and women have different but equally valid styles of thinking and responding to their experiences. She described a man who performs certain unnecessary activities to avoid letting others know he has made a mistake. His wife is amazed at this response, saying that she would have just blurted out her mistake. She would have been upset about making the mistake, but not about people knowing. This story prompted another woman to remark that her husband had advised her that when she was in a group discussion and had a question, she should wait until she got home and ask him, rather than let others know what she did not know. The woman stated that this had always puzzled her. ''I would rather let others be aware of my lack of knowledge than to lose the gist of the conversation because I was afraid to ask. My husband feels just the opposite.''

A similar example involves a male physician (Bill) and a female physician (Ann). Ann states, ''I noticed that whenever we are in conference and someone quotes from a journal article, Bill's response clearly indicates that he has read the work. Finally, one day I asked him how he had time to read so much. He laughed and said, 'Oh Ann, I don't read it all; I have just learned to nod and look knowingly.''' Ann laughed as she told this story, saying that physicians are always insecure. The work of Gilligan and other female researchers might suggest that it was the maleness, rather than the physician in Bill, that was insecure.

Belenky, Clinchy, and Goldberger (1986), in their book *Women's Ways of Knowing,* described the development of the self, voice, and mind of the female. They pointed out that women through the ages, as a whole, have been silent rather than face rejection because their views were considered incorrect or unimportant. Their research indicates that "listening to women's voices" will change the future of education and the further study of human development (p. 229). Women, they indicated, work more effectively in collaboration than in debate, which affirms Gilligan's (1982) work described earlier.

A popular mystery writer (Clark, 1992) described a female child, Laurie, who is kidnapped and abused. Laurie "forgets" this period of her life entirely, but develops multiple personalities for coping with what she knows is wrong but is helpless to stop. One personality, a female, grows up with her and is disgusted at her weakness and inability to deal with the experience. Another personality is a boy who is protective, authoritative, and can withstand some of the abuse. Based on Gilligan's comments earlier in the chapter, we can speculate as follows. The boy portion of the female child has the ability to distinguish right from wrong, based on some beginnings of logical thinking, and can be stern and authoritative with others who try to harm Laurie. The girl portion also knows right from wrong, but is concerned with relationships and is unable to cope with the overwhelming wrongness.

These ideas can remind us, as we use the theories cited in this chapter to plan care for all our clients, that we await further research involving the development of both the male and the female in our world. It is important to recognize that we are not to overgeneralize about how males and females are either alike or different until the research is done.

*N*ursing *Implications*

The theory of cognitive development as described by Piaget helps nurses recognize how children develop intelligence and learn to think. The theory suggests that certain approaches to teaching are more effective at different times. For example, we recognize that stress also affects how our adult clients think and learn, and may cause them to revert to earlier ways of processing information. Moreover, the response to learning under stress may vary according to the individual. Some persons learn when alarmed or aroused because of a critical need for information, whereas others are unable to concentrate on the task at hand. The nurse will want to assess how stress affects a particular person's ability to learn.

Piaget (1973) described intelligence as the indispensable instrument for interaction between the subject and the universe. Feeling directs behavior by assigning a value to its end; feeling provides the energy necessary for action, and knowledge gives a structure to it. Piaget stated that every action involves an energetic or affective aspect and a structural or cognitive aspect (pp. 4–5).

However, the ages stated for each level are somewhat arbitrary. That is, a child may be either slower or faster than suggested in reaching a new level; the range of normal is broad.

Nurses also note that adults demonstrate great variance in the ability to use formal operations of thought. This becomes apparent when we help adult clients to learn about their health needs. Those who are more comfortable with concrete thought operations may take longer to understand and apply new information; those who have used formal thought processes may understand more quickly. Therefore, nurses contemplating health teaching and care planning will need to assess both age level and the client's ability to grasp and apply information.

In summary, reconsider how nurses can use the theories of Erikson, Piaget, and Maslow together when planning nursing care. For example, we know that persons use their intelligence as well as their emotions to solve problems and to develop skills toward the resolution of developmental tasks. Infants learn to trust, in part, because they use their beginning cognitive skills of recognition and memory to know who the parent is. The adolescent or young adult uses the ability to think conceptually and to make relationships among the pieces of information he or she receives. This ability assists the individual to make good decisions about how to take care of himself or herself and how to plan the direction the individual wishes his or her life to take. If we consider Maslow's theories, we know that a person's ability to meet the basic needs may also influence the decisions the person makes about self and his or her life.

From Developmental Theory to Clinical Application

We have drawn from the works of Maslow and Erikson to talk about the control persons have in realizing their potential. Nurses view persons as individuals with the potential to take care of themselves and to achieve a high level of health. Carl Rogers has provided several important "learnings" (as he called them) that give support to the concepts of person-centered nursing care and self-care (discussed in Chapter 6). He developed a person-centered therapy throughout his many years as a counselor and psychotherapist. According to Rogers (1961),

> It is the *client* who knows what hurts, what directions to go, what problems are crucial, what experiences have been deeply buried. It began to occur to me that unless I had a need to demonstrate my own cleverness and learning, I would do better to rely upon the client for the direction of movement in the process (pp. 11–12).

Rogers described how he learned to listen to and accept himself and his own feelings about a particular person or a situation. He believed that to act one way on the surface while feeling another way underneath becomes more of a hindrance than a help in developing a therapeutic (healing) relationship. According to Rogers, it is important for a person not to try to be something he or she is not.

Although Carl Rogers (1961) did not use the word *empathy* (which appears in Chapter 9), he nevertheless described it in another of his learnings: "I have found it of enormous value when I can permit myself to understand another person'' (p. 18). He used the word *permit* because he believed that too often we respond immediately to another person's ideas as right or wrong, good or bad, moral or immoral. We respond because of our own value system and out of fear that if we really understand the person, it might somehow change us or our way of thinking—a distressing notion. We do not want to lose a part of ourselves in response to another person. He pointed out, however, that rather than changing, we become enriched and can grow when we truly understand the ideas and feelings of others.

Rogers (1961) believed strongly in learning from his own experience and in trusting what he had learned. He stated,

> I can only try to live by my interpretation of the current meaning of my experience, and try to give others the permission and freedom to develop their own inward freedom and thus their own meaningful interpretation of their own experience. If there is such a thing as truth, this free individual process of search should, I believe, converge toward it (p. 27).

These words provide for nurses the essence of the person-centered approach to nursing care and can, if we return to them repeatedly, assist us in developing and delivering effective and relevant care to the persons nurses seek to help toward the healthy state.

Other Theoretical Views of Person

The material presented so far offers humanistic and varied views of person that are not exclusive to the discipline of nursing: the view is generic and applicable to all persons as suggested earlier in the Erikson discussion. Nursing, however, is unique among the health professions in claiming the holistic biopsychosocial person as the client of its care. Also, there are other theorists—nurse–theorists—who present a somewhat different view of the concept of person.

Within the science of nursing, various theorists have suggested refinements of the concept of person based on their particular conceptual models. According to Fawcett (1995), each conceptual model provides a ''distinctive'' frame of reference regarding how an important phenomenon such as person is defined and described. A discussion of nursing theorists' views on the person can be found in Chapter 3. As you consider these views, note how well they flow with those of Maslow, Erikson and Piaget. Also, consider how well the views of these theorists, the views of the nurse–theorists, and the models of health discussed in Chapter 6 blend. Together, they all improve our understanding of both individual persons and groups such as families, communities and cultures.

As these and other theoretical views of person are refined, they will undoubtedly influence both future nursing research and care delivery. Many aspiring professionals are strongly attracted to nursing because of the opportunity to work closely with persons in all aspects of their being: biologic, psychologic, social, cultural, and spiritual.

This Incredible Being: The Person

We have briefly explored the essence of this incredible being called the person, whose subsystems interrelate and produce a being greater than the sum of the parts. What causes the person to be strong in the face of weakness, healthy in the face of illness, and brave in the face of grief? How is it that the person can continue to grow and flourish through a lifetime, and even during periods of great strife? The very nature of the unique person is perplexing, and our understanding, although developing, is still limited. In her book *Heartsounds,* Lear (1980) described her husband, who lived through a cardiac crisis despite medical expectations to the contrary:

> An intern recalled, "We got a guy with an infiltrated intravenous. So he wasn't getting dopamine, the drug to maintain blood pressure. He had no palpable blood pressure and yet he was able to talk to us. This in itself was unusual. He was in cardiac shock: blood pressure too low to maintain life; no urine; decreased mentation; clammy extremities. I would have thought his chances of coming through were very, very small."

And after Lear's husband had improved, the cardiologist came out to tell his family: "He's better. He wants to know every detail of treatment. He's driving them all crazy in there. It's unbelievable. It's something spiritual, that fight, that fight that keeps him alive."

Lear went in to see her husband and described him as follows:

> He lay still panting, his eyes closed, his face remote behind the [oxygen] mask, and I wondered *Better*? but surely they are wrong. How can anyone who looks like this be *better*? And I bent down again . . . and whispered, "Darling, you're much *better*. You've got to *fight*. You're going to *make it*. You're going to *make it*. . . ."
>
>   And with one sudden swift move he ripped the mask off his face and turned to confront me directly. His eyes consumed me. *"I've already made it"* he said (pp. 338–339).

KEY CONCEPTS

Holism is basically a theory in which the universe, and especially living nature, is seen in terms of interacting wholes that are greater than the sum of their parts.

The **Person** is a living system who contains many subsystems with energy that flows among each, thus affecting the larger system (the person) as a whole.

In A Different Voice (Carol Gilligan, 1982) suggests for our consideration that males and females may view life from different perspectives and should be studied separately as well as together.

Basic Need Theory (Abraham Maslow, 1970) declares that both a deficit and a being state are inherent in all of us as persons, and that our behavior is motivated by the degree of satisfaction of the basic needs of each state.

The **Person's Perception of Self** is the larger concept that includes components such as self-concept, self-ideal, self-esteem, body image, and values.

The **Developmental Tasks** (Erik Erikson, 1963) describe eight stages of the person's growth and development, each containing a nuclear conflict that, when resolved to some satisfaction, facilitates progress to the next stage.

Cognitive Development (Piaget, 1973) is described as cumulative, with the understanding of new experiences evolving from what was learned during earlier ones.

The concept of the **Incredible Being** denotes the person whose subsystems interrelate and produce a being greater than the sum of the parts, who grows and flourishes over a lifetime—in the face of strife as well as bounty.

CRITICAL THINKING QUESTIONS

1. Consider the following situation: A 45-year-old man is in the hospital recovering from a heart attack. His wife divorced him one year ago, leaving their three teenage children in his care. The children are alone while he is in the hospital. Consider the biopsychosocial needs of this man and discuss how the concept of holism applies in this situation.

2. Explain the terms *open system* and *closed system*, and discuss how they occur within the person.

3. Describe the notion of energy movement between systems and subsystems.

4. Discuss the categories of basic needs on Maslow's hierarchy and give an example of each.

5. Consider yourself as a person. How do terms such as *self-concept, self-ideal, self-esteem,* and *body image* apply to you?

6. Consider the following situation: A 40-year-old woman is hospitalized for a radical mastectomy (surgical removal of the breast). Throughout her recovery, she wears a large heavy robe, even though it is summer. She is aloof to the female nurses and openly rude to her male doctor. She stares out the window when her husband visits and shows little interest in the activities of her children. Analyze this woman's response using the concepts discussed in the section on the person's view of self (Erickson et al., 1983, p. 123).

7. Discuss the notions of *value* and *value judgment.* What kinds of experiences influence how we develop value systems? How would you feel about a person who refuses chemotherapy for cancer? If you were unable to assist that person, how would you feel about yourself?

8. Discuss how the terms *growth, maturation,* and *development* are pertinent to each person.

9. State the age, the developmental task, and the basic virtue of each age of humans according to Erikson. Describe how these factors would influence the nursing care of a variety of persons.

10. Consider several persons in different stages and assess their resolution of the Erikson developmental tasks. Describe the balance they have attained between the favorable and unfavorable outcomes for their particular level.

11. Define the terms associated with Piaget's theory of cognitive development. Describe how you would use this theory when giving safety tips to first graders.

12. Identify "learnings" according to Carl Rogers, and suggest an application for such ideas.

13. Suggest personal examples from clinical or social experiences to demonstrate how males and females may respond differently to life experiences.

14. Indicate how the need for caring changes across Erikson's stages of development.

15. Select a biologic, psychologic, sociologic, or spiritual variable that interests you and read a professional article on this topic.

REFERENCES

Abbey, J.C. (1978). General systems theory: A framework for nursing. In A. Putt (Ed.), *General systems theory applied to nursing* (pp. 19–29). Boston: Little, Brown.

Belenky, M.F., Clinchy, B.M., & Goldberger, N.R. (1986). *Women's ways of knowing: The development of self, voice, and mind.* Philadelphia: Basic Books.

Chekhov, A. (1904). The cherry orchard. In Young, S. (translator), *Best plays by Chekhov.* New York: The Modern Library.

Clark, M.H. (1992). *All around the town.* New York: Simon & Schuster.

du Maurier, D. (1957). *The scapegoat.* Garden City, NY: Doubleday.

Erickson, H.C., Tomlin, E.M., & Swain, M.A. (1983). *Modeling and role-modeling: A theory and paradigm for nursing.* Englewood Cliffs, NJ: Prentice-Hall.

Erikson, E.H. (1963). *Childhood and society* (2nd ed.). New York: W.W. Norton.

Fawcett, J. (1995). *Analysis and evaluation of conceptual models of nursing* (2nd ed.). Philadelphia: F.A. Davis.

Gilligan, C. (1982). *In a different voice: Psychological theory.* Cambridge, MA: Harvard University Press.

Hall, A.D. & Fagen, R.E. (1968). Definitions of systems. In W. Buckley (Ed.), *Modern systems research for the behavioral scientist* (pp. 81–92). Chicago: Aldine.

Klir, G.J. (1972). Preview: The polyphonic general systems theory. In G.J. Klir (Ed.), *Trends in general systems theory.* New York: Wiley.

Kohlberg, L. (1987). *Child psychology and childhood education: A cognitive-developmental view.* New York: Longman.

Lear, M.W. (1980). *Heartsounds.* New York: Simon & Schuster.

Lee, H. (1960). *To kill a mockingbird.* Philadelphia: J.B. Lippincott.

Maslow, A.H. (1970). *Motivation and personality* (2nd ed.). New York: Harper & Row.

Murray, R.B. & Zentner, J.P. (1993). *Nursing assessment and health promotion: strategies through the life span* (5th ed.). Norwalk, CT: Appleton and Lang.

Norris, K. (1996). *The Cloister Walk.* New York: Riverhead Books.

Piaget, J. (1973). *The psychology of intelligence.* Totowa, NJ: Littlefield, Adams.

Polit, D. & Hungler, B. (1995). *Nursing research: Principles and methods* (5th ed.). Philadelphia: J.B. Lippincott.

Rogers, C.R. (1961). *On becoming a person.* Boston: Houghton Mifflin.

Roy, C., & Andrews, H.A. (Eds.). (1991). The Roy Adaptation Model: The definitive statement. Norwalk, CT: Appleton & Lange.

Schaef, A. (1990). *Meditations for women who do too much.* San Francisco: HarperCollins.

Singer, D.G. & Revenson, T.A. (1996). *A Piaget primer: How a child thinks.* (Revised edition). New York: Plume, a division of Penguin Books.

Smuts, J.C. (1926). *Holism and evolution.* New York: Macmillan.

Stuart, G.W. & Sundeen, S.J. (1995). *Principles and practice of psychiatric nursing.* St. Louis: C.V. Mosby.

Tannen, D. (1990). *You just don't understand: Women and men in conversation.* New York: Ballantine Books.

Tolstoy, L. (1988). *Childhood, boyhood, youth.* London: Penguin Books.

von Bertalanffy, L. (1968). General systems theory: A critical review. In W. Buckley (Ed.), *Modern systems research for the behavioral scientist* (pp. 11–30). Chicago: Aldine.

5

Environment

Asepsis
Boundaries
Climate
Community
Cultural healing
  beliefs
Cultural variables
Culture

Ecology
Epidemiology
Ethnicity
Family
Geography
Group
Noise
Norms

Nosocomial
  infection
Pathogens
Positions
Person–environ-
  ment fit
Roles
Sensory deprivation

Sensory overload
Social support
Societies
Subculture
Universal
  precautions
Values
Violence

Objectives

After completing this chapter, students will be able to:

Define the environment.

Identify the relationship of person–environment interaction to health.

Describe how nursing views the concept of environment.

Discuss factors within the immediate physical environment and the physical environment of the community that affect health.

Discuss how the social environment affects health.

Identify the relevance of cultural factors to health care.

The relationship of the environment to health has been recognized by nurses since the time of Florence Nightingale. Nightingale was one of the first health professionals to emphasize the importance of a healthy environment in the prevention of illness and maintenance of wellness. During the past several decades, chronic disease and pollution have become significant threats to health. Thus, we have seen increased investigation of environmental influences on health within a variety of disciplines, including nursing, medicine, public health, and sociology.

Nursing, which emphasizes the care of holistic persons, continues to be concerned with the phenomenon of human interaction with the environment in clinical practice, research, and theory development. This chapter examines the interactions between persons and their environments from the perspectives of systems and nursing theories. Physical, social, and cultural aspects of the environment, as well as their relevance for nursing, are also described. The concept of caring discussed in Chapters 1 through 4 is extended to caring for the environment. Throughout the chapter, the role of nursing in providing an optimum environment for the maintenance of wellness is emphasized.

The Concept of Environment

Environment is an important concept in nursing because healthy environments lead to healthy people. Traditionally, nurses have used the concept of environment to describe the effect of the immediate physical surroundings on an individual's well-being. Recently, the influences of social, political, and economic factors have been examined as significant aspects of the environment that affect health. Kleffel (1991) stated that focusing on the relationships of social, political, economic, and cultural conditions that produce health and illness emphasizes the precursors of poor health rather than the illness resulting from these conditions.

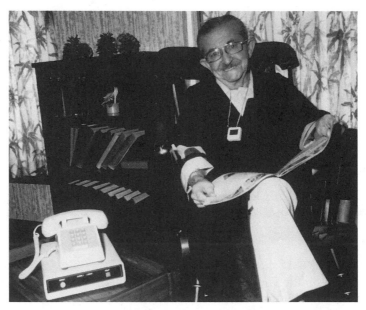

A pleasant and comfortable environment has a significant relationship to health.

For example, examining social and political factors that are related to mental health enables nurses to focus on correcting societal conditions that can lead to mental illness, with an emphasis on prevention. The environment can be considered a system comprising subsystems and their variables, whether they are sociocultural, physical, economic, or political.

The social environment consists of other humans with whom persons interact in the family, the community, and society. The physical environment includes both natural and humanmade factors such as weather, natural resources, and shelter. The economic environment includes variables such as the availability of goods and services. The political subsystem consists of governmental and other power structures and influences. Examples of environmental variables that influence health are listed in Table 5-1. This chapter limits discussion to physical, social, and cultural environments. Political and economic systems affecting health care are discussed in Chapter 7.

Because both persons and environment are open systems, both are constantly interacting, each affecting and being affected by the other (Fig. 5-1). Although we would like to think of ourselves as masters of the environment, we are changed by our surroundings even as we try to alter them. For example, when we use pesticides to kill disease-bearing insects, those chemicals enter the food chain and may predispose us to cancer. Humans have changed the courses of rivers and restructured the land, yet we are prone to the effects of barometric pressure changes and lunar cycles, as evidenced by fluctuations in crime rates shown in Moos's (1973) classic study. The following display is a clinical example of the importance of environment during patient recovery.

The Physical Environment

The physical environment refers to factors that exist in the external environment, such as air, water, food, furnishings, noise, and lighting. The physical environment consists of natural phenomena such as climate and geography, and humanmade

TABLE 5-1 *Examples of Environmental Variables*

Social Variables	Physical Variables	Economic Variables	Political Variables
Roles	Water	Business	Laws
Education	Plants	Industry	Political power
Family	Weather	Transportation	Health policy
Marriage	Pollution	Availability of services	Governmental structure
Norms	Light	Payment for services	Interest groups
Life-style	Noise	Technology	Economic policy
Religion	Shelter	Economic growth	Litigation

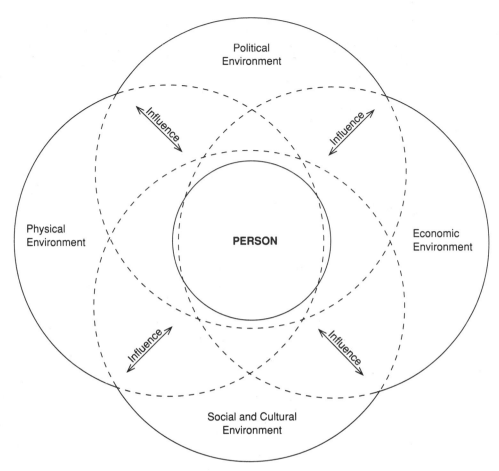

FIGURE 5-1 A reciprocal interaction exists between person and environment.

phenomena such as buildings and industry. The 1989 oil spill in Prince William Sound, Alaska, the environmental destruction during the Gulf War, the nuclear accident at Chernobyl, and the toxic chemical disaster in Bhopal, India, have increased public awareness of environmental issues. Environmental pollution caused by human activities is becoming increasingly significant as a health hazard. In 1992 the Earth Summit, an international conference on global environmental problems, gave greater visibility to environmental concerns. **Ecology** is the study of the relationship between humans and the external environment. An intimate interdependency exists between living things and the environment, which the field of ecology seeks to explain. Consider the next display about one patient's condition, Mrs. Rush.

Mrs. Rush is a 72-year-old woman who had a leg amputated. While she was recovering from surgery, the nurses and physical therapists noted her abilities to walk with her walker and the occupational therapist obtained a description of her home environment. Mrs. Rush, her husband, and the health team decided on changes that would accommodate her current level of mobility. Because Mrs. Rush could not negotiate stairs, they decided to move her sleeping quarters to the first floor. After Mrs. Rush was discharged, the community health nurse assisted her to arrange her cooking supplies and furniture so that she could perform her usual activities with her walker. These environmental adaptations helped her to maintain optimum independence despite her mobility changes.

Ecology is an important science for nurses because it provides insight into factors that affect health. For example, ecologic studies might examine the high incidence of malignancy in areas of heavy toxic waste discharge by an industry. Obviously, such health hazards are of concern to nurses, particularly those in community and occupational health nursing. What follows considers the physical environment of the community and the immediate physical environment, examining factors that influence health.

Physical Environment of the Community

The physical environment of the community comprises many factors, both natural and humanmade. They include climate, geography, air quality, water quality, soil quality, and food purity.

Climate

Climate refers to the average weather conditions at a place over a period of years, including factors such as average temperature, humidity, precipitation, and wind velocity. Climate is related to the incidence of particular health problems. For example, malaria and encephalitis are serious health problems in tropical climates that support the breeding of disease-bearing mosquitoes. Climate can exacerbate or relieve chronic health problems. You may have known someone with chronic respiratory disease who moved to another region because the dry, pollen-free climate helped relieve symptoms. The weather has also been shown to affect persons' behavior: for example, there is an increased incidence of violent behavior when temperatures are high.

Geography

Geography describes the physical features of an area, that is, the land, sea, and air, and the plant and animal life supported by these physical features. Like climate, the geography of a region is related to the health status of the population residing there. For example, the Japanese and indigenous people of Alaska have a low incidence of cardiac disease. Both groups live in oceanic regions and eat a diet rich in seafood. It is believed that this diet, abundant in fish oil, may confer protection against heart disease.

Rural and mountainous regions make access to health care difficult. Health care providers need to be creative in assisting people in these areas to reach their services. Mobile health centers and helicopter transportation for emergency victims may be used to provide health care.

Air Quality

Air quality, particularly in urban areas, is a leading global health concern. **Air pollution,** the introduction of impurities into the air, is a major problem in many urban areas. Air pollutants can be classified as particulate matter, organic gases, or inorganic gases. Two major sources of air pollution are automobile emissions, which contain nitrous oxides, and industrial smoke discharge, which emits sulfur oxides. Coal-burning factories are significant sources of sulfur oxides that are converted to sulfuric acid in the atmosphere. The resultant acid rain has caused incalculable losses to crops and forests. Fossil fuels are predicted to cause a greenhouse effect and global warming, with unknown effects on agriculture and health.

Air pollution can exacerbate symptoms in persons with cardiac and respiratory diseases and allergies. Industries may release noxious chemicals into the atmosphere as by-products of manufacturing. Substances such as asbestos and vinyl chlorides (by-products of plastics manufacturing) are carcinogenic and are suspected to be a factor in the increased incidence of malignancy in communities where these chemicals are produced. These substances are also depleting the ozone layer, leading to increased exposure to harmful radiation and diseases such as skin cancer and cataracts.

Water Quality

Water quality is a major concern as industrialization increases and population spreads into new regions, creating new demands for water. Local water treatment plants are responsible for purifying the water supply for their communities. Residential and commercial growth may strain the ability of treatment plants to adequately treat water, and inadequate treatment facilities are a source of pollution. Industries that discharge toxic wastes are another source of pollution. Among the growing list of hazardous wastes are radioactive substances. Agriculture is also responsible for pollution resulting from runoff of pesticides and fertilizers into the water supply.

Water pollution may be responsible for illness related to bacterial or parasitic contamination (e.g., hepatitis or giardiasis, a waterborne gastrointestinal disease). Industrial contaminants such as mercury may enter the food chain, tainting fish and causing illness in humans who consume them.

Soil Quality

Soil quality has become a concern with the discovery of the effects of careless toxic wastes dumping. Radioactive materials, by-products of plastics manufacturing, and pesticides have been implicated in the increased incidence of birth defects, miscarriage, and cancer.

A well-publicized example of these problems occurred in 1978 at Love Canal in New York. One hundred homes were built on a former toxic dump site. The miscarriage rate in the area was 30%, a number of cancer deaths occurred, and children and animals were burned by contact with the toxic ooze from the soil. In other instances, inadequately disposed substances have seeped into the groundwater, making the drinking water unsafe in entire communities.

Food Purity

The safety of the food supply is of great concern to health professionals. The food chain may be contaminated when additives and flavorings with unknown long-term effects are introduced to food; when pesticides are inappropriately used in agriculture; when animals ingest contaminated water; or when air or soil pollutants come into contact with crops, livestock, or fishing grounds. A disastrous example occurred in Michigan in the mid-1970s, when polybrominated biphenyls **(PBBs)** were accidentally mixed with livestock feed during production. The contaminated feed was ingested by cattle, which, in turn, were consumed by Michigan residents before the accident was discovered. The contamination was so widespread that PBBs could be found in human breast milk. It may be decades before the effects on human health can be identified.

Food also can be contaminated by bacteria or other organisms. *Salmonella*, *Staphylococcus*, and *Shigella* are common culprits in illnesses caused by ingesting contaminated food. Contamination of beef with *E. Coli* was responsible for hundreds of illnesses and several deaths in the Pacific Northwest in 1993. *Clostridium botulinum* (which causes botulism) is a microorganism that produces a deadly toxin. Because it survives in anaerobic environments—that is, those without free oxygen—it is a dangerous contaminant of canned foods.

Nursing Implications: Caring for the Environment

Community health nurses are actively involved in identifying or intervening with environmentally caused health problems. **Epidemiology** is the study of the incidence, distribution, and control of disease in a human population. Nurses in the community may be involved in case-finding or health-screening programs that produce data for epidemiologic studies. For example, nurses may identify a large number of cases of giardiasis. They then report their findings to the local water treatment authorities, who test the community's water supply and confirm the presence of the parasite. The nurses implement a program of preventive education in the area to curb further incidence of the disease.

TABLE 5-2 *Suggestions for Caring for the Environment*

Three basic principles of conservation are reduce, reuse, and recycle.

In the Hospital

Establish a hospital recycling program

Use fewer disposable items for client care

Take own beverage cup to meetings and meals rather than use disposable cups

Work with hospital purchasing department to urge suppliers to minimize packaging of hospital equipment and supplies

Dispose of hazardous materials appropriately (including toxic and biohazardous waste)

Establish an ecology committee in the hospital to identify changes in policy, purchasing, and operations that conserve environmental resources

In the Home

Recycle whenever possible

Establish a community recycling program

Reuse scrap paper, plastic, and glass containers

Avoid disposable products and polystyrene products

Buy earth-friendly products

Conserve water when washing dishes, showering, laundering, brushing teeth, and flushing toilets

Avoid use of toxic chemicals in cleaning, gardening, painting, and wood finishing

Participate in beach or stream cleanup

Plant trees

Conserve energy by minimizing automobile use, buying energy efficient products, turning off lights, reducing use of air conditioning and heating

Additional suggestions can be found in a publication by the Earthworks Group (1991), an environmental group.

Caring for the environment is a theme that is growing in importance in nursing literature. Schuster (1990) noted that nursing theories based on human care should be extended to environmental concerns. Although nursing has focused on the care of the immediate physical environment, current concerns about the health effects of the global environment require nurses to take a broader view (Smith & Whitney, 1991). Nurses and nursing students can take many actions to care for the environment. For example, Dysart (1990) noted that hospitalized clients generate 11.35 kg of waste per day. Nurses can urge hospitals to use earth-friendly products and establish recycling programs. Table 5-2 contains other suggestions for caring for the environment.

The Environmental Protection Agency (EPA), established in 1970, is the federal body responsible for establishing standards and regulations related to air and water purity, noise, solid waste disposal, and control of toxic substances. State and local governments also have authority in matters of air and water purity, solid waste disposal, and control of toxic substances. Political activity can be a useful tool for nurses in influencing these governmental agencies.

Immediate Physical Environment

The immediate environment may involve a variety of settings. The most important for health status are the home and work environments, and for ill individuals, the hospital. Nurses often can influence the health of the immediate environment in all of these settings. Of particular relevance to health are safety factors, temperature, lighting, noise, and room arrangement.

Safety Factors

One of the biggest health-related concerns for nurses is environmental safety. Many safety factors can be directly influenced by nurses. Accidents are ranked as the fifth leading cause of death in the United States for all ages and the leading cause of death up to age 45 (U.S. Department of Health and Human Services, 1996). Injuries, often classified according to their source, include mechanical, thermal, electrical, radiation, and chemical.

MECHANICAL INJURY

Falls are one of the most common injuries in the home and hospital. In the client, factors such as poor eyesight, dizziness, confusion, and weakness may be involved, and the elderly are at particularly high risk for falls. Physical hazards in the environment also may contribute to falls: for example, standing water on floors, loose rugs, objects cluttering stairs and floors, and electrical cords in pathways. Infants and toddlers, another group at high risk for falls, should never be left unattended on high places—such as changing tables—and stairways should be blocked. Mechanical injury in the workplace may include lacerations, back injury, and eye trauma. Motor vehicle accidents are a leading cause of injury-related death, with adolescents and young adults at particularly high risk (U.S. Department of Health and Human Services, 1996).

THERMAL INJURY

Burns are another common source of injury in the hospital, home, and workplace. Burns in the hospital can be caused by improper use of therapeutic heat, such as hot water bottles or heating pads, or from faulty electrical devices. In the home, fires are a dangerous source of thermal injury. Scalding liquids, improper use of flammables such as gasoline, woodstoves, and kerosene heaters, and faulty electrical appliances are all potential sources of burns in the home. Children and elderly persons are the age groups at high risk for injury from burns. In the workplace, caustic chemicals, sparks from welding devices, and hot machinery are a few of the possible sources of burns.

ELECTRICAL INJURY

Hospitals use a variety of electrical devices for diagnostic and therapeutic purposes. Electrocardiographs, mechanical ventilators, defibrillators (devices that use electric current to restore normal cardiac rhythm), and electrical cauterizing equipment are examples of electrical devices used in client care. Because the hazards of electrical shock are always present, nurses must carefully protect themselves and their clients from injury. Although electrical devices are housed in insulating material that reduces the flow of leakage current, a small amount of leakage does occur. When a nurse touches an appliance and a client simultaneously, a small amount of current flows from the electrical device, through the nurse, and into the client. Although this current is usually harmless, certain clients, such as those who have abraded skin or are attached to monitors, may sustain injury. Other hazards include frayed electrical cords, overloaded circuits, and improperly grounded equipment.

In the home, electricity can be a hazard if circuits are overloaded; electrical cords become frayed, thus losing their protective insulation; three-pronged plugs are bypassed, causing loss of grounding; or electrical devices are used near water sources (such as using hair dryers while bathing). Uncovered electrical outlets can be hazards to toddlers who may try to insert fingers, keys, pencils, and the like into them.

RADIATION

Like electricity, radiation has many diagnostic and therapeutic uses in the hospital. X-rays are a common tool used in diagnosis, particularly now that computer technology has increased the range of information that can be obtained. Radioactive cobalt or cesium is used to treat cancer. However, this invaluable tool may be hazardous to all who are exposed to it. The effects of radiation depend on the length of exposure, the proximity to exposure, the adequacy of shielding, and the sensitivity of organs to radiation effects. Side effects of radiation exposure include radiation sickness, change in bone marrow function, burns, sterility, and skin ulcers. Long-term exposure to radiation can be carcinogenic. Unborn babies are at high risk from radiation, particularly during the first 3 months of development. Effects of fetal exposure include miscarriage, birth defects, and childhood leukemia. Pregnant women should be extremely cautious about exposure to sources of radioactivity. Pregnant nurses need to take careful precautions against exposure to radiation at work.

Radiation is becoming an important hazard in the home and workplace as well. Industrial uses of radiation include electric power generation, lasers, and radioisotopes used for measuring, testing, and processing. In the home, electronic devices such as microwave ovens may yield exposure, although minimal, to radiation. Another source of radiation is radon, a radioactive gas that enters the home through dirt floors, openings in foundations, and sewers. Radon has been implicated in lung cancer, and the EPA recommends home detection. Nurses in occupational and community health have the important tasks of reviewing home and work environments for radiation hazards and implementing safety programs.

CHEMICAL HAZARDS

In the hospital, the most significant source of chemical injury is also one of the most important therapeutic agents: medications. Because nurses are responsible for most medication administration in the hospital, they have a responsibility to protect their clients from harmful effects of medications. Nurses monitor their clients for side effects and signs of drug toxicity. Nurses also are responsible for administering drugs cautiously so medication errors are avoided. Poisoning can occur when substances are not labeled or labels are not read carefully. For example, liquid soap may look like medicine, and the client may mistakenly swallow it if left unlabeled at the bedside.

Chemical injuries are also a concern in the home and at work. Workers in many industries come into contact with chemicals that may be hazardous if inhaled or if prolonged skin contact occurs. For instance, anesthetic gases are an occupational hazard for health care workers in the operating room. Poisoning is a potential danger in households with small children. Cleaning agents, medications, and paint supplies are just some of the hazardous items that should be stored safely out of reach.

Infection Control

Infections are a serious source of concern for hospitalized persons. **Nosocomial infections** (those acquired in the hospital) can add time and expense to a person's hospital stay. For infections to develop, the following components must exist:

❒ A significant number of microorganisms entering the host
❒ A virulent microorganism (one that is efficient at causing disease)
❒ A susceptible host

Hospitals, by nature, house many pathogenic (infection-causing) microorganisms. **Pathogens,** microorganisms that are capable of causing disease, prefer warm, moist, dark environments. Hospitalized persons have increased susceptibility to infection because of weakened natural defenses, such as breaks in the skin, and decreased or altered immune systems. Prevention of infection requires knowledge of principles of asepsis. **Asepsis** means freedom from infectious agents. One of the most important techniques in asepsis is hand washing. This is one of the first skills that nursing students learn and the technique that is most often neglected in practice. Graham (1990) studied hand washing in an intensive care unit (ICU) and found that recommendations for frequency and duration of washing were not being met.

Infections also are likely to spread in day-care centers. Both children and workers need to be careful to wash hands before preparing food or eating, after toileting or changing diapers, and after sneezing. Much opportunity exists for nurses to do health teaching related to infection control in these agencies.

Other Factors in the Immediate Environment

TEMPERATURE AND HUMIDITY

Comfortable room temperature ranges from 68°F to 74°F; comfortable humidity is approximately 30% to 60%. In illness, many factors, such as presence of fever, joint disease, and respiratory symptoms, may require adjustments in room temperature and humidity for clients to feel comfortable. Elderly persons often prefer higher room temperatures.

LIGHTING

Lighting contributes to clients' safety in the hospital. Lighting should be adequate to allow persons to navigate safely, particularly at night. Lighting should follow natural cycles, that is, brighter in the day hours, dimmer at night. Constant exposure to bright lights is uncomfortable, inhibits sleep, and can be disorienting. This possibility is a concern in ICUs, which often use bright lighting day and night.

Elderly persons may experience visual changes that make them susceptible to discomfort from glare. They also may need greater illumination. Nurses need to provide indirect but sufficient lighting when the elderly are reading or learning self-care skills in the home or the hospital.

NOISE AND ODORS

Noise is defined as unwanted sound. It is a problem that is becoming increasingly significant as a health hazard, particularly on the job. Noise exposure can lead to permanent hearing loss, interference with job performance, sleep interference, and psychological stress. Noise-induced hearing loss affects 10 to 20 million U.S. workers alone. The Occupational Safety and Health Administration (OSHA) has set standards for the level of noise and length of exposure at the workplace. Nurses may be involved in case finding for auditory problems by conducting hearing tests at the workplace. Occupational health nurses may see other noise-related problems such as stress and interference with job performance. These nurses are often responsible for assisting with noise abatement programs as well as caring for individual workers.

Although the fictional television hospitals all bear signs proclaiming, "Quiet! Hospital Zone," real-life hospitals are notoriously noisy. Sleep interference is a common complaint of hospitalized persons. Hospital noise can also induce stress in ill persons and can contribute to **sensory overload,** a perceptual disturbance caused by excessive sensory stimulation.

Hospitals also can contain sources of unpleasant odors such as drainage, excreta, and cleaning agents. Sick persons are often quite sensitive to odors. Even pleasant smells such as food, fragrant flowers, or the nurse's perfume can be offensive to ill individuals.

LAYOUT AND DECOR

Many health problems are associated with changes in functional ability. Fatigue, shortness of breath, cardiac problems, neurologic changes, and bone or joint changes can affect a person's ability to function in his or her environment. Nurses, along with other health team members such as occupational or physical therapists, assist persons to adapt their living quarters to suit their altered abilities.

Health care institutions have found that homelike environments can reduce psychological stress and have positive effects on clients' health. In psychiatric units, the use of homelike layout and decor diminishes the sense of institutionalization and eases the transition between hospital and home when the client is discharged. In obstetrics, birthing centers have become a popular choice for prospective parents. A birthing room resembles a hotel suite, in contrast with the typical labor room with its hospital bed, hard, straight-backed chairs, and display of technical equipment. Some practitioners believe that a homelike environment can actually encourage the normal progress of labor and contribute to healthier mothers and babies. Other settings where the environments are becoming more homelike include hospices (where dying persons are cared for) and pediatric units.

Whether the setting is the home or the hospital, decor is a matter of personal preference and nurses should not alter the clients' immediate environments without consulting them. In the hospital, clients' bedsides become their personal space at a time when many possessions and routines have been given up (e.g., privacy, usual clothing, personal furnishings, decisions about mealtimes). Thus, it is particularly important to arrange bedside articles according to clients' preferences to the fullest extent possible.

Nursing Implications

Nursing care in relation to the immediate physical environment has four major goals:

1. To promote safety
2. To control communicable disease
3. To provide comfort and appropriate sensory stimuli
4. To maximize the person–environment fit

Nurses have the knowledge and ability to implement a wide range of actions that promote healthy environments. These actions include alteration of environmental factors and client teachings.

SAFETY PROMOTION

Surveillance is an essential component of nurse caring with relation to the environment. Surveillance means looking for potential safety concerns. In the hospital, nurses constantly observe the environment for hazards such as malfunctioning electrical equipment; cords or items on the floor (over which persons could trip); inadequate lighting; or improperly labeled medications. Table 5-3 lists categories of hazards in the hospital and nursing actions to prevent client injury.

Accidents are a frequent cause of injury in the home and workplace. Nurses can be instrumental in helping clients to survey the home and work environments and plan appropriate protective measures. Occupational health nurses have a key role in identifying health hazards in the workplace, providing assessment and nursing care for work-related injuries, and developing safety programs for employees. These nurses also assist with implementing standards and record keeping for federal programs, particularly OSHA regulations.

Accidents are the leading killers of children (U.S. Department of Health and Human Services, 1996). Community health, pediatric, and school nurses can help prevent such tragedies by implementing safety teaching for children and parents. Nurses also assist parents to survey their homes for possible safety hazards and make appropriate changes. A summary of actions to promote childhood safety is found in Table 5-4.

TABLE 5-3 *Potential Injuries in the Hospital and Preventive Actions*

Potential Injury	Prevention
Falls	Wipe up spilled liquids promptly
	Remove objects in clients' pathways
	Use siderails and place call lights within reach
	Never leave infants unattended
	Keep beds in lowest position
	Avoid dangling electrical cords and drainage tubing
	Use brakes on beds and wheelchairs
	Accompany clients who are susceptible to dizziness, confusion, or weakness when they are ambulating
	Use safe transferring techniques when moving clients
Electrical Shock	Check line cords and plugs for defects
	Remove cords from sockets by grasping the plug
	Be sure that clients who are attached to electrical devices are properly grounded
	Check electrical equipment for proper functioning
Poisoning or Medication-Related Injuries	Remove harmful substances from clients' bedsides when not in use (e.g., disinfectants, antiseptics, liquid soaps)
	Never put hazardous substances in drinking or medication cups
	Never leave medications at bedside
	Carefully check labels on medications and verify correct dosage before administering
	Identify clients correctly before administering medications
	Watch for side effects; check for drug allergies
	Chart medications promptly after administering
	Keep medication supplies out of reach (especially in pediatric units)
Burns	Check temperature of bath water or hot compresses before client use
	Use heating pads and heat lamps cautiously (pay attention to length of time used, distance from heat source, and temperature of device)
	Caution clients from smoking in bed (particularly confused or drowsy clients)
	Avoid smoking near oxygen sources
	Know agency policy regarding fire procedures
	Avoid overloading electrical sockets
Radiation	Watch for signs of radiation injury in clients receiving radiation therapy
	Use proper shielding; limit exposure time near clients who have radioactive implants
	Know hospital policy regarding radiation therapy

TABLE 5-4 *Potential Childhood Injuries and Preventive Actions*

Potential Injury	Prevention
Burns	Teach child the meaning of "hot"
	Lock up matches
	Keep hot liquids, electric cords from hot appliances out of reach
	Turn pot handles away from reach when cooking
	Place guards around heat sources (e.g., fireplaces, barbecue grills, portable heaters)
Falls	Block stairways safely
	Never leave children unattended on high surfaces
	Keep crib rails up
Drowning, Suffocation	Never leave child unattended in bathroom (can drown in bathtub or toilet)
	Never leave child unattended in swimming or wading pools
	Toys should be too large to swallow; small parts should be securely fastened
	Keep buttons, coins, small candies, and so forth off floor and out of reach
	Avoid toys or objects with long cords
	Keep plastic bags out of reach
Poisoning	Keep medications, household cleaners, other hazardous substances out of reach
Vehicle Accidents	Use approved car seats for young children
	Use safety belts for older children
	Teach traffic safety to children
	Use approved helmets when riding motorcycles, snowmobiles
	Teach bicycle safety

General Safety Precautions

* Keep emergency numbers for fire, police, medical care, and poison control posted in a conspicuous place.
* Teach older children what to do in emergency situations

Accidents continue to be a leading cause of death in adulthood. Health teaching and environmental alterations can prevent many accidents from occurring. Teaching clients how to establish environments that promote motor vehicle safety, prevent fires, promote electrical safety, and—especially for the elderly—prevent falls is an important nursing activity. Specific suggestions include the following:

❐ Avoid overloading electrical circuits or outlets.
❐ Use caution with hot liquids, particularly oils.
❐ Label hazardous substances clearly and leave them in their original containers.
❐ Store flammable substances away from heat sources.
❐ Never smoke in bed.

❏ Discard all unused medications and always leave medications in their original containers.
❏ Keep pathways clear of toys, slippery rugs, and so forth.
❏ Use caution when climbing ladders.
❏ Keep stairways well lit and uncluttered.
❏ Check electrical cords for fraying.
❏ Use grounded plugs correctly; avoid adapters.

CONTROL OF COMMUNICABLE DISEASE

Pathogens are transmitted through several modes, including:

❏ Contact route, that is, direct (person-to-person) or indirect (through inanimate objects)
❏ Vehicle route (contaminated food, water, medications, serum)
❏ Airborne route (droplets or dust)
❏ Vectorborne route (insects, vermin)

Interrupting these routes of transmission is one means of infection control. Hand washing is the most important measure that prevents the transmission of microorganisms. Use of running water, soap, and friction for at least 30 seconds is essential to good hand washing. In the hospital, hands should be washed before and after any direct client contact, before handling food or medications, and after handling used equipment and supplies. Teaching good hand washing technique to clients can control the transmission of pathogens in the home, workplace, schools, and day-care centers. Even toddlers are capable of learning to wash hands at mealtimes and after toileting.

Along with hand washing, personal hygiene measures interrupt the transmission of infection. Years ago, maintaining personal hygiene was as uncomplicated as bathing, covering the mouth when sneezing, and disposing of body wastes appropriately. In today's era of sexually transmitted diseases and acquired immunodeficiency syndrome (AIDS), teaching personal hygiene measures includes discussing the dangers of sharing drug paraphernalia and indiscriminate unprotected sexual intercourse. Fear of AIDS is a national concern, and nurses can do much to relieve anxiety by discussing how the disease is spread and how to protect against contracting it.

Taking sanitation measures is a second means of preventing communicable diseases. Community health nurses can educate people about proper disposal of trash and wastes. In the hospital, nurses are responsible for proper disposal of used supplies such as contaminated dressings, hypodermic equipment, and linens. Isolation technique, which involves special precautions such as private rooms, gowns, masks, and gloves, may be implemented when caring for persons with certain communicable diseases. **Universal precautions,** special techniques for handling and contact with blood and body fluids, are recommended by the U.S. Centers for Disease Control and Prevention to prevent the transmission of the human immunodeficiency and the hepatitis B viruses.

Modifying the environment is a third means of infection control. Two special means of altering the environment for microorganisms are disinfection and sterilization. Disinfection removes all pathogenic organisms from an object. An example is disinfection of a hospital room after a client is discharged. Sterilization removes all microorganisms and their spores. Heat, chemicals, and radiation are methods used for disinfecting and sterilizing equipment and supplies.

A fourth means of reducing communicable disease is altering factors related to host susceptibility. One important method is immunization, a process whereby antibodies or weakened antigens are administered to produce immunity to specific diseases. Nurses are responsible for planning and implementing community immunization programs. Nurses also maintain persons' resistance to disease by ensuring good nutrition, providing skin care that prevents breaks in the integument, and promoting adequate rest. Certain persons are particularly susceptible to infection and require careful protection from microorganisms. The elderly and newborns, persons receiving immunosuppressive drugs (e.g., following organ transplants), persons receiving chemotherapy for cancer, and persons who have wounds (including postoperative clients) are among those who require careful precautions against infection.

PROVISION OF COMFORT AND SENSORY STIMULATION

Maintaining a comfortable environment is an important caring activity, particularly for ill or hospitalized persons. These individuals often lack control over stressful environmental factors such as noise, bright lights, and odors. Nursing actions to promote a comfortable environment include the following:

- ❏ Turn off bright task lighting after completing nursing procedures.
- ❏ Adjust curtains or doors to provide the desired level of privacy.
- ❏ Reduce irritating noise sources such as monitor sounds, staff conversations, or radio and television noise.
- ❏ Provide clients with controls for lighting, television, and radio so that they can adjust these to their preference.
- ❏ Mask undesirable odors with room deodorants; remove odor sources such as soiled dressings or bedpans promptly.

In addition to factors of lighting, temperature, noise, odor, and privacy, decor can enhance the comfort of an environment. Displaying photographs, gifts, or meaningful items from home is one means of providing a more individualized environment for the hospitalized person.

Appropriate sensory stimulation in the environment is essential to health. Lack of appropriate stimuli can cause boredom and depression. At the extremes, too much or too little environmental stimulation can lead to **sensory overload** and **sensory deprivation,** syndromes that are characterized by altered perception and disorientation. Provision of normal day-to-night patterns of lighting, clocks, calendars, opportunities for socializing, and reduction of noise are nursing actions that provide appropriate sensory stimulation for clients. For infants and children, adequate stimuli are essential to normal development. In the hospital, nurses provide stimuli by talking and playing with children and using mobiles, music boxes, or favorite toys from home. Nurses can influence sensory environments in the home by teaching parents about child care, nurturing, and play activities that stimulate normal development. Much of this education can occur when the child comes to the health care setting for checkups.

MAXIMIZING PERSON–ENVIRONMENT FIT

A basic premise of this chapter is that persons are constantly interacting with their environments, and these interactions influence health. Nurses are concerned with the nature of these interactions. **Person–environment fit** is the match between the needs and resources of the individual and the demands and resources of the environment. Fit is unique for each person–environment system and can be maximized by modifying the needs or demands and the resources of either the person or the environment.

The example of Mrs. Rush (presented in an earlier display) shows how health care professionals can assist clients to modify their environment to fit altered functional ability following an illness. Another example is the nurse who is caring for a client with newly diagnosed emphysema. The nurse counsels the client regarding his or her cigarette smoking and teaches breathing techniques. These actions modify the needs and resources of the client. In addition, the nurse discusses ways of adding humidity to the home, and explores means of obtaining an air filter for the furnace. The focus of these interventions is modification of the environment. By examining the client's situation in the context of his or her environment, the nurse can provide broader and more individualized strategies that are more likely to be successful in optimizing health.

The Social Environment

Societies are groups of people sufficiently organized to carry out the conditions necessary to live together. The social environment consists of the social systems with which a person interacts. These social systems may include the person's family, school, neighborhood, social or hobby club, or community. The interaction of a person with the social environment is becoming increasingly recognized as a factor affecting health. Likewise, a social system such as a family or community may be the "client" for whom nurses care. For these reasons, it is essential for nurses to have an understanding of the various social systems and the structures and processes that compose them.

Structure of Social Systems

Social systems are characterized by structural components, among which are boundaries, norms, roles, and positions.

Boundaries separate the members of a social system from the environment. They distinguish members from nonmembers. Boundaries may be rigid and highly defined, such as those of a nuclear family, or flexible, such as those of a drop-in support group for new parents. Boundaries of social systems vary in their permeability. Some are relatively impermeable, meaning that the system interacts minimally with its environment. An example might be an alcoholic family whose members keep to themselves and do not accept outside assistance.

Norms are expected behaviors. They provide rules about standards of appropriate behavior in particular situations. Norms flow from cultural values about what is important in various situations. Church attendance on Sunday may be a norm for a religious group.

Roles are sets of expected behaviors that are normatively defined. Roles serve to make behavior predictable, and *role enactment,* the carrying out of a role, makes social interactions run smoothly. The role of motherhood in the United States is associated with nurturing and child-rearing behaviors. A mother who relegates these behaviors to her husband or a baby sitter might run the risk of being labeled an "oddball" or a "deviant." Some roles are explicit and formal; others are implicit (not readily apparent) or informal. For example, in a family, a man might have a formal role of "breadwinner" and an informal role of "dominator." Inability to perform one's role (i.e., role deprivation) leads to diminished self-esteem, anxiety, or depression. Nurses often deal with these concerns when they care for ill persons.

Positions are syntheses of related roles and represent the locations of persons in a social system. Positions have many associated roles. For example, the position of staff nurse in a hospital may involve roles of bedside caregiver, hospital employee, client advocate, committee member, and mentor to inexperienced nurses.

Processes of Social Systems

Three major processes of social systems are input, throughput, and output. *Input* is the process of taking energy, information, or matter into the system. *Throughput* involves using this energy, information, or matter to fulfill its functions and produce *output,* the products of the social system. A family might take in information on child rearing and use it to raise a child who can become a productive member of society. To carry out these processes, social systems need a communication system, a decision-making system, and a means of allocating power.

Types of Social Systems

Social systems are of many types, from informal recreational groups to defined communities. The social systems with which nurses are most concerned are families, groups, and communities.

Families

The basic unit of organization in every society is the **family.** The concept of family is changing rapidly in this country. Whereas earlier a definition would have specified the nuclear family (mother, father, and dependent children), such a description would not allow for arrangements encountered today: unmarried couples and their unrelated children, homosexual families, the person who lives alone, and extended families, among others. Friedman (1992) defined family as "two or more persons who are joined together by bonds of sharing and emotional closeness and who identify themselves as being part of the family" (p. 9). Because the definition of family is so variable, it is important to ascertain whom the client identifies as significant family members.

The health of individuals depends heavily on family influences. The family socializes individuals, that is, influences them to take on the norms and values of society. Acquisition of attitudes, beliefs, and behaviors related to health is part of this process. Families also nurture individuals, enabling them to grow and develop normally. Persons who have healthy physical and psychosocial development are better able to withstand stressors and maintain wellness. The economic status of one's family also influences health status; it affects ability to obtain health care, good nutrition, safe living conditions, and so forth. Family structures and processes such as norms, roles, decision making, and communication all affect the health of the family and its individual members.

Family structures that have importance for nurses include boundaries, positions, roles, and norms. Boundaries that are too rigid may inhibit a family who needs help from accepting it. The roles and norms associated with family positions are changing rapidly. Many mothers now hold jobs, assuming a "breadwinner" role, and fathers are taking on child-rearing roles by becoming more involved in caretaking activities. Nurses cannot assume that family roles are assigned in a traditional manner and need to identify which roles are threatened by the health problems of a family member.

Many functions of the family have been identified, including the following:

❏ Physical functions, for example, providing food, shelter, and health care
❏ Affectional functions, for example, generating affection and providing a sense of security and companionship
❏ Social functions, for example, developing a sense of responsibility for behavior and social values and preparing members to assume productive societal roles

Processes of communication, decision making, and power allocation are essential to fulfilling these functions. Nurses who are working with families evaluate these processes as they affect the health status of family members. For example, in many Arab families, the male members assume power and make decisions for females. If a nurse were teaching an Arab woman about a health problem, it would be essential to include her husband.

Groups

A **group** is an assembly of people who share specific functions or goals and who interact over time. Health-related groups are a relatively recent phenomenon, but it is possible to find an appropriate resource group for almost every health concern. Nurses have opportunities to work with groups such as childbirth preparation classes, cancer support groups, bereavement support groups, postmastectomy groups, and psychotherapy groups. It is obvious that groups are a component of the social environment with the potential to influence health.

Groups possess structure consisting of boundaries, roles, norms, and positions, and are characterized by processes of communication, decision making, and power allocation. In examining a group's boundaries, a nurse might identify the members and how the group defines its membership. For example, a support group for women who are having infertility problems might feel uncomfortable or angry with a group member who becomes pregnant. The members may ask her to leave the group despite her continued need for emotional support.

The relationships of group members to each other in terms of roles, duties, and responsibilities are another important consideration. Roles may be formal, such as note-taker, or informal, such as mediator or scapegoat. The position of leader may be formal; in "leaderless" groups, informal leaders develop. When a group is having difficulty performing its functions, the difficulty may be related to conflicting roles within the group.

A group's communication process affects its ability to fulfill its functions. For example, a formal, structured communication process—such as going from one member to another for ideas—is unlikely to encourage spontaneous expression of thoughts and feelings in a new mothers' support group. Power and decision-making processes also affect a group's ability to achieve its goals. Leadership styles are related to how a group makes decisions. Autocratic group leaders determine their groups' functions and roles with little input from members. Democratic leaders share power and facilitate decision making with group members.

Nurses often function as leaders of health-related groups, and need to develop effective leadership styles that suit the purposes of the group. Some characteristics of an effective group leader include the following:

- ❏ Appears comfortable with own limits; in turn, accepts others and helps them feel secure
- ❏ Demonstrates friendliness, trust, and concern for others
- ❏ Listens for nonverbal as well as verbal messages
- ❏ Values freedom within the group
- ❏ Demonstrates a sense of humor
- ❏ Handles dissent among members respectfully
- ❏ Does not use or permit blaming of members
- ❏ Uses conflict within the group as an opportunity for learning interpersonal skills
- ❏ Does not use or permit manipulation
- ❏ Does not assume superiority

Communities

A **community** is a group of people living in the same locality and having common characteristics, interests, and needs. A community has an enormous impact on the health status of individuals by providing and allocating health care resources, influencing access to health care, and affecting living conditions related to health. Nurses can learn much about the wellness of a community by examining its structures and processes, including those related to decision making, information sharing, power allocation, production and distribution of goods and services, and social control. The following are examples of factors that influence a community's health:

- ❏ The economic climate—unemployment affects ability to pay for health care, and poverty is related to poor health status.
- ❏ Cultural, racial, and ethnic backgrounds of residents—cultural variations affect health beliefs, and racial and ethnic backgrounds affect susceptibility to specific health problems.
- ❏ Types of industries within the community's boundaries—industrial pollutants and occupation-related injuries are significant health hazards.
- ❏ Crowding and adequacy of housing—substandard housing and crowding are associated with increased incidence of communicable disease and accidents; crowding is also linked to high incidence of mental illness.
- ❏ The type and variety of health care agencies present—availability of major hospitals, emergency and specialty care (such as obstetrics, mental health, or rehabilitation), and services of physicians, nurses, and other health care professionals all affect the quality of health care in a community.
- ❏ The presence and adequacy of government programs for financing personal health care—the ability to obtain Medicare or Medicaid affects access to health care for the poor and elderly.

Healthy People 2000: National Health Promotion and Disease Prevention (1991) is a report that describes objectives for the health of persons in the United States. Community health concerns such as teen pregnancy, violence, and minority health needs are outlined in this document.

Nurses can do much to affect the community environment. Community health is a nursing specialty concerned with the well-being of populations, or the community at large. One tool used by community health nurses is the *community assessment,* an examination of variables such as statistics about residents, physical size and characteristics, medical services and facilities, economic status, and health status. Such information provides insights into the health needs of the community. On the basis of these findings, nurses engage in health promotion and health maintenance programs, health education activities, program planning, and political activities. Examples of specific nursing actions include providing a screening program for hypertension, health education for high-risk mothers and infants, or a rural clinic for a medically underserved community.

Political activity is an important tool for influencing the health of the community environment. Although nurses cannot directly relieve problems such as crowding, lack of funding for health care, or a depressed community economy, they can take indirect action through politics. For instance, nurses can lobby local political leaders for development of community housing or drug abuse programs.

Nurses can support political candidates who support the community's health needs by working on election campaigns and voting for these individuals.

Violence

Violence is a social systems problem that has emerged as a major health concern (Healthy People 2000, p. 150). **Violence** includes any nonaccidental act that results in physical or psychological injury including homicide, assault, rape, sexual abuse, emotional abuse, and physical abuse. Many factors are believed to influence the rise in violence, including social isolation, stressful lifestyles, breakdown in the family system, unemployment, poverty, and overcrowded living conditions. Violence is a nursing concern because it is a major cause of injury and mortality. Nurses often care for victims of violence who seek medical treatment. Because nurses may work directly in the home or community settings, they are in a key position to detect persons who are at risk for violence, either as perpetrators or victims.

Nurses may be particularly effective in the assessment and intervention of family violence. Because violence is a common social problem, nurses need to be aware when they are dealing with a possible victim. Children and the elderly may be victims of abuse. Partner abuse is another form of family violence. While victims of partner abuse are more likely to be women, mutual abuse and husband or male partner abuse also occur. Some ways in which nurses in many settings can address the problem of family violence include the following:

The primary care nurse screens for risk factors related to violence during routine health examinations.

The emergency room nurse follows up clients who come for treatment with suspicious injuries.

The home health care nurse assesses a family at risk for violence regarding how they deal with stress, and teaches stress reduction techniques.

The school nurse reports children with injuries that indicate potential abuse.

The community mental health nurse conducts a support group for victims of violence.

Social Support

An important function of the systems that compose the social environment is social support. Classic definitions of **social support** include:

❑ Information leading a person to believe he or she is cared for and loved, esteemed and valued, and belongs to a network of communication and mutual obligation (Cobb, 1976, p. 300)

❑ Support accessible to an individual through social ties to other individuals, groups, and the larger community (Lin, Ensel, Simeone, and Kuo, 1979, p. 109)

❏ A flow of emotional concern, instrumental aid, information, or appraisal between people (House, 1981, p. 26)

❏ Interpersonal transactions that include one or more of the following elements: expression of positive affect; affirmation of another person's behaviors, perceptions, or views; giving aid to another (Norbeck, Lindsey, & Carrieri, 1981)

The positive effect of social support on health was first identified in the 1970s. Nurses have contributed a great deal to the understanding of social support (Stewart & Tilden, 1995). Nuckolls (1972), who conducted the first study of social support, is a nurse. Jane Norbeck and Virginia Tilden are two others whose works on social support are excellent examples of nursing scholarship.

Functions and Sources of Social Support

Pender (1996) identified four ways that social support may positively affect health. Social networks may:

❏ Create an environment that enhances self-esteem and well-being.
❏ Decrease the likelihood of stressful life events.
❏ Provide feedback regarding the consequences of one's actions for health and well-being.
❏ Buffer the negative effects of stressful events.

Social support has many sources. If you consider persons to whom you feel close and share confidences, or on whom you can rely during difficult times, you will have identified your personal support network. Sources of support that have been identified in the literature include family, neighbors, friends, coworkers, religious organizations, self-help groups, and helping professionals (e.g., social workers, physicians, or nurses). For many individuals, the family provides the most significant source of support. The informal sources (family, peers, recreational groups, and so forth) are often identified as the most important by individuals, a factor related to the mutual sharing and spontaneity that characterize informal helping relationships.

Nursing Implications

Because social support is clearly related to the person's health status, this concept is an important nursing concern. Nurses find it useful to identify the significant sources of support in the client's social environment and enhance the effectiveness of the support systems. An examination of the client's support systems includes identifying the following factors:

❏ Who provides support: Does the client have a confidant? Are the spouse, family, and friends supportive? Does the client participate in organizations or activities?

❏ What helping behaviors are important to the client: financial assistance, emotional support, information sources, and so forth?

❏ Is the support system adequate from the client's perspective: Is there enough support of the kind desired by the client?

Once the support system has been identified, nurses provide help to maintain its adequacy or to alleviate deficits that may involve working directly with the support persons.

Nurses can also assist persons to extend their sources of support or make better use of sources currently available. Possible ways of assisting clients to develop or strengthen social support include the following:

❏ Teaching effective parenting skills
❏ Counseling to improve marital relationships
❏ Teaching assertiveness
❏ Encouraging clients to join interest groups (e.g., leisure activities or political work)
❏ Setting up lay or professional support networks (e.g., self-help groups)
❏ Establishing a telephone support system to obtain self-help for health concerns
❏ Using computers in client's homes to provide linkages to support groups and health care personnel

The following example illustrates one nursing student's creative interventions to provide social support to his young client.

For more than a month, J's only glimpse of the outdoors was through a hospital window. The teenager said that the sterile environment, intended to protect her during her recovery from a bone marrow transplant from leukemia, felt more like a holding cell than a hospital room. I used low cost video conferencing over the internet to link J. with her friends and classmates at home. Through two personal computers, one in J's hospital room and one in her school, J and her classmates were able to see and talk to each other. Imagine being isolated in a hospital room, nauseated, weak, and uncertain about the future. This is a time when support is needed the most. Hopefully the computer will allow people to talk with others at home or who are going through the same thing. (Adem Arslani, SN[4]).

Each person's need for social support is unique; what one person finds helpful might not be useful for another. The need for social support varies with personal differences and the degree and type of crisis. Remember that the *person's*—not the nurse's—appraisal of the adequacy of available support is critical. Refrain from making personal judgments about clients' social support without validating these impressions with them.

Social support is a phenomenon that appears to have a significant relationship to health. Because nurses focus their care on the whole person, they have a unique ability to assist clients to maximize the support available from the social environment. Using this holistic approach, nurses can aid in the prevention of illness and in the achievement of optimum health.

The Cultural Environment

Like the social environment, cultural influences have an enormous effect on health. All of us are members of a cultural group. Culture affects how we define health, how illness is manifested, and the way in which we deal with health problems. In the past two decades, the nursing profession has become acutely aware of cultural variations and their impact on providing person-centered care. The trend toward a global community means that nurses will be exposed to many different cultures and health beliefs that differ from their own. Nurses from developed countries increasingly have the opportunity to provide care to medically underserved nations, as illustrated in the example below. To give meaningful nursing care to clients from various cultural backgrounds, it is necessary to gain some insight into culture as a component of the person's environment and its influence on health and illness. Working with clients from various cultural groups can be as rewarding to the nurse as it is to the client.

Through a church organization, I was on a team of eighteen people who brought equipment for an eyeglass clinic to a church in Accra, Ghana. In five days we fitted 1200 people with eyeglasses. The people of Ghana gave us much more than we gave them. Their warmth and hospitality was apparent from the moment we landed in Accra, where we were greeted by church members with a wonderful supper. Although the poverty and sanitary conditions in this country were heartbreaking, I was amazed that, no matter how little they had, the people of Ghana were the kindest, most generous people I have ever met. (Mary Beth Pohanka, R.N.)

Definitions and Characteristics of Culture

Numerous theories and definitions of **culture** exist. A classic definition of culture is "the acquired knowledge that people use to interpret experience and generate social behavior" (Spradley, 1979, p. 5). In every society, people create systems of meaning to organize their behavior to understand themselves and others and to make sense out of the world in which they live. These meaning systems constitute their culture.

Leininger (1991), a nurse anthropologist, defined culture as the "learned, shared, and transmitted values, beliefs, norms, and lifeways of a particular group that guides their thinking, decisions, and actions in patterned ways" (p. 47). Every culture holds beliefs and behaviors that deal with how to maintain health, treat illness, give birth, and die. These are the very situations in which nurses care for people. Leininger stated that cultural knowledge is essential for nurses to provide care that is meaningful to their clients.

Culture has four characteristics. Culture is:

1. Learned through socialization and through language acquisition. The knowledge acquired through this learning process is often tacit and not easily identified or described directly. For this reason, students often

have difficulty recognizing and describing their own cultural beliefs. For example, many of us would have difficulty describing how far apart people should stand when they are having a conversation. However, we can tell when someone is standing too close for our comfort. Hall (1966), in a classic study of communication, noted that the appropriate distance for social conversation varies among cultural groups. His concept of *proxemics*, the use of space in interpersonal relationships, has been studied in a variety of cultures. Some cultural knowledge is explicit and stated directly. "Wash your hands before you eat" is an example of explicit cultural knowledge.

2. Shared by members of the same cultural group, and these shared beliefs and patterns give identity to the group. Communication systems, means of economic and physical survival, family systems, social customs, and religious beliefs are examples of shared patterns that may be culturally determined. It is important to recognize that such patterns are unequally shared among group members. Knowing cultural group norms does not allow us to predict the behavior of any individual within that group.

3. Dynamic and ever changing. Although cultural patterns are usually stable, they evolve over time. For example, in the early part of the 20th century, it was the norm for mothers to assume all of the child-care responsibilities and for fathers to assume the breadwinning role in two-parent families. These norms have evolved in response to economic and societal changes. Finding mothers and fathers sharing breadwinning and child-care roles in two-parent families currently is not unusual.

4. Contextual. Cultural patterns are understood in terms of their influencing factors. The context of a culture may include historical, political, social, economic, and geographic features. For example, people may use folk healing remedies because they do not have access to formal health care systems.

Subcultures

Many societies are multicultural—societies in which various groups live in close proximity and yet maintain somewhat different cultures. A **subculture** is a system of patterns and meanings that has shared characteristics of a larger culture but also has characteristics that are unique. Group members of a subculture may be distinguished by characteristics such as speech patterns, dress, gestures, etiquette, forms of worship, foods, and life-styles. Subcultural groups may be identified by features such as geographic region, religion, age, sex, occupational role, or ethnic identity. Nurses might be considered a subculture of the health care system because the profession is associated with a certain set of values, behavioral norms, and language. Although these patterns share some commonalities with health care workers in general, they have some differences that are unique to nursing.

Many countries have people from different subcultures. Subcultural group members may have varying relationships with the dominant culture. Some members may have the goal of assimilation, taking on the values and behaviors of the dominant culture, while others may desire separatism, identifying with values and behaviors that differ from the larger culture. A third group may have the goal of plurality, holding some norms from the larger group along with those of the subculture (Coleman-Burns, 1992). Nurses need to be aware of the subcultural groups that are served by their health care agency. It is important that nurses not assume that because a client is a member of a particular subculture, he or she holds a particular set of beliefs. For example, a person of Japanese descent who has lived in the United States for 50 years may have different beliefs and behaviors than a person who has recently relocated from Japan, although they share a common ethnicity. Likewise, Mexican-Americans, Cubans, and Puerto Ricans may all speak Spanish but have different cultural patterns.

Cultural Variables

Cultural variables refer to those characteristics that a person exhibits or identifies with from a particular cultural group. These variables may or may not be exhibited by every person from a cultural group. Any individual, depending on personal experience, may have all, none, or any combination of these variables.

Ethnic and Racial Identity

Ethnic origin and racial background have a great influence on how a person reacts and is reacted to by others in the health care environment. **Ethnicity** refers to affiliation within a group because of shared linguistic, religious, geographic or cultural background. Persons may identify their ethnicity by any of the following:

❐ Geographic origin
❐ Language
❐ Racial background
❐ Shared traditions, values, and symbols such as folklore or religion

In North America, blanket terms such as "Asian," "Hispanic," and "Native American" have been used to label ethnicity. If a nurse were caring for someone of Hispanic background, a distinction among Mexican, Cuban, or Puerto Rican would be important as the nurse attempts to relate to the person . Likewise, the nurse would need to distinguish between Iroquois and Navaho Native Americans. The Chinese-American who has lived in the United States for many years has little in common with the recent immigrant from Cambodia. These groups have different social, historical, and geographic backgrounds, affecting their health and illness beliefs, health behaviors, value systems, and communication processes.

Value Orientations

Values are intrinsic beliefs or ideals about desirable conduct, customs, and other entities. As such, they provide the basis for each person's attitudes and behaviors, and they assist in establishing hierarchies of needs and goals. Kluckholn and

Strodtbeck (1961), in their classic work, defined *value orientations* as principles that assist in the solution of common human problems. Among the value orientations that may differ across cultures are those concerning human nature, human-to-nature and human-to-human relationships, and time.

Kluckholn (1976) described three different value orientations toward time:

1. Past: Focus is on ancestors and traditions
2. Present: Time is "now"; little concern for past or future
3. Future: Orientation is toward progress and change; not content with present; past is "old-fashioned"

For example, while planning and goal-setting (future orientation) are valued in the dominant culture in the U.S., other cultural groups emphasize existing in the world as it is now (present orientation). Similarly, some people value punctuality and clock time; others value flexibility and lived time. A nurse who adheres to fixed schedules for appointments, baths, meals, and sleep may find conflict with a client who has a flexible time orientation. It is important not to assume that clients share the nurse's value orientation or that the nurse's values are inherently better.

Language and Communication

Communication is a dynamic process involving the exchange of messages and meanings, both verbal and nonverbal. Cross-cultural communication occurs whenever a message producer is a member of one culture and a message receiver is a member of another. Persons from two different cultural groups will make meaning of a message from their own cultural frameworks. For instance, perceptions of pain, complaints of illness, symptoms, and reactions to death and dying are all influenced by a person's cultural framework.

Cultural differences can be responsible for communication problems. For example, Spector (1996) described how some persons from Native American groups place high value on nonverbal communication and privacy. These persons may say little during visits to a health care setting and may be offended by direct questioning and note-taking. If a nurse expects clients to talk directly and openly about health problems, misunderstandings can occur.

Nonverbal communication behavior is culturally determined. Behaviors such as touch, interpersonal distance, eye contact, and handshakes may be interpreted differently depending on the cultural expectations of the nurse and client. Sensitivity to the client's responses to the nurse's nonverbal behavior can avert misunderstanding.

Family System

Traditionally, the family serves many functions. It provides for the physical and emotional well-being of its members, including health needs, it provides financial resources, it produces and rears children, and it transmits social beliefs and socially prescribed behaviors. The way in which families carry out these functions is culturally prescribed. For example, among many Arab-American Muslims, family care and support is an obligation and responsibility. If a family member is ill, others are obliged to stay and care for that person (Luna, 1989).

Family values are influenced by culture and are an important consideration for nurses. For example, it is useful to identify how family decisions are made and who is involved in decision making. Traditional Filipino culture holds elders in great respect, and deference is shown for their decisions. If a nurse is working with a family who holds this value, it can be helpful to seek out the elder regarding care of an ill family member.

Family structure is another variable that is culturally influenced. In the United States, the nuclear family is often held up as the ideal in areas such as government policy and advertising. Yet in some groups, extended family networks are the norm. Yoos, et al. (1995) noted that strong kinship systems are often found in African-American families. Mexican-Americans are likely to value the needs of the family over the needs of the individual (Friedman, 1990). These strong family networks can be a resource the nurse can use for the client's benefit.

Cultural Healing Beliefs and Practices

Cultural healing beliefs are beliefs that reflect a specific cultural orientation toward health and illness. They include definitions of health and illness, cause and prevention of illness, healing practices and remedies, types of health care practitioners, and methods of health promotion. What is recognized as illness and wellness is determined by one's culture. For example, Western medicine identifies demonstrable physiologic abnormalities as illness. When a client's symptoms cannot be linked to a physical cause, the client's illness may be discounted by Western practitioners. Yet, other cultural groups may believe in supernatural causes of illness. For example, Spector (1996) explained that many cultures believe in the evil eye, that is, harm caused by gazing or staring at another or another's belongings.

Although North American nurses attribute authority to traditional medical beliefs, it is important to recognize that North American medical theories have not always been rigorously tested. For example, North American nurses traditionally positioned newborns on their abdomens to prevent choking. Japanese mothers traditionally place newborns on their backs to prevent suffocation. The North American practice recently has been associated with sudden infant death syndrome.

Nurses must be aware of how cultural healing beliefs affect a person's response to the health care system. A person may reject the formal health care system because of differences in beliefs. Health professionals, when feasible, should use a treatment plan that demonstrates respect for and reflects a person's cultural healing system. Nurses can combine traditional medical practices with the client's healing beliefs to promote wellness. Munet-Vilaro and Vessey (1990) described how traditional chemotherapy was used with culturally-based treatments for Puerto Rican children diagnosed with leukemia. Lay healers, foods, and protective objects and rituals may be part of any client's cultural healing beliefs and usually can be incorporated into the medical and nursing plan of care.

Religious Beliefs and Practices

Religion may influence a person's concept of health and illness, treatment programs, and recovery. Religion also can act as a resource in facing crises related to critical illnesses or death. However, it must not be assumed that all persons from certain ethnic or cultural backgrounds have the same or similar religious belief systems. Andrews (1995) described several religious belief systems and their characteristics as related to birth, death, health crisis, diet, and special beliefs. For instance, the Islamic religion has specific practices related to care of the body after death that must be adhered to. Donation of body parts after death is unacceptable among Jehovah's Witnesses. The nurse should assess the characteristics in a person's religious belief system and determine their influence on the health state.

There may be a thin line between religious and cultural beliefs that makes it difficult to separate the two. For example, the Filipino culture is associated with a strong sense of destiny related to Asian heritage, and a deep faith in God drawn from Spanish influence. Filipino clients may be reluctant to complain, particularly about pain, attributing it to God's will (Leininger, 1995) and may need careful pain assessment by nurses. Some religious groups may object to medical interventions, as shown by the refusal of Jehovah's Witnesses to allow blood transfusions or the avoidance of drugs by Seventh Day Adventists unless they are absolutely necessary (Andrews, 1995).

Nutritional Behavior and Cultural Influences

The kinds of foods eaten, the way they are prepared, and the manner in which they are consumed are practices that are embedded strongly in the behavioral systems of each culture. When people enter the health care system, they bring all of their cultural beliefs and practices about food with them. For example, the typical North American diet is high in fat and sodium. If a client's preferences and manner of consumption differ from those of the health care system, conflict can occur. For example, Schubin (1980) described the incident of a Mexican-American client who disappeared from his hospital room soon after undergoing major surgery; he had gone home to obtain specific cultural foods—tacos, tortillas, and beans. Later he returned, believing that these foods would speed his recovery.

Cultural food practices also involve which foods are regarded as edible. For instance, North Americans regard milk as a good food, but Southeast Asians do not. Some cultural groups may eat insects or dogs, foods which are considered inedible in North America. Infant feeding practices are also influenced by cultural beliefs, as illustrated in the example below:

Rosa, a young Mexican mother, had indicated her wish to breastfeed her infant. Imagine the nurse's surprise when Rosa pulled the baby away from the breast as soon as he was brought to her for the first feeding, immediately after birth. The nurse continued to urge Rosa to feed her baby right away to establish successful breastfeeding. I spoke Spanish and was asked to be an interpreter. As I sat with Rosa and gently questioned her about her distress, I learned that some Mexican women believe that first milk (colostrum) is "bad milk" and might harm the baby. Although the nurse meant well, trying to force Rosa to feed her baby colostrum resulted in an unnecessary power struggle. Establishing trust, including with family members, and negotiating health care with her are more effective ways of dealing with differing health beliefs. (Katie Winnell, 3rd year nursing student)

Religious beliefs and practices may strongly influence nutritional behavior. For example, African Americans who are Muslim are prohibited from alcoholic beverages, pork, and foods such as cornbread and collards that are traditionally eaten by many African Americans. Orthodox Jews who observe strict kosher dietary laws will not eat pork and shellfish or combine meat and milk at the same meal.

When assessing nutrition, nurses may gain knowledge of clients' cultural patterns of food intake that may have implications for health teaching. Although it would be difficult to have knowledge of all existing food habits, nurses can learn about the cultural food preferences of the people who are served by their health care agencies. It is difficult to change food patterns that have been established over a lifetime. Nurses can be helpful by assisting clients to modify preparation of familiar foods to meet the requirements of a prescribed diet.

Biophysical Variations

Biophysical variations among ethnic and racial groups influence findings on health assessment, health concerns, and growth and development patterns. *Mongolian spots,* which are areas of bluish-black pigmentation of no clinical significance, are common in blacks, Asians, and Native Americans. They may be mistaken for bruises by some health care practitioners. Also, skin color changes that signify disease such as jaundice and cyanosis may be difficult to detect in dark-skinned individuals.

Certain cultural groups are at higher risk for development of specific diseases. Some reasons include environmental influences, genetic factors, and inadequate health care resources. For example, African-American males have a high incidence of hypertension, and Jews of northeastern European descent are at risk for Tay-Sachs disease. The infant mortality rate for African-American infants is significantly higher than that of white infants and has been attributed to lack of access to prenatal care. This information is significant for nurses who are involved in health screening and preventive health programs.

Ethnic differences in responses to and metabolism of drugs have been identified in many research studies (Andrews, 1995). For example, Asians are more sensitive to pharmacologic effects than Caucasians. Keltner and Folks (1992) noted that African-Americans are more likely to show delirium during therapy with psychotropic drugs. Nurses need to be aware of these ethnic differences when monitoring the effects of drug treatment in their patients.

A final factor related to physical differences is growth and development patterns (Andrews, 1995). For example, studies have shown African-American children to be taller and heavier than white children between ages 5 to 14. African-American children have thinner skin folds than white children. Asian children tend to be smaller than Caucasian children. It is important that school nurses or pediatric nurse practitioners be aware of these variations when doing physical assessments of children.

*N*ursing *Approaches to Cultural Differences*

The need for nurses' awareness of cultural patterns is emphasized in this section. Knowledgeable nurses can greatly assist clients who are struggling with differences between their own cultural norms and those of the health care system.

Nurses also need to develop an openness to beliefs and behaviors that differ from theirs. Nurses are often unintentionally guilty of *ethnocentrism,* the belief that one's own cultural or ethnic group is superior to others. Whenever a nurse labels a client's food practices as "strange" or his or her beliefs about folk remedies as "worthless," the nurse is acting from ethnocentrism. *Stereotyping,* assigning preconceived and untested beliefs to people, can lead to faulty assessments and inappropriate care. For example, nurses who believe that physical abuse or substance abuse is a problem of poor people may miss these problems when they are present in middle-class clients. Leininger (1991) described three modes of action that lead to meaningful nursing care:

1. Cultural care preservation, which helps people retain cultural values to enable well-being, recovery, or peaceful dying
2. Cultural care accommodation, which helps people negotiate with health care providers for satisfying or beneficial health outcomes
3. Cultural care repatterning, which helps clients modify or change lifeways for new, different, and beneficial health care patterns while respecting the client's cultural values and beliefs

All three modalities require the mutual participation of the nurse and clients, who work together to achieve culturally congruent care.

Nursing students may find it hard to accept that the client's health beliefs and behaviors have as much validity as their own. It is helpful to think of belief systems as different colored eyeglasses that one can try on to temporarily view the world from the client's perspective. Flexibility, open-mindedness, willingness to learn, and the ability to establish trust are all important attributes when caring for clients from different cultural groups.

As a summary, a nursing professor who specializes in multicultural issues listed the principles that she uses to maintain sensitivity to people's beliefs. Her interventions are found in the display.

The ever growing role that culture has in the care we provide our clients means that we cannot have all that we need at our fingertips. However, several general interventions that can be useful when working with clients follow:

1. Approach clients and families as if they may have cultural needs that are not obvious (for example, even if they do not appear to come from a specific cultural group).
2. Recognize that clients from the same racial or ethnic group may not have the same needs and issues as others from that group.
3. Provide the same respect for all clients and families.
4. Recognize that there are many kinds of diversity among our clients. Approach people gently, respectfully, and politely question them about their needs.
5. Do not make assumptions about roles or relationships among the persons who are with the client. For example, do not assume that a couple are husband and wife.
6. When you recognize that clients are of a particular cultural group, acknowledge this openly and ask for assistance or explanations about their way of viewing their situation.
7. Empower your clients by engaging them in their care.

Use of these guidelines will assist nurses to learn more about their clients and to demonstrate that we recognize value in all persons.
Patricia Coleman-Burns, Ph.D.

KEY CONCEPTS

✔Environment is the physical, social, and cultural world outside the person.

✔Persons and their environments are constantly interacting, each changing and being changed by the other.

✔The interactions between persons and their environments affect health.

✔The physical environment consists of the community environment with related ecologic issues, and the immediate environment with concomitant concerns of safety, function, and comfort.

✔The social environment comprises the social systems of family, group, and community.

✔Violence is a growing social problem that negatively affects health.

✔Social support has been shown to be positively related to health.

✔Culture is learned, shared, and transmitted values, beliefs, and lifeways of a group that guides thinking, decision-making and action.

✔Cultural differences between clients and health professionals in health and illness beliefs, language, nutrition, and so forth affect clients' experiences as they seek health care.

✔An important aspect of nursing care is making appropriate environmental alterations.

CRITICAL THINKING QUESTIONS

1. Review the newspaper or a news magazine for one week. What environmental issues are receiving media attention? What action could you take to affect these problems?

2. Examine your home environment for safety hazards. Now look again and identify hazards if the following people came to visit your home:
   a. A toddler
   b. A person who uses a cane or a walker
   c. An elderly person with poor vision

3. How can nurses control infection in the following situations:
   a. A day-care center?
   b. Caring for a person in the home?
   c. Caring for clients in the hospital?

4. Ask several people to define their family. How do their responses differ from the definitions presented in this chapter?

5. Examine a group to which you belong for the following factors:
   a. Roles of group members
   b. Communication patterns
   c. Decision-making processes

   What changes would strengthen the functioning of your group?

6. Examine the community where you live for the following factors:
   a. Do most employers provide health insurance for their employees? What is the level of unemployment?
   b. Is there a hospital in your community? What kinds of services does it provide? Where do people go for specialty care?
   c. What kinds of industries are present in your community? Do any present health hazards?
   d. What health care services are provided by the local government? How do these factors in the community system affect health care?

7. Interview a nurse who works in an emergency room setting. How does this nurse intervene when a client is a suspected victim of abuse?

8. What is social support? Why is it important for nurses to identify the adequacy of social support for their clients?

9. What cultural factors should be considered in caring for the following clients?
   a. A 40-year-old African-American man who is a middle manager in an automobile firm, and has been diagnosed with high blood pressure.
   b. A 20-year-old Lebanese woman who is pregnant with her first child and has recently moved to the U.S.

c. A 65-year-old Native American who lives on a Navajo reservation, who has diabetes.

REFERENCES

Andrews, M.M. (1995). Transcultural nursing care. In M.M. Andrews & J.S. Boyle, *Transcultural concepts in nursing care* (2nd ed., pp. 49–96). Philadelphia: J.B. Lippincott.

Cobb, S. (1976). Social support as a moderator of life stress. *Psychosomatic Medicine, 38,* 300–314.

Coleman-Burns, P. (1992, July). *Social and political thought of African Americans.* Paper presented at the Closing Conference of National Council of Black Studies, Columbus, OH.

Dysart, J. (1990). Rethinking the earth. *Canadian Nurse, 86*(7), 6–17.

Friedman, M.M. (1992). *Family nursing: Theory and assessment* (3rd ed.). Norwalk, CT: Appleton & Lange.

Friedman, M.M. (1990). Transcultural family nursing: Application to Latino and black families. *Journal of Pediatric Nursing, 5*(3), 214–222.

Graham, M. (1990). Frequency and duration of handwashing in an intensive care unit. *American Journal of Infection Control, 18*(2), 77–81.

Hall, E.T. (1966). *The hidden dimension.* Garden City, NY: Doubleday.

(1991). *Healthy people 2000: National health promotion and disease prevention objectives.* Washington, DC: U.S. Department of Health and Human Services.

House, J.S. (1981). *Work stress and social support.* Reading, MA: Addison-Wesley.

Keltner, N.L., & Folks, D.G. (1992). Culture as a variable in drug therapy. *Perspectives on Psychiatric Care, 28*(1), 33–36.

Kleffel, D. (1991). Rethinking the environment as a domain of nursing knowledge *Advances in Nursing Science, 14*(1), 40–51.

Kluckholn, F.R. (1976). Dominant and variant value orientations. In P.J. Brink (Ed.), *Transcultural nursing: A book of readings* (pp. 63–81). Englewood Cliffs, NJ: Prentice-Hall.

Kluckholn, F.R., & Strodtbeck, F.L. (1961). *Variations in value orientations.* Evanston, IL: Row, Peterson.

Leininger, M.M. (1995). Phillipine-Americans and culture care. In M.M. Leininger (Ed.), *Transcultural nursing: Concepts, theories, research, and practices* (2nd ed., pp. 349–363). New York: McGraw-Hill.

Leininger, M.M. (1991). *Culture care diversity and universality: A theory for nursing.* New York: National League for Nursing.

Lin, N., Ensel, W.M., Simeone, R.S., & Kuo, W. (1979). Social support, stressful life events and illness: A model and an empirical test. *Journal of Health and Social Behavior, 20,* 109–119.

Luna, L. (1989). Transcultural nursing care of Arab muslims, *Journal of Transcultural Nursing, 1*(1), 22–27.

Moos, R. (1973). Conceptualizations of human environments. *American Psychologist, 28,* 652–665.

Munet-Vilaro, F., & Vessey, J.A. (1990). Children's explanation of leukemia: A Hispanic Perspective. *Journal of Pediatric Nursing, 5*(4), 274–282.

Nightingale, F. (1859). *Notes on nursing: What it is and what it is not.* London: Harrison. (Facsimile ed., Philadelphia: J.B. Lippincott, 1966)

Norbeck, J.S., Lindsey, A.M., & Carrieri, V.L. (1981). The development of an instrument to measure social support. *Nursing Research, 30,* 264–269.

Nuckolls, K.B., Cassel, J., & Kaplan, B.H. (1972). Psychosocial assets, life crisis, and the prognosis of pregnancy. *American Journal of Epidemiology, 95,* 431–441.

Pender, N.J. (1996). *Health promotion in nursing practice* (3rd ed.). Stamford, CT: Appleton & Lange.

Schubin, S. (1980). Nursing patients from different cultures. *Nursing '80, 10*(6), 78–81.

Schuster, E.A. (1990). Earth caring. *Advances in Nursing Science, 13*(1), 25–30.

Smith, M., & Whitney, G. (1991). Caring for the environment: The ecology of health. In P.L. Chinn (Ed.), *Anthology on caring* (pp 59–69). New York: National League of Nursing.

Spector, R. (1996). *Cultural diversity in health and illness* (4th ed.). Stamford, CT: Appleton & Lange.

Spradley, J.P. (1979). *The ethnographic interview.* Fort Worth, TX: Harcourt Brace Jovanovich.

Stewart, M.J. & Tilden, V.P. (1995). The contributions of nursing science to social support. *International Journal of Nursing Studies 32,* 535–544.

U.S. Department of Health and Human Services (1996). Advance Report of Final Mortality Statistics, 1993. *Monthly Vital Statistics Report, 44*(7). Washington, DC: US DHHS.

Yoos, H.L., Kitzman, H., Olds, D.L., & Overacker, I. (1995). Child rearing beliefs in the African-American community: Implications for culturally competent pediatric care. *Journal of Pediatric Nursing, 10,* 343–353.

6

Health: A Nursing Perspective

Key Words

Adaptation	Situational (accidental)	Health-promotion	Maladaptation
Anxiety	crisis	behavior	Quality of life
Behavior	Maturational (normative or	Health-protection	Self-care
Coping	developmental) crisis	behavior	Stress
Crisis	Environment	High-level	Stressor
	Health	wellness	

Objectives

After completing this chapter, students will be able to:

Develop a nursing perspective of health.

Recognize various models of health.

Discuss the relationship between health and adaptation.

Describe the phenomena of change, stress, crisis, anxiety, and coping, and their effects on persons.

Identify theories of adaptation as they relate to persons and their environment.

Describe the experience of health using nursing models.

Describe the concept of health behavior.

Identify ways the professional nurse promotes health.

As a nurse, you will be in a unique position to learn how to help yourself at the same time you learn how to help others. You will be privileged to assist persons in dealing with some of their most difficult and intimate life experiences. As a health professional, you will make decisions affecting clients' well-being in collaboration with clients, their families, and other health professionals. Nurses need to know a great deal about life and persons and health.

Nursing was described in Chapter 3 as the health science of caring. Many changes have occurred in the past few decades that raise questions about former ideas of health. Persons with chronic disease now live longer, life expectancy has increased, and technology has enabled many persons to survive critical illness with questionable quality of life. The influx of people from other countries into the U.S. and Canada challenges nurses to consider cultural influences on health. A nursing definition of health must be meaningful for the diverse situations in which nurses care for people. Is health the absence of disease, or is it something more? Is it possible for persons who have chronic disease to be healthy? Is the young adult's level of functioning the standard against which we determine the health of the elderly? Is there a definition of health that encompasses the health concerns of technologically advanced countries as well as those that are still developing? The answers to these questions will influence the way that nurses provide service to clients.

This chapter explores the concept of health and presents several models. Nursing perspectives of health are explored and applications to nursing practice are also discussed. In response to increased concerns about the cost of illness-related care and increased focus on wellness, the concept of health promotion is explored in relation to nursing care.

Models of Health

Health means different things to different persons; nevertheless, the term is familiar. Identifying our own concept of health is accomplished by recalling past experiences of illness as well as those activities we perform to keep well. Some consider health the opposite of illness. Others view health as a personal asset, as shown in these statements: "When you have your health you have everything." "I lost my health when. . . ." Health may be viewed as an outcome of careful lifestyle or as an aspect of life over which one has little control.

These examples illustrate a variety of individual perspectives about the concept of health. The scientific community has been engaged in defining health for decades. One commonly accepted definition, developed by the World Health Organization in 1947, is ". . . a state of complete physical, mental, and social well-being, not merely the absence of disease or infirmity"(p. 29). Smith (1983) identified four different models of health based on extensive reviews of theoretical literature. They are the (1) clinical, (2) role-performance, (3) adaptive, and (4) eudaimonistic models. Additional perspectives of health include the primitive, epidemiologic, and experiential models. This section explores these viewpoints and discusses their applicability to nursing.

Primitive Model

In the primitive model, health and illness are controlled by forces external to humans. Ancient humans viewed natural phenomena, including illness, as the work of gods or spirits, and religious and health practices were often closely interwoven. Medicine men or priests dispelled evil spirits from the unfortunate sick. Even today, nurses may encounter many persons who view their illness as a punishment for wrongdoing or as an autonomous, amorphous force that attacked without provocation. "Why me?" may be a concern when these individuals become ill. When caring for these individuals, nurses may need to work with religious healers or healing practices in addition to traditional medical treatment.

Ecological Model

The ecological model is based on person–environment relationships. The three components of this model are (1) a host or susceptible individual; (2) an injury- or disease-producing agent; and (3) the **environment,** which if poor or un- healthy may predispose persons to disease. Illness is a directly observable aberra- tion caused by the interaction of these factors. One advantage of this model is its focus on the health of populations rather than on individual health.

Clinical Model

The clinical model represents the biomedical perspective of health. Health is the absence of disease or the opposite of illness. The concept of the health–illness continuum, with health at one end of the scale and illness at the other, is consis- tent with this model. The focus of care in this model is "primarily the elimination of morbid physical or mental conditions and relief from concomitant pain" (Smith, 1981, p. 46). The health care provider's role ends when symptoms of disease are no longer present and relief is obtained.

Most nursing definitions of health reject this model because it oversimplifies illness. Many illnesses are related to multiple factors rather than a single cause. Furthermore, the clinical model does not acknowledge a holistic view of persons.

This model is important, however, because it has been the dominant model in the North American health care system, particularly in hospitals, where nurses traditionally have practiced. Many health care consumers also adhere to this model of health. But with the trend toward preventive and health-promoting care and consumer concerns about quality of life, the clinical model of health has a limited focus.

Role-Performance Model

The role-performance model represents health as the ability of a person to perform his or her roles effectively. It is based on the work of medical sociologists and the writing of Parsons (1972). Roles can include wage earning and parenting, among many others. Illness is viewed as an incapacity to perform social roles and tasks based on feelings of not being well. Illness may be difficult to define in this model, because persons may perform some roles and yet fail to perform others.

Role performance is included in two nursing theorists' (King, 1981; Orem, 1995) descriptions of health. It also may be the model that clients use to define their health. For example, Lantz et al. (1994) found that, for economic reasons,

Hispanic farm workers reported reluctance to engage in behaviors that reduced their exposure to cancer-causing pesticides. In this study, workers delayed seeking health care because of the need to work and also because of long workdays.

*A*daptation Model

Adaptation is the process in which persons faced with new, different, or threatening experiences change throughout life without loss of health, wholeness, or integrity of self. Adaptation includes the concepts of persons as biopsychosocial beings, interaction with the environment, change, and health as the goal of adaptation.

The essence of adaptation is change; it is a process of dynamic equilibrium that is vital for survival. In broad terms, adaptation consists of biologic, psychosocial, and spiritual facets. Adaptation moves a person toward health and growth.

When change occurs in the environment, the person must adapt. This process requires energy, and rapid change may require more energy than the person has available. When the rate or amount of change exceeds our capacity to adapt, illness may occur; however, successful adaptation may strengthen integrity of self or lead to an even higher level of functioning.

The adaptive model has been widely used in nursing and is the basis for several nursing theories. Levine's Conservation Model (1973), the Roy Adaptation Model (1991), Erickson et al.'s Modeling and Role-Modeling Theory (1983), and the Neuman Systems Model (1995) are nursing theories that incorporate adaptation. (See Chapter 3.)

Historical Development of the Adaptation Concept

The development over the past 150 years of the adaptation concept is reflected in Table 6-1 and summarized as follows.

BERNARD (STEADY STATE)
Claude Bernard, a 19th-century physiologist, was one of the pioneers in the study of the body's attempts to achieve a steady state while dealing with change. He pointed out that the internal environment of all organisms remains fairly constant even though the external environment changes. For example, the body maintains a stable core temperature despite changes in the weather.

CANNON (HOMEOSTASIS)
In the early part of the 20th century, Walter B. Cannon (1939), another physiologist, introduced the concept of homeostasis. *Homeostasis* means the maintenance of equilibrium or a steady state of the body. For instance, the oxygen concentration within arteries remains fairly constant, even though carbon dioxide is continually given off by cells and oxygen is taken in by the lungs. Cannon identified many mechanisms, particularly neurologic and endocrine responses, that preserve equilibrium in the body. Cannon recognized that this steady state was not completely fixed; rather, it varied within certain limits.

TABLE 6-1 *Historical Development of Adaptation Concept*

Scientist and Profession	Contribution
Claude Bernard, physiologist	Identified that the internal environment of all organisms remains fairly constant even though the external environment changes
Walter B. Cannon, physiologist	Defined *homeostasis* as the ability of living organisms to maintain their own equilibrium
Hans Selye, endocrinologist	Described the general adaptation syndrome: The body's response to stress of any kind occurs as a unified defense mechanism with specific structural and chemical changes; The reaction elicits resistance by the body to stressful agents and protects against disease; when the reaction is too long or faulty, disease or death may occur.
Rene Dubos, biologist	Defined *health* or *disease* as the expression of the success or respectively, failure, by persons in their efforts to respond adaptively to environmental challenges
T. H. Holmes and R. H. Rahe, psychiatrists	Developed the Social Readjustment Rating Scale, which demonstrates a correlation between stressful life events and illness and may be a predictor of illness
Richard Lazarus, psychologist	Described the influence of appraisal on coping; daily stresses may be more significant than major life events for overall coping

SELYE (STRESS)

The work of Hans Selye (1956) stimulated great interest in the concepts of stress and adaptation. Selye, an endocrinologist, defined **stress** as the nonspecific response of the body to any demand placed on it, and a **stressor** as anything that induces stress. Selye discovered that the body responds to stressful stimuli with specific physiologic mechanisms, and called this the general adaptation syndrome (GAS). The GAS response elicits resistance by the body to stressful agents, enhancing its ability to ward off those stressors. However, if this reaction is faulty or prolonged, disease or death may result.

The GAS has three phases: (1) alarm reaction, (2) resistance, and (3) exhaustion. The responses in each stage are as follows:

Alarm—Defenses mobilize to respond to stressor.

Resistance—Body tries to adapt to stressor.

Exhaustion—If stressor persists or is severe, or if the person has limited adaptive capacity, the body loses ability to adapt; exhaustion and death follow.

DUBOS (ADAPTATION)

Another perspective is that of biologist Rene Dubos, a 20th-century biologist and philosopher. Dubos (1965) wrote, "Health or disease is the expression of success or failure by persons in their efforts to respond adaptively to environmental challenges." (p. xvii). Within his model, health is a reaction of the whole organism—the consequence of factors including internal and external stimuli and the predisposition of the individual. Health care focuses on restoring the ability to cope with environmental changes. Dubos' adaptive model focuses on the ability of persons to respond to changes in the environment; the goal is stability of the individual.

HOLMES AND RAHE (LIFE EVENTS AND ILLNESS)

T.H. Holmes and R.H. Rahe (1967) stimulated well-known research on the relationship between adaptation and health. They developed the Social Readjustment Rating Scale to demonstrate the correlation between stressful life events and serious illness. The ranking of life events is the result of perceived changes in lifestyle following the events. The life events identified are not necessarily undesirable; rather, they include any experience that requires some degree of adaptation. Their list of life events included positive changes such as marriage, as well as negative circumstances such as death.

Studies have shown that the number of life changes and subsequent alterations in the lifestyles of persons negatively affect health. For this reason, persons experiencing too many life changes (multiple stressors) in a short time span may be suitable candidates for intervention to prevent serious illness.

LAZARUS (APPRAISAL AND COPING)

Richard Lazarus, a psychologist, contributed to stress and adaptation theory by developing the concept of appraisal in relation to **coping**. Lazarus believed that responses to stress were related not only to the nature of the stressful event but also to how the person perceived the event. Lazarus (1984) focused on psychological coping, believing that coping was a cognitive process rather than merely the reflection of personality traits. He also believed that coping was contextual, meaning that it was influenced by people's appraisal of the actual demands and resources in the specific stressful situations they encountered. Lazarus stated that adaptation was a construct, that is, a broad concept with many related variables. Lazarus also disagreed with Holmes and Rahe's Social Readjustment Rating Scale. He believed that daily "hassles" were more significant stressors than life events. He developed the Everyday Hassles Scale to measure the stress produced by daily events.

Nursing Models of Adaptation

The adaptation concept has been the focus of work by professional nurses in education, research, and practice. Common themes about adaptation in nursing are summarized below, based on the work of Myra Levine (1973), Sister Callista Roy (1991), Betty Neuman (1995), and Helen Erickson (1983):

- ❐ Persons continually interact with their environments.
- ❐ Adaptation is the person's response to a change in the environment.
- ❐ Environmental changes occur constantly, so adaptation is a continuous process.

❏ The goal of nursing is to promote adaptation.
❏ As we help persons to adapt, we are helping them to maintain or to achieve health.

The adaptation model is used by many nurses in education, research, and clinical practice. The following section gives an overview of key concepts related to the process of adaptation.

Process of Adaptation

To understand the process of adaptation, nurses must be familiar with several of its subconcepts:

❏ Stress and stressor
❏ Anxiety
❏ Coping
❏ Crisis

None of the subconcepts is a synonym for the others; yet, each is related to the others, as indicated in the following statement (subconcepts are italicized):

Wear and tear from *stressors* may produce disequilibrium and *stress*, especially if persons are unprepared or unskilled to manage (*cope* with) the event. The failure to regain equilibrium will lead to *anxiety*, and excessive anxiety that remains unrelieved may lead to a *crisis*.

STRESS

Stress has been defined as a stimulus, a state, and a response by various researchers. In this discussion, stimuli that place a demand for change on persons are termed stressors. Stressors may be physical, such as an injury or pain, or psychological, such as the loss of a loved one or the birth of a child. Stressors are not necessarily negative. Stressors identified in the Social Readjustment Rating Scale by Holmes and Rahe included unhappy and happy events. Persons themselves define whether stimuli are positive or negative, because perceptions of such events are an individual matter. For this reason, how persons perceive and respond to stressful events is critical to health.

Stressors result in a state of stress that includes physiologic, psychologic, and social responses. Nurses need to obtain information about their clients' strengths that protect the clients from stressors as well as their responses to stress.

ANXIETY

Any threatening situation can produce anxiety. **Anxiety** is a diffuse, unpleasant, vague feeling of apprehension, nervousness, or dread expressed both somatically and psychically. Like fear, it is a reaction to a threat; however, unlike fear (which is a response to a known, definite, external, and immediate danger), anxiety is felt as a future threat from something unknown, vague, and internal.

Anxiety is a normal response to a stressful event; everyone experiences it. Caplan's (1964) classic work describes anxiety in a crisis situation: "When the individual's usual problem solving methods fail, and the problem persists, he or she experiences a rise in inner tension, unpleasant emotional feelings, and disorganized functioning"(pp. 38–39).

Because an individual needs to relieve the discomfort (anxiety) of a stressful situation, he or she will use coping behavior to protect against disorganization or an unstable state of physical and emotional health. Therefore, some kind of adaptation or reorganization occurs; the result may be either growth or regression.

Nurses need to understand the phenomenon of anxiety when working with persons in crisis. Individuals who are experiencing a high level of anxiety often have a limited ability to solve problems and, therefore, to adapt. These persons need assistance to lower their anxiety to a functional level. A mild degree of anxiety may be beneficial, because it motivates persons to make needed changes in their behavior. Determining the level of anxiety is essential for choosing successful nursing actions.

COPING

Coping refers to the way we deal with stressors. Lazarus (1984) defined *coping* as behavioral and cognitive efforts to manage specific internal or external demands that are appraised as exceeding the resources of the person (p. 141). As defined by Allport (1965), *coping* is characteristically

- ❐ Purposive.
- ❐ Determined by the needs of the moment and situation.
- ❐ Formally elicited rather than spontaneously emitted.
- ❐ More readily controlled.
- ❐ Aiming to change the environment (p. 243).

Coping implies action in response to our environment; effective coping leads to wellness. Lazarus (1984) identified two types of coping: problem-focused and emotion-focused coping (p. 150). *Problem-focused coping* is directed at managing or altering the problem causing the distress. It may include problem-solving or information-seeking activities. *Emotion-focused coping* is directed at regulating emotional responses to the problem. Avoiding feelings through escapist activities, blaming others, venting anger, or looking for emotional support are examples of emotion-focused coping.

Adaptive Versus Maladaptive Coping. Coping behaviors may be either adaptive or maladaptive. Roy (Roy & Andrews, 1991) states that an adaptive response is behavior that promotes the integrity of the individual. An ineffective response is one that does not maintain integrity and may threaten survival, growth, reproduction, and mastery. **Adaptation** is successful when the person responds to stressful events in a way that maintains or enhances integrity.

Maladaptation occurs when a person uses inadequate or ineffective methods of coping to maintain equilibrium. In the adaptation model, illness may be the result of maladaptive coping. However, maladaptive coping is not to be considered a fault, because a person is never prepared for all the contingencies of change. On occasion, individuals find themselves in new situations for which previous coping methods may not be effective, and their attempts to survive in the situation may fail. Under such circumstances, they may need to seek help and learn coping methods. Unfortunately, many times persons who cope maladaptively with changes in their environment may not be aware that they need help. Some persons may find it extremely difficult to seek help, even when they recognize their problems. For instance, a woman who discovers a breast lump may delay seeking help because she cannot cope with the possibility of having cancer.

When circumstances warrant help, nurses, as well as other professionals, become resources in the environment; nurses assist persons to cope adaptively. Behaviors considered maladaptive in one culture may be adaptive in another. Consequently, nurses need to understand a person's sociocultural beliefs before making plans to intervene.

CRISIS

The phenomenon of **crisis** is universal; no one escapes crisis because no one escapes change. The term *crisis*, like the term *stress*, has been used frequently to imply something that is positive and desirable as well as something that is negative or undesirable. Also, stress and crisis have been used interchangeably by some. The word crisis often connotes personal failure and inability to handle stressful events. Erik Erikson (1963), however, used *crisis* to describe a turning point, a crucial period of increased vulnerability and heightened potential. Thus crises have the potential to lead to personal growth and reorganization for healthier functioning.

A crisis is temporary and usually lasts no longer than 4 to 6 weeks. Because a person's usual coping mechanisms do not work, this period may be both a time of danger and an opportunity for learning new coping patterns. Whereas a crisis may be overwhelming to some—for example, a woman who considers suicide after the death of her husband—others may use this time as a period of growth. Whether a crisis has a positive or negative outcome depends on its nature and the person's coping abilities and resources.

Situational Versus Developmental Crisis.   Crisis may occur as the result of a sudden and significant change in a person's life. During crisis, a person may be helpless and less able to find a solution; his or her functioning becomes disorganized.

Crises are of two types: situational (or accidental) and maturational (normative or developmental). A **situational (accidental) crisis** occurs when the sense of biologic, psychologic, and social integrity is threatened due to unexpected events such as death, illness, divorce, loss of job, moving, unexpected pregnancy, or natural disaster.

A **maturational (normative or developmental)** crisis occurs when a person is unable to make appropriate changes in response to new life situations, such as marriage, beginning school, adolescence, or parenthood. Crises can potentially occur during stages of social, physical, and psychological change that are

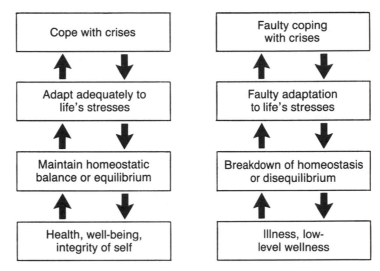

FIGURE 6-1 Balancing factors for health. (Harms, M. B. [1983]. Adapted in Lindberg, J. B., Hunter, M. L., Kruszewski, A. Z. *Person-Centered Nursing*, [p 86]. Philadelphia: JB Lippincott.)

experienced in the normal growth and development process (Aguilera, 1994). During periods of maturational crisis, the person learns to develop coping strategies for these new life situations.

Coping With Crises. Figure 6-1 describes the balancing factors that determine health. The paradigm illustrates how health, well-being, and integrity of self depend on the person's ability to cope with crisis, adapt to life stresses, and maintain a stable state. Likewise, the person unable to cope with crisis and adapt to stress suffers disequilibrium and potential illness.

Figure 6-2 is a paradigm of the development of crisis (Aguilera, 1994). Figure 6-3 is an illustration of the paradigm using two men's responses to the same event: the appearance of cancer symptoms and the need for diagnostic tests. This example shows how a stressful event experienced by two individuals can lead to different outcomes, depending on which coping mechanisms each person uses. Note that maladaptive coping hinders problem solving, whereas adaptive coping enhances it. The coping behaviors used may make the difference in whether a stressful situation becomes a crisis.

The positive outcome of crisis is that persons may function at a higher level than before. Therefore, the nurse focuses on the person's strengths and abilities to change and adapt, and provides positive reinforcement by pointing out the person's past successes. Nurses often provide support during crises. In a situational crisis such as acute illness, they identify a person's strengths and provide emotional or physical support (e.g., being a sounding board or giving physical care).

(*text continues on page 178*)

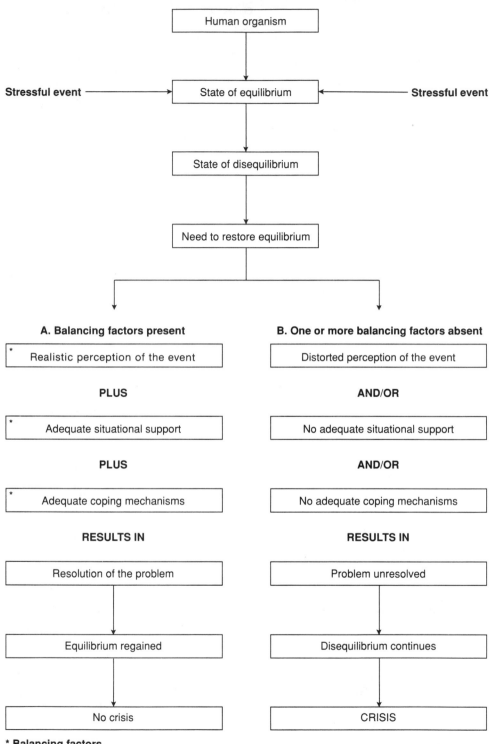

FIGURE 6-2 Effect of balancing factors in a stressful event. (Aguilera, D.C., [1990]. *Crisis Intervention: Theory and Methodology,* [6th ed., p 66]. St. Louis: CV Mosby.)

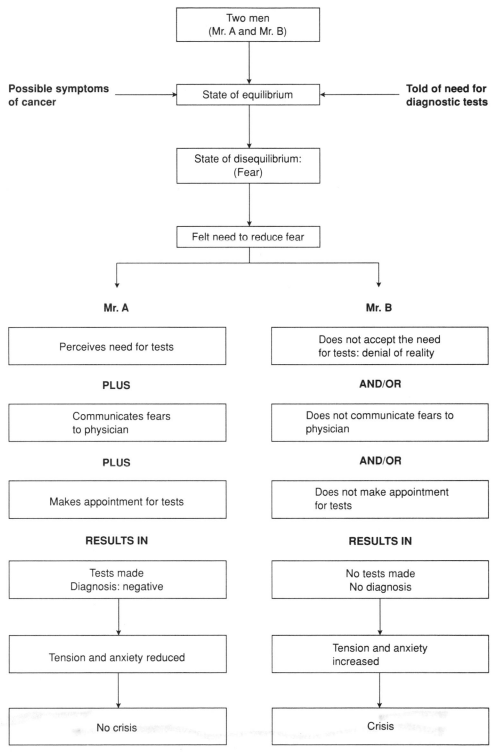

FIGURE 6-3 Paradigm applied to case study.

During developmental crises, nurses provide guidance to give persons the necessary skills for helping themselves.

*A*daptation Model: Implications for Nursing Practice

The display at the end of this chapter is an example of a client who has experienced a situational crisis. The elements of health and adaptation are evident in this situation. The client has experienced a crisis and has begun to cope with it.

Several elements of the adaptation process that are affecting Jan's health can be identified in this situation. Jan is currently experiencing several stressors, including her parent's increasing dependence on her, her own health problems, and hospitalization. She is undergoing a situational crisis because her usual coping methods are ineffective in helping her deal with these stressors. Notice that when Jan felt totally unable to cope with stress, she developed a physical symptom (blurred vision). This point illustrates the relationship between health and adaptation. Jan had inadequate energy to cope with psychological stress; she drew energy from her biologic subsystem, causing it to become less healthy also. Jan has an absence of balancing factors, as described in Figure 6-2. She has little situational support from her family, and few effective coping mechanisms to deal with this situation. Her usual coping mechanisms include overeating, controlling situations through strict schedules or routines, and problem solving.

When the nurses interfere with one of her most important coping mechanisms (control), Jan has no way to deal with anxiety, as evidenced by her reaction of anger. Nursing care is focused on assisting Jan to resolve her crisis. Jan's nurse will use Jan's coping resources to help her become independent. This aid requires knowledge of Jan's strengths, her current level of anxiety, her past methods of coping, and the current stressors in her life. Because Jan is in a moderate state of anxiety, her nurse can help her to think of new ways to deal with the situation. The nurse and Jan set goals together for crisis resolution. Because control is the coping mechanism that Jan is currently using, her nurse develops ways of returning a sense of control. These methods involve teaching her to care for her infected wound, following her schedule as closely as possible, and encouraging her to make her own decisions about her hospital care. In this way, Jan's nurse supports the development of healthy adaptive mechanisms and wellness. The nurse might also talk with Jan about how she can use her social supports to help her deal with her parent's health needs. Other resources, such as a community health nurse or social worker, might be called to give additional support after Jan's discharge from the hospital.

*E*udaimonistic Model

Eudaemonia, from which this model's name is derived, refers to a state of happiness as the result of an active life governed by reason. This model is represented by the work of humanistic psychologists, particularly Abraham Maslow. Humanistic psychologists based their work on a belief in the uniqueness and wholeness of persons, and recognized qualities such as potential for growth, individuality, autonomy, self-realization, and productivity. As a result of the humanistic movement, perspectives of health began to broaden; perceptions of human potential expanded. Health was defined as actualization or realization of one's potential. Illness was defined as a condition that prevented self-actualization.

H.L. Dunn (1959), a physician with the U. S. Public Health Service for many years, reflected the views of the humanistic psychologists when he wrote,

> Good health can exist as a relatively passive state of freedom from illness in which the individual is at peace with his environment—a condition of relative homeostasis. Wellness is conceptualized as dynamic—a condition of change in which the individual moves forward, climbing toward a higher potential of functioning (p. 447).

He defined **high-level wellness** as "an integrated method of functioning which is oriented toward maximizing the potential of which the individual is capable within the environment where he is functioning" (p. 447). High-level wellness involves the following:

- ❏ A continuing improvement in the way we function
- ❏ Continuing progress in our ability to respond to life's challenges
- ❏ Increasing oneness of our whole being—mind, body, and spirit—in the way we function

This model has been integrated into many of the nursing definitions of health. Within the eudaimonistic model, the client is a rational and free-thinking person capable of self-determination and autonomy. Persons are responsible for their own health care. Health is a process of growth or becoming. Realization of one's potential rather than stability is the essence of health. Change is desirable and even necessary to achieve one's potential. Madrid and Winstead-Fry (1986) wrote that health is "participation in the life process by choosing and executing behaviors that lead to the fulfillment of a person's potential"(p. 91). This view is consistent with many clients' views of health. Woods et al. (1988) studied the meaning of health for 528 women from diverse economic and ethnic backgrounds, and found a predominance of images that were consistent with actualization. The role of nurses and other health professionals within this model is to assist clients to achieve self-actualization.

Recently, this model has been criticized for focusing exclusively on individual health. For many persons, well-being is defined in terms of the health of the family or the community. This model also has been criticized for being biased toward Western values. The goal of high-level wellness may be irrelevant to nurses in undeveloped countries, where adequate food and safe drinking water are the most significant health concerns.

Experiential Model of Health

In the past decade, nurses have questioned the premises of existing models of health, particularly their focus on equilibrium and stability and the assumption that there are universal norms for wellness. Recent nursing theories view health as a life experience. In this view, nursing focuses on the experience of health for clients and the meanings given to this experience. Some nursing theorists who have developed these ideas include Martha Rogers (1990), Jean Watson (1988), and Madeleine Leininger (1991). From the writings of these theorists, and other nurses who share their assumptions about health, several themes emerge.

Health is the experience of well-being. Rogers believed that persons and environments are engaged in a continuous mutual process that is directed toward change and growth. Leininger described health as a state of well-being that is culturally defined, valued, and practiced. Jean Watson viewed health as unity and harmony among the mind, body, and soul that leads to self-awareness, inner strength, and transcendence. In the experiential model of health, care is directed toward the whole person. The focus is on dealing with the experience and expressions of illness or health.

Health is characterized by patterns and meanings for individuals and groups. Rather than focusing on coping processes and client responses, the experiential model of health focuses on understanding health from the client's perspective. How people live with illness and suffering, and the personal experience of feeling well, provide the basis for meaningful care. Benner and Wrubel (1989) call the discovery of meanings "understanding the lived experience of the illness"(p. 9). Pender (1990) identified five categories of expressions of health (affect, activity, attitudes, aspirations, and accomplishments) from person's descriptions of their own well-being in the United States.

Health is defined by its context. There are no universal norms for health; health depends on the client's situation. Leininger and Rogers make this point when they consider how various societies define wellness and illness. What is wellness in one culture may not be valued as such by another. What is health for the dying person is different than health for a newborn. Even physiologic norms vary depending on factors such as age, gender, and ethnic origin. Nurses risk giving inappropriate care if they have a normative view of health.

There is a distinction between illness and disease. Illness is subjective; only the person experiencing it can describe it. Disease is defined by objective parameters such as behavioral manifestations. Watson (1988) stated that illness is the experience of disharmony within the spheres of the person, and can lead to physical or behavioral manifestations of disease. Nurses are concerned with both illness and disease. Knowing how persons live day to day with health-related concerns provides the basis for nursing care that is relevant to the client as an individual.

The experiential model of health encompasses emerging concerns about **quality of life** as an outcome of health care. Quality of life is defined as the subjective experience of well-being that includes physical, mental, and social dimensions. Before the 1970's, assessments of health outcomes focused on length of survival, regardless of quality of life. In the past several decades, clients' *experiences* of health after treatment have received increased attention. Quality of life issues imply that a treatment must be evaluated for its detrimental effect on social, emotional, and physical functioning in addition to its effect on survival. This approach is consistent with nursing's emphasis on the day-to-day experience of health and illness. See Chapter 11 for a discussion of ethical concerns regarding quality of life.

Clinical Example

The following example illustrates some of the common themes of experiential models of health. The situation is described by an experienced intensive care unit (ICU) nurse in the following display.

Jan is a 42-year-old female client who underwent a hysterectomy 1 month ago. After leaving the hospital, she noticed that her surgical wound reddened, swelled, and began to drain pus. She was re-admitted with a wound abscess. Jan also has been diabetic for 12 years and takes daily insulin injections. She is knowledgeable about her disease and has developed a strict schedule for herself to control it.

Jan has a difficult family life. She states that her mother has a history of emotional problems and relies on Jan to make even the simplest decisions, and her father is experiencing memory loss due to aging and often forgets where he is. Jan expresses concern about caring for her parents. Jan is very close to her sister and a niece and has many friends in her church group. She also has a dog whom she describes as "almost human. . . we really understand each other."

Jan weighs 242 pounds. She says she often feels lonely, depressed, or anxious and overeats to "feel better." She is trying to change by recognizing her eating habits and developing new eating behaviors.

In the hospital, Jan's infected wound is cleaned and dressed three times daily. Jan will need to clean and dress her wound herself after discharge. She experienced blurred vision soon after this hospital admission, for which no physical cause could be found. She states, "I realized that I was probably feeling overwhelmed at having to take care of my parents and their problems after I went home, on top of doing all those dressing changes and watching my diabetes. I guess my vision problem was a way to get out of all the demands on me. As soon as I recognized this, my blurred vision went away."

Jan has established a strict routine in the hospital. When this routine is followed, she feels comfortable in the hospital environment. However, if the nurses do not include her in planning her own care, such as determining times for dressing changes, she becomes visibly anxious and angry. Jan is open and expresses her feelings readily. She can identify her own weakness and strengths and is usually able to solve problems. She assumes responsibility for as much of her own care as possible, yet asks for assistance when she needs it.

The client was a 43-year-old man who had experienced a massive myocardial infarction (heart attack) during a cardiac catheterization. I attended the cardiac arrest as the ICU nurse on code duty for that day. When I arrived, I saw a failing cardiac pattern on the electrocardiogram monitor, doctors of various levels of expertise yelling at each other, and a pharmacist mixing drugs quickly. A medical student was doing chest compressions, and the patient was still conscious, with a look of wild terror in his eyes.

(continued)

Observing that the patient's physical needs were being attended to, I spoke to him in soft tones that contrasted with the general chaos in the room. I rubbed his arm and told him that he was having a heart attack, but that we would take good care of him. I told him that he would lose consciousness, but that we would be there with him helping him breathe until the doctors were able to get his attack under control. As a seasoned nurse, I knew his chances of survival were nil, yet none of what I told him was an untruth. As I spoke to him and touched him, the fear left his eyes and he was able to focus on my face. He too, knew that he wasn't going to survive, but in the moment that we looked at each other, we shared hope and gratitude that enriched us both. I continued to talk to him until he lost consciousness and was intubated. In the course of 1 hour, he died. I performed all the technical tasks I had been trained to do, but my real work had been accomplished in the first few minutes.

Mary Gail Blazier, RN.

This example illustrates several themes from nursing models that focus on the experience of health. The nurse viewed health as a process of actualization. For the dying man, realization of his potential meant death with dignity. Using reassurance, touch, and giving information, the nurse focused on her client's humanity rather than just the medical emergency at hand.

The nurse in the example also defined health from the client's perspective. As she attempted to understand his personal experience of the emergency, she observed the terror on his face and his ability to comprehend his own imminent death. In a brief time, she was able to understand the fear of dying unexpectedly among strangers. Her assurance that the health care team would not abandon him illustrates ''understanding the lived experience of the illness.''

The nurse also differentiated between the client's illness and the disease. Although the client was ill with a massive heart attack, the significant disease in this situation was his fear of dying. This nurse knew that nothing could be done about this patient's disease; his death was inevitable. However, the nurse knew she could care for him in his illness, to promote a peaceful death. Her nursing care demonstrates a consideration for the whole client—body, mind, and soul. Death was not a failure for her, because she was able to help this client end life with dignity and serenity, thus accomplishing an important and meaningful goal.

Analysis of Models

The various models of health pose several questions. Using the clinical model, how do we explain the variety of responses we see among persons exposed to the same organisms or traumas? Not everyone becomes ill when exposed to the same environment. The ecological model describes the susceptibility of individuals to illness. Yet, how do we evaluate who is susceptible and who is not when all other factors are present, as in the ecological and clinical models? The adaptive model focuses on the organism as a whole, but does not consider health as a growth process. The experiential model of health is emerging in nursing as a view that encompasses both growth and holism.

These models suggest a number of perspectives about health. Today, nurses

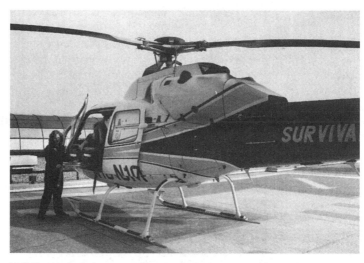

Holistic care includes responding to physical emergencies.

encounter many views about health held by persons from different cultures in the United States and elsewhere. Therefore, it is important that nurses understand the biologic, psychologic, sociocultural, and environmental facets of persons who may be patients or clients. Nursing theorists have noted the importance of defining health to identify the unique services that nurses provide. Nursing has often distinguished itself from medicine by claiming to have a focus on health rather than on disease. This distinction challenges us to continue to develop definitions of health from a nursing perspective.

Health Behavior

Efforts by some theorists to define health have been directed toward objective criteria, namely behavior. **Behavior** refers to an emitted response (action or reaction); it is overt, observable, and measurable. Consequently, scientists in the health care fields have begun research to define and clarify behavior as outcomes that can be measured and evaluated.

The concept of health behavior is quite complex and extensive, as evidenced by the literature on the subject. Pender (1996) noted that it is important to differentiate between behavior that is directed toward illness prevention and behavior that is oriented toward health promotion. **Health-protection behavior,** or preventive behavior, aims to decrease the probability of illness, emphasizes early diagnosis and treatment of disease, or may be focused on rehabilitation following disease. **Health-promotion behavior** is directed toward increasing the level of well-being and actualizing the health potential of individuals, families, communities, and society.

Health-Protection Behavior

Three types of health protection behavior have been described: primary prevention, secondary prevention, and tertiary prevention. Primary prevention emphasizes protection against the occurrence of specific diseases, and might include actions such as immunizations and air pollution control. Secondary prevention focuses on early detection and treatment of disease in susceptible persons. It includes efforts such as cholesterol screening and breast or testicular self-examination. Tertiary prevention is directed toward reducing disability following disease. An example is rehabilitation after an acute disease episode such as a spinal cord injury.

The Health Belief Model (Becker, 1977) is a framework for explaining a person's motivation to take action to prevent illness. (See Figure 6-4.) In this model, beliefs about personal susceptibility and the seriousness of a disease increase the perceived threat of disease. Other factors such as knowledge level and influence of significant others also affect perceived threat. Perceived threat and perceived benefits and barriers to action are factors that increase the likelihood of taking preventive action. For example, a middle-aged female may decide to stop smoking because she has read several articles that state that the risk of heart disease increases as women approach menopause, thus raising her perceived susceptibility and the perceived threat of heart attack.

The Health Belief Model can be useful in explaining clients' adherence to treatment recommendations such as diet changes or medications. As an example, if a medication to reduce blood pressure is expensive and produces unpleasant side effects, the perceived barriers to taking pills will outweigh the threat of hypertension, a disease in which there are few symptoms. These factors may explain why a client neglects to take antihypertensive medication.

Health-Promotion Behavior

Health-promotion behavior involves actions that enhance health. Unlike preventive-behaviors, they are not motivated by threat. In the 1980's, Nola Pender, a nurse, developed a framework to explain motivation to engage in health-promotion behaviors, as illustrated in Figure 6-5. In her model, factors such as prior related behavior and personal factors influence behavior-specific thoughts and feelings. These thoughts and feelings are related to the commitment to a plan of action and the actual performance of health-promoting behavior. For example, a college student who begins a regular exercise program may have been influenced by enjoyable sports participation in high school, perceived benefits such as weight control, a belief that she can successfully carry out her program, and the influence of her best friend who asked her to exercise with her.

Self-Care and Health Behavior

Self-care is a nursing concept that is related to health-behavior. Self-care has been defined as activities individuals perform that are directed to themselves or their environments to regulate their own functioning and development to

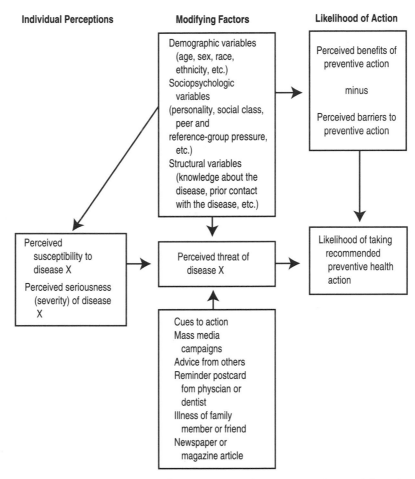

Individual Perceptions   **Modifying Factors**   **Likelihood of Action**

FIGURE 6-4 Health Belief Model. (Becker, M. H., Haefner, D. P., Kast, S. V., et al., [1977]. Selected psychosocial models and correlates of individual health-related behaviors. *Medical Care, 15,* p. 27-46.

maintain or enhance life, health, and well-being (Orem, 1995). The tremendous growth in the number of self-help groups in the past two decades is evidence of clients' increased role in maintaining or recovering their health. Alcoholics Anonymous and Weight Watchers are some of the many self-help groups.

Orem's definition of self-care implies that nurses assist clients with health care practices and activities of daily living when clients are unable to care for themselves. Thus, nurses have long been supportive of clients' health-related self-care activities. Helen Erickson's (Erickson et al., 1983) concept of self-care incorporates the belief that individuals know the kind of help they need to mobilize their own strengths and resources. Erickson has said that those who are ill know what has made them ill and what will make them well. Caring (well) for

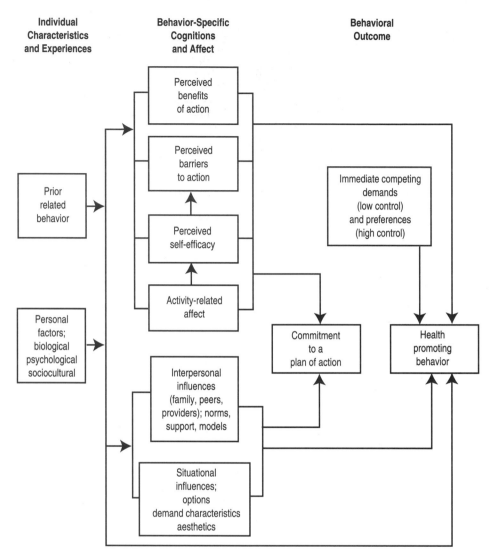

FIGURE 6-5 Revised Health Promotion Model. (Pender, N. J., [1996]. *Health promotion in nursing practice* [3rd ed., p. 67]. Stamford: Appleton & Lange.

oneself, taking (good) care of oneself, and "self-care for health" involve learning to know and exercise one's power to choose, as well as creating conditions within one's relationships with persons and one's environment wherein personal growth and development toward an even healthier state occur. These definitions suggest that nurses assist clients with their health-promotion and preventive activities as a means of empowering clients toward health. See Chapter 3 for more information on these concepts.

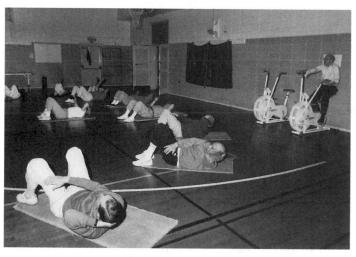

Persons enhance their sense of well-being by engaging in healthy activities.

Nurses' Role in Health-Protection and Health-Promotion

Because chronic diseases are the major causes of morbidity and mortality in developed countries, nurses are involved in increasing health protection and health-promotion behaviors in their clients. Behaviors such as exercise, good nutrition, and stress management can maximize a person's physical energy and sense of well-being. Both health-protection and health-promotion are important goals for nursing care.

Nurses participate in preventive and health-promoting activities in many settings, such as schools, clinics, the workplace, community health fairs, and the hospital. The following are examples of nursing roles:

Health-screening and wellness assessment. Nurses evaluate clients for risk factors for disease (such as sexual practices that pose risks for AIDS) and examine their lifestyle for habits that enhance health (e.g., good nutrition, exercise, and safety practices).

Health education and counselling. Nurses teach clients about health risks, self-management of chronic disease, and stress-management to enhance health. They also counsel clients about lifestyle changes and how to incorporate them—such as how to plan meals that are low in fat and high in fiber.

Implement wellness or preventive programs. Nurses may run immunization clinics, smoking-cessation programs, and parenting classes as ways of enhancing health and preventing problems.

Disseminate information. Nurses may be consultants or planners for media programs regarding health risks such as child abuse, alcohol use, and seat-belt practices. Newspaper articles, health fairs, and pamphlets are among the ways that nurses disseminate information to a community.

Summary

Ideas about health may be summarized in the following statements:

❏ Health is a dynamic process.
❏ Health is determined subjectively and objectively.
❏ Health is a goal.
❏ Health is being able to take care of yourself.
❏ Health is optimal functioning in body, mind, and spirit.
❏ Health is integrity of self.
❏ Health is a sense of wholeness.
❏ Health is coping adaptively.
❏ Health is a subjective experience.
❏ Health is growing and becoming.
❏ Health is a broad concept.
❏ Health is both an individual and societal issue.

Nurses will encounter a variety of health beliefs among clients. The challenge of promoting and protecting health is one of collaboration between nurse and client. The subject is a broad and engrossing one, and we encourage you to take advantage of the readings listed at the end of this chapter.

KEY CONCEPTS

The primitive model of health suggests that health and illness are controlled by forces external to humans

The ecological model of health includes concepts of a host, a disease-producing agent and an environment which interact to produce illness.

In the clinical model, health is the absence of disease or the opposite of illness; the focus is elimination of illness symptoms.

The role performance model represents health as the ability of a person to perform his or her roles effectively.

The adaptation model of health involves concepts of stress, anxiety, crisis, and coping.

The eudaimonistic model describes health as actualization or realization of one's potential.

The experiential model views health as the experience of well-being.

Nursing theorists have used the adaptation and experiential models to develop nursing perspectives of health.

Health behavior is the measurable and observable outcomes of health, which includes both health-protection and health-promotion.

Health promotion is preventive behavior that is directed toward increasing well-being of individuals, families, groups, and communities.

✓ Health protection is action that aims to decrease probability of illness, detect disease, or rehabilitate following disease.

✓ Self-care is activities that individuals perform to enhance health, is related to health behavior.

✓ Nurses protect and promote health by developing and implementing individual and community-based programs such as health screening and education in a variety of settings.

CRITICAL THINKING QUESTIONS

1. What is your personal definition of health? Of illness?

2. Discuss the various perspectives on health described in this chapter. What are the strengths and weaknesses of each view?

3. Describe the differences between the concepts of crisis, anxiety, stress, and coping.

4. Give three examples of life events that may lead to
   a. situational crisis.
   b. maturational crisis.

5. Think about some of your own experiences with health problems. Which of the models of health were your health care providers using to provide care? Which model best fits with your personal definition of health?

6. Mr. Raymond has been caring for his wife at home since she developed symptoms of dementia four years ago. His wife is becoming increasingly confused, but he believes that she is best managed in their own home. Mr. Raymond has had a long history of high blood pressure and reluctantly admits that it is becoming difficult for him to be the only care-provider for his wife. How could you use one of the models of health to design nursing care for this family?

7. Define health behavior, health-promotion, and health-protection. What are your own preventive and health-promotion practices?

REFERENCES

Aguilera, D.C. (1994). *Crisis intervention: Theory and methodology* (7th ed.). St. Louis, MO: C.V. Mosby.

Allport, G.W. (1965). *Pattern and growth in personality.* New York: Holt, Rinehart & Winston.

Becker, M.H., Haefner, D.P., Kast, S.V., et al. (1977). Selected psychosocial models and correlates of individual health-related behaviors. *Medical Care,15*, 27–46.

Benner, P.E., & Wrubel, J. (1989). *The primacy of caring: Stress and coping in health and illness.* Menlo Park, CA: Addison-Wesley.

Cannon, W.B. (1939). *The wisdom of the body.* New York: W.W. Norton.

Caplan, G. (1964). *Principles of preventive psychiatry.* New York: Basic Books.

Dubos, R. (1965). *Man adapting.* New Haven, CT: Yale University Press.

Dunn, H.L. (1959). What high level wellness means. *Canadian Journal of Public Health, 50,* 447–457.

Erickson, H.C., Tomlin, E.M., & Swain, M.A. (1983). *Modeling and role-modeling: A theory and paradigm for nursing.* Englewood Cliffs, NJ: Prentice-Hall.

Erikson, E. (1963). *Childhood and society* (2nd ed.). New York: W.W. Norton.

Holmes, T.H., & Rahe, R.H. (1967). The Social Readjustment Rating Scale. *Journal of Psychosomatic Research, 11*(2), 213–218.

King, I.M. (1981). *A theory for nursing: Systems, concepts, process.* New York: Wiley.

Lantz, P.M., Dupuis, L., Reding, D., Krauska, M. & Lappe, K. Peer discussions of cancer among Hispanic migrant farm workers. *Public Health Reports, 109,* 512–520.

Lazarus, R.S. (1984). *Stress, appraisal and coping.* New York: Springer.

Leininger, M.M. (1991). The theory of culture care diversity and universality. In M.M. Leininger (Ed.), *Culture care diversity and universality: A theory of nursing* (Publication No. 15-2402, pp. 5–68). New York: National League for Nursing.

Levine, M.E. (1973). *Introduction to clinical nursing* (2nd ed.). Philadelphia: F.A. Davis.

Madrid, M., & Winsted-Fry, P. (1986). Rogers' conceptual model. In P. Winsted-Fry (Ed.), *Case studies in nursing theory* (pp. 73–102). New York: National League for Nursing.

Neuman, B. (1995). *The Neuman Systems Model* (3rd ed.). Norwalk, CT: Appleton & Lange.

Orem, D.E. (1995). *Nursing: Concepts of practice* (5th ed.). St. Louis, MO: Mosby Year Book.

Parsons, T. (1972). Definitions of health and illness in light of American values and social structure. In E. Jacob (Ed.), *Patients, physicians and illness* (2nd ed., pp. 107–137). New York: Free Press.

Pender, N.J. (1990). Expressing health through lifestyle patterns. *Nursing Science Quarterly, 3*(3), 115–122.

Pender, N.J. (1996). *Health promotion in nursing practice* (3rd ed.). Stamford, CT: Appleton & Lange.

Rogers, M.E. (1990). Nursing: Science of unitary, irreducible, human beings: Update 1990. In E.A.M. Barrett (Ed.), *Visions of Rogers' science-based nursing* (Publication No. 15-2285, pp. 5–11). New York: National League for Nursing.

Roy, S.C. & Andrews, H.A. (1991). *The Roy Adaptation Model: The definitive statement.* Norwalk, CT: Appleton & Lange.

Selye, H. (1956). *The stress of life.* New York: McGraw-Hill.

Smith, J.A. (1983). *The idea of health.* New York: Teachers College Press.

Smith, J.A. (1981). The idea of health: A philosophical inquiry. *Advances in Nursing Science, 3*(3), 43–50.

Watson, J. (1988). *Nursing: Human science and human care.* New York: National League for Nursing.

Woods, N.F., Laffrey, S., Duffy, M., Lentz, M.J., Mitchell, E.S., Taylor, D., & Cowan, K.A. (1988). Being healthy: Women's images. *Advances in Nursing Science, 11*(1), 36–46.

World Health Organization, Interim Commission. (1947). Constitution of the World Health Organization. *Chronical of the World Health Organization, 1,* 29.

Part Three

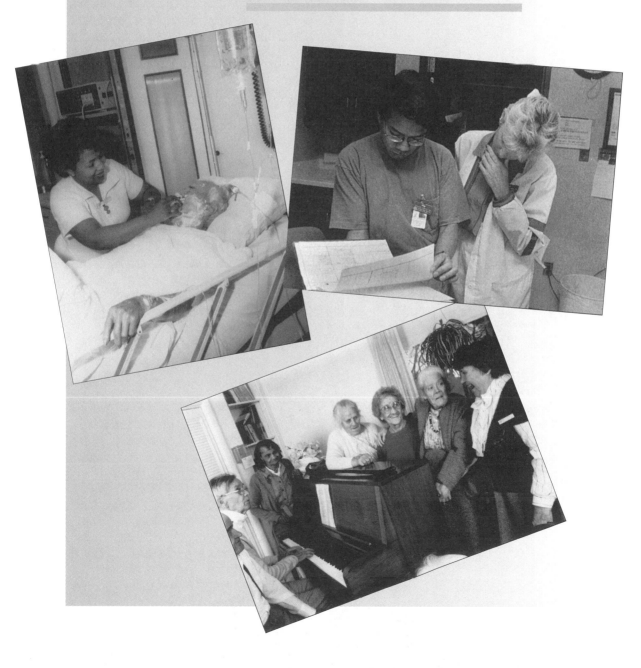

7

Health Care Delivery

Objectives

After completing this chapter, students will be able to:

Identify the major problems of health care delivery.

Discuss the contribution of nursing to health care delivery.

Discuss several ways in which government and the private sector have attempted to manage health care delivery.

Identify health problems of persons in the United States.

Discuss the consumer movement in health care.

Health care delivery has changed remarkably in the last decade. Some observers call the change revolutionary; others, sensing the magnitude of change needed, call the changes to date merely evolutionary. Regardless of perspective, most observers expect future changes of geometric proportions. For example, gene therapy suggests as yet incomprehensible possibilities. At the same time, wide-ranging entitlements such as Medicare and Medicaid threaten to bankrupt the system that created them. Whatever changes ensue in the next millennium, understanding health care delivery as it has developed during the present century is basic to understanding future changes, related issues, and their implications for all health professionals.

Health care delivery in the United States is a huge and heavily stressed system. Health care services frequently are inconsistent, but miraculously lifesaving and curing. The needs of the people within our large and diverse nation are often beyond the resources of this system that deals fairly well with immediate crises, but less well when longer-term, consistent care is needed. For example, in the past 20 years, major advances in life-support systems, transplant programs, and chemotherapy have saved thousands of lives. However, new health care challenges such as substance abuse, AIDS, and Alzheimer's disease, which require long-term solutions, have surfaced. Premature newborns, as well as others who come through grave injuries from motor vehicle and work-related accidents, are treated well at the critical moments, but virtually abandoned when life-long and expensive care is needed. We see longer but not always healthier life spans, as persons with major disabilities survive. These serious but chronic problems do not fare well with current programs.

In addition, millions of homeless persons, as well as the victims of violence throughout U.S. cities, have presented health problems largely ignored by the current focus of health care delivery. As the costs of programs to solve these various problems escalate, our abilities to intervene are severely limited. Moreover, health care is simply inaccessible to many because they do not have the ability to pay. During the current decade, an estimated 31 million people have been uninsured. While we may assume that these are people living below the Federal poverty level, only 25% actually do (Hess, 1993). Many people with reasonable incomes do not receive health insurance benefits at work and cannot afford to buy benefits themselves. Students are often within this group, particularly when they are no longer carried on their parents' insurance. Small business owners, those who work for them, and the elderly or others on adequate (if nothing goes wrong) but fixed incomes are also part of this group. Considering this problem, Munson (1996) states, ''The result then is likely to be the emergence of a three-tier system in which the rich get the care they need, the middle class the care they can afford, and the poor the care we are willing to give them'' (p. 611). As Norling (1996) stated, ''Our society has failed to address social problems until they become medical problems, which is why they now account for a significant portion of our health care expenditures'' (p. 54). Nurses have always known that economic and social concerns are often the predecessors of poor physical and emotional health. As a nation, and as a profession, we must now come to terms with the health care crisis.

We are all consumers of health commodities and health services. Although we want to spend money wisely and receive value in return, we may settle for less than the best because of the expense involved or a lack of awareness about other available products. During an illness, it is especially difficult to make effective decisions concerning health care. Moreover, nurses who understand the characteristics of the health care consumer and the variables that influence health behavior can act as client advocates and assist clients to participate in promotional and preventive health care.

Health Care Delivery as a System

An exploration of **health care delivery** in the United States today may help us to understand the problems. Current literature on health care often describes it as a "system." As indicated in Chapter 4, a *system* is an organized unit with a set of components that mutually react and function as a whole or total entity. Health care delivery comprises many smaller systems, or subsystems. For example, in some communities clinics, pharmacies, and the community hospital may function as components of a larger system of health care. Agencies such as heart or diabetic associations, the Visiting Nurses Association (VNA), and the United Way may work together with other smaller system components. In that case, overall health care delivery in the community can be described as a system.

However, when persons in that community are referred to a large medical center, they may find themselves in an unfamiliar and "unsystematic" environment. Too often, persons entering large health care facilities feel overwhelmed by the system. They encounter specialists from several professions, many clinics, painful diagnostic procedures, long waits, and difficulty finding their way around.

Consider the experiences that you, your family, or friends have encountered in the health care system. Perhaps you have known someone who needed several services in the course of one illness. This person started with a family physician, and then was sent to a large hospital. There, he or she was referred to the social services department for financial assistance, given physical therapy, and provided with nutritional counseling from a dietitian. After returning home, the person was visited by a community nurse, and bought medicines and supplies from the nearest pharmacy. Consider this example and the following questions:

Is there a common philosophy of health and health care among the agencies and caregivers?

Are the person's basic needs considered when care is planned, and does the person participate in this plan?

Is there effective transfer of records and appropriate data about the person among agencies, caregivers, and the person seeking health care?

Do nurses function as coordinators of care?

You may note from these questions that the concept of "system" does not apply well to health care delivery, either economically or philosophically. Solutions to these problems require that health care professionals and governmental agencies collaborate and base health care delivery on a common philosophic framework.

Problems in Health Care Delivery

Current health care is actually an industry that sells products and services, often emphasizing illness rather than health. Consider the following problems associated with our current structure of health care:

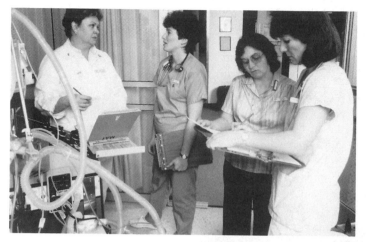

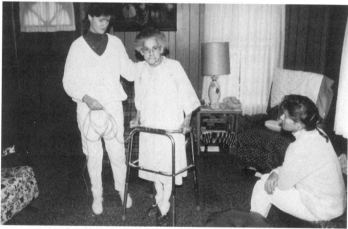

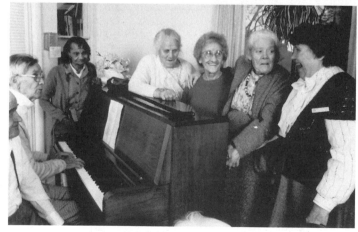

Health care delivery takes place in the hospital, the home, and the community.

❑ Emphasis on illness rather than on health promotion
❑ Insufficient standards to ensure quality
❑ Minimal consumer participation
❑ Poor coordination and inequitable distribution of services
❑ Inadequate collaboration among providers of services
❑ Extremely high costs

Health Care Providers

Health care providers constitute a major component of the health care delivery system, with the largest groups being registered nurses (RNs), physicians (with doctor of medicine or doctor of osteopathy degrees), pharmacists, and dentists. During the early 1990s, nurses (RNs) constituted the largest group, with about 1.8 million members. In addition, there were approximately 555,000 licensed practical nurses (LPNs) and 1.1 million assistive nursing personnel. Other groups included physicians, with 600,000 members; pharmacists, with 175,000 members; and dentists, with 150,000 members (U.S. Department of Health and Human Services [HHS], 1993). Although the number of nurses will increase through the mid-1990s, it will begin to decline during the early 21st century. The supply of RNs per 100,000 people will increase to a maximum of 713 in 2000, and will then decline to 558 by 2020. In general, other professional groups will follow similar trends. Although nursing numbers may drop below the needs of the nation, it is thought that "the ratio of physicians to the population will continue to increase into the next century as the supply of physicians grows faster than the population" (U.S. Dept. HHS, 1993, p. 53). Unfortunately, certain desirable geographic areas may have an overabundance, whereas cities and rural areas may be lacking.

The preceding figures indicate that the nursing profession is twice the size of any other health profession. Clearly, nursing ought to have a great effect on the health of this nation. However, health and illness care provided by nurses is often difficult to quantify. Significantly, nursing is the only group to provide regular, consistent, around-the-clock care. For real changes to occur in the health care delivery industry, nursing leadership in collaboration with other professionals must be as evident as the numbers indicate it should be.

Other health care professionals and providers include nutritionists, dietitians, physical and occupational therapists, optometrists, and audiologists. These persons also contribute many skills to health care delivery. Other professionals closely associated with the health care industry assist with rehabilitation (e.g., social workers, psychologists, speech therapists, and vocational rehabilitation counselors).

The health professions and the federal government frequently conduct studies to determine whether current personnel supplies are meeting society's needs. This information helps with plans to raise or lower the number of professionals in a particular group. Changes in one group may have an impact on the functions of another. For example, if there are not enough physicians to meet medical care needs, nurses may suddenly be considered capable of performing tasks and procedures previously thought to be medical in nature. As the number of physicians increases, nurses may be considered less competent for those duties.

Consider also the functions, as well as the supply, of health care providers. For example, the team approach is believed essential for effective care. Each professional has a set of skills seen as necessary to provide quality care. Unfortunately, we can overwhelm our clients when we ask them to relate to a team that may consist of nurse, physician, pharmacist, dietitian, physical therapist, social worker, and chaplain. Clients' needs will vary, and they may indeed need direct care from these professionals. However, as nurses, we consider all of our varied skills. As the professional having the most direct contact with the client, the nurse acts as a **coordinator of care.** The nurse relates to the team, whereas the client relates to the nurse as caregiver. Nurses can assist the client in making more effective use of other professional resources. The trend for clients to seek nurses as primary health care providers is growing. Note the discussion in Chapter 12 related to nurse practitioners and nurses in advanced practice.

Hess, RN (1993), writing for The Department of Health and Human Services, indicates the following important points in planning for the nurse workforce appropriate for current and future health care delivery:

- ❐ Increase the supply of baccalaureate trained nurses and master's prepared advanced practice nurses for non-hospital settings.
- ❐ Meet the continuing challenge of attracting the best and brightest of our youth to a nursing career.
- ❐ Strengthen enrollments in baccalaureate programs of students from racially and ethnically diverse backgrounds.
- ❐ Prepare students entering associate degree programs for the need to continue their education and achieve a baccalaureate degree.
- ❐ Increase opportunities for students to develop and master the skills needed in high technology environments.
- ❐ Develop partnerships between schools of nursing and practice institutions to meet the high technology demands of all settings.
- ❐ Provide more tools for systematic problem-solving and autonomous practice in community.
- ❐ Meet the demand for advanced practice nurses and nurse practitioners to function in primary health care provider roles.
- ❐ Recruit nursing faculty with advanced practice nursing expertise (p. 43–45).

Historical Influences in Health Care Delivery

Several changes have occurred in the United States since World War II (Table 7-1). Advances in science and technology, with the accompanying movement from rural to industrial areas, have resulted in changing needs for health care. However, some needs may have existed long before they were recognized. For example, a growth in the number of indigent persons was followed by an increased incidence in the health problems for this segment of the population. Yet, this phenomenon may reflect the improvement in census activities rather than an increase in actual numbers.

Changes in family structure, civil rights demonstrations, and the emergence of the consumer movement have affected our current method of health care delivery. For example, older persons stay productive and are able to maintain their own homes longer than was previously true. They often continue working at their careers or engage in more meaningful recreational, social, and charitable activities. Many older adults are more independent than their forerunners and, as a result, often do not live with their adult children. When these persons become ill or disabled, their long-term needs greatly increase the costs of national health care.

Although substance abuse, eating disorders, and sexually transmitted diseases (STDs) have existed for years, they have increased greatly in the past 5 to 10 years. In particular, cocaine addiction and AIDS have presented a series of new challenges similar to those of infectious diseases and mental illness in the early part of the 20th century.

As indicated in Chapter 3, changes in nursing also have influenced health care delivery. As nurses pursue professional development, they are recognizing their unique contributions to the health needs of society; they are beginning to influence health care legislation and the politics of health care delivery. (See legal and ethical issue discussion in Chapter 11.)

Legislation represents another historical influence on health care. For example, legislation has provided monies for physical facilities, resulting in a prominence of tertiary care. **Tertiary care** is care that occurs in highly specialized institutions that provide sophisticated diagnosis and treatment. Although persons may receive care in either the hospital or the ambulatory-care setting, it is generally considered to be long-term care.

Legislation also has attempted to place controls on the accessibility, quality, and cost of health care. Legislation has been enacted to ensure the safety and efficacy of the drugs that are developed and distributed for general use in society. Specific legislation is discussed later.

Ethical issues are more prominent now than ever before in our history. Perhaps most issues are actually very old, but they are resurfacing at a faster rate than in the past. For example, even as recently as twenty years ago, abortion was barely mentioned in public. Even though now it is a common discussion, and while many have always been against it, there has been a recent and passionate upsurge of activity denouncing abortion. Issues such as who should receive scarce resources, (e.g., organs, or expensive treatments), who should live (e.g., the deformed or very premature infant, the severely handicapped and the elderly) and who should have the right to die, are debated daily in many forums. One major question in many circles today is whether people have the right to receive health care if they cannot pay for it.

Health Problems of Persons in the United States

Despite the many problems discussed in this section, we should emphasize that Americans are a healthier people and have become progressively more so since 1900.

(*text continues on page 202*)

TABLE 7-1 *Historical Influences in Health Care Delivery*

Changes	Influences
Population dynamics since 1940	Increase in 　General population 　Nonwhite population 　Life expectancy and birth rates among nonwhite persons 　Proportion of foreign-born persons
Urbanization	Movement into suburbs
	Increase in 　Marriage and divorce rates 　Illegitimacy and teenage pregnancy 　Pregnant women who do not receive prenatal care 　Unemployment rate 　Adult crime and juvenile delinquency 　Violence in cities 　Numbers of persons living in substandard housing 　Numbers of persons living at the poverty level 　Homelessness 　Older adult population 　Automobile accidents, homicides, and suicides 　Infant mortality rate and birth defects 　Violence in the workplace and at home
Industrialization	Decrease in 　Farming 　Self-sufficiency once common among rural population
Literacy and education	Increases in 　Knowledge about health care 　Demand for more higher-quality care 　Demand for more knowledge 　Information technology
Economic status	Wider range between high and low economic status
	Increase in government and private health insurance programs
	Major changes in health care delivery structures
	Capitation
	Managed care
	Shorter hospital stays
	Ambulatory surgery
	Increases in co-payments
Advances in science and technology	Control of infectious diseases
	Development of drugs for control of many serious illnesses
	New and lifesaving surgical techniques
	Life-maintenance techniques and equipment
	Hazardous industry
	Pollution resulting in increase in lung cancer and heart disease
Family structural changes	Breadwinner other than father
	New family structures (e.g., communal living)
	Single-parent families
	Working mothers
	Grandparents in own homes, far from adult children
	Same sex partners
Civil rights movements	Equality in health care as a right
	Equality regardless of race, creed, gender
	Women's liberation movement

(continued)

TABLE 7-1 (Continued)

Changes	Influences
Consumerism	Change in consumer concept of health and illness
	Self-help groups
	Increase in litigation
	Ethical dilemmas
	Gene therapy
	Invitro fertilization
	Who should live and who should die?
	Right to die
	Physician-assisted suicide
Nursing profession	Increase in sense of accountability and responsibility
	Greater independence and autonomy
	More involvement in health policies and politics
	Nurse practitioners
	Advanced practice nurses
Legislation	Hill–Burton Act of 1946
	Amendments of the Federal Food, Drug and Cosmetic Act of 1938
	Durham–Humphrey (1952)
	Kefauver–Harris (1962)
	Department of Health, Education, and Welfare (1953)
	Community Mental Health Centers Act (1963)
	Regional Medical Program (1965)
	Comprehensive Health Planning Program (1966)
	Social Security Amendments
	Title XVIII Medicare (1966)
	Title XIX Medicaid (1966)
	Comprehensive Drug Abuse Prevention and Control Act of 1970
	Health Maintenance Organization Act of 1973
	Professional Standards Review Organization Act of 1973
	Child Abuse Prevention and Treatment Act of 1974
	National Health Planning and Resources Development Act of 1974
	Generic and Brand Names for Drugs Legislation (1977)
	The Tax Equity and Fiscal Responsibility Act of 1982–TEFRA (Introduced DRG)
	Social Security Amendment of 1983: Medicare prospective payment, P.L. 98–21
	National Organ Procurement Act of 1984
	Consolidated Omnibus Budget Reconciliation Act of 1985–COBRA
	The Medicare Catastrophic Coverage Act of 1988
	Americans with Disabilities Act (1991)
	Legislation before World War II
	U.S. Public Health Service (1798)
	Pure Food and Drug Act of 1906
	Social Security Act of 1935
	Federal Food, Drug and Cosmetic Act of 1938
	Omnibus Budget Reconciliation Act (1987)
	National Case Management Task Force (1995)
	Kassenbaum-Kennedy Bill (1996)

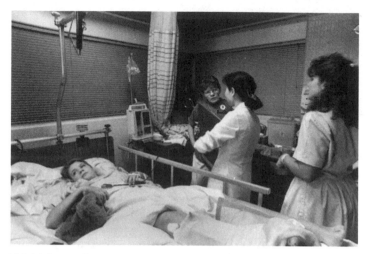

Maintaining quality in an era of diminishing resources requires a collaborative approach.

Diseases such as tuberculosis (TB), gastroenteritis, diphtheria, and poliomyelitis—major causes of disability and death early in the development of this country—are nearly nonexistent today. However, with the increase in homelessness and the number of persons below the poverty level, TB is again on the rise.

With the advent of antibiotics, bacteria-related diseases have become readily treatable—however, it is also wise to note that with the increased use of antibiotics, new strains of bacteria have developed that are resistant to many of our most potent antibiotics.

In 1900, the death rate per year was about 17 per 1000 persons, compared with 9 per 1000 persons recently.

Since World War II, the mortality rate for children aged 1 through 14 years has been cut in half.

Life expectancy has increased throughout the 20th century, from 47 years to 73 years. Cancer chemotherapy and new approaches to cardiac disease have had major positive effects on the cure rate of these health concerns (U.S. Dept. HHS, 1995-1996).

Advances in our national health resulted from a variety of developments: improvement in sanitation, housing, and nutrition; the advent of antibiotics and immunization programs, as well as the development of numerous drugs to control diabetes, hypertension, and other diseases; a growing awareness that certain lifestyles and habits impact on our health; and the emergence of more self-help groups and stress reduction techniques. However, in our complex society, with its diverse populations, we have barely begun to address the health needs of our people.

As these needs are being further considered, note the following goals and objectives described in the publication *Healthy People 2000: National Health Promo-*

tion and Disease Prevention (1995-1996). This publication indicates the following three goals for special focus over the next several years: increasing the span of healthy life for Americans, reducing health disparities among Americans, and achieving access to preventive services for all Americans. These objectives will be implemented through programs aimed at tobacco, cigarette smoking, substance abuse, highway safety, violence in the workplace, and firearms. In addition, other health problems such as diabetes, peptic ulcer disease, AIDS, and birth-related neurological anomalies will be targeted. These programs will be available in workplaces, neighborhood clinics, and other areas close to the people. They will consist of health education and counseling services, will have a certain amount of federal funding, and will establish linkages between current programs and primary care clinics (pp. 1–2).

Selected Contemporary Health Problems

Although many health problems cannot be described in this chapter, we have elected to discuss two contemporary problems—homelessness and AIDS—to help students view the issues these problems present. While health problems may have social, moral, and financial implications, other issues involved do not present themselves as readily. For example, assumptions are sometimes made that jobless people could find work; yet, if they do, they may lose their Social Security benefits while earning less money at a new job. Persons with STDs may be seen as irresponsible or immoral, yet they may be unwitting partners or patients infected by other persons. Furthermore, those who unsuccessfully attempt suicide can create more problems for themselves and society with a bullet than those with life-threatening illnesses related to substance abuse. Moreover, issues of personal rights such as sexual preference and the right to smoke must also be considered.

Homelessness

Homelessness arises from a variety of causes. A primary cause is the closure of many state and federal mental hospitals. In 1963, Congress passed President John F. Kennedy's Community Mental Health Centers Act. The purpose of the act was to deinstitutionalize the mentally ill and move them into the warmth and caring of the community. In general, communities responded well initially and instituted effective programs. In addition, many people were able to live independently or with minimal supervision, and some returned to their families. However, over time, systems became overloaded and funds were reduced, currently leaving many who are both homeless and mentally ill with minimal resources. Although a few mentally ill persons with health problems are violent, they are more likely to be treated poorly by others than to commit crimes themselves.

Other causes of homelessness are the rising cost of living and the loss of jobs. Car companies, which long have provided jobs, have closed some of their big plants, leaving people jobless and unable to pay their rent and maintain health care protection. Sometimes whole families live in an old car for shelter. Homelessness presents issues of illness, lack of health promotion, and limited access to health care, and contributes to devaluation of persons and decreased quality of life.

AIDS

AIDS is a complex of infectious diseases caused by a severe infection with the human immunodeficiency virus (HIV). AIDS was first recognized in the United States in New York and San Francisco in 1981, and nearly 1.5 million people in the United States are now infected with HIV. Among the many issues related to AIDS are the following: the threat of a global epidemic, intensive and expensive care demands, loss of human resources and talent, and the stigmatization of those infected.

Although AIDS presently is a serious public health risk, its spread can be limited by using the current knowledge we have about prevention. *AIDS is spread only through the exchange of blood or sexual secretions with an infected person.* There has been absolutely no transmission of an HIV infection through casual contact, which includes touching; talking; riding in a car; or sharing food, towels, cups, swimming pools, work areas, or bathrooms.

High-risk groups include homosexual, bisexual, and heterosexual persons who have had many sexual partners. Lesbian couples rarely have transmitted the virus, and transmission is more common from a man to a woman than from a woman to a man. It is also more likely that a patient will transmit to a caregiver than that a caregiver will infect a patient. Other high-risk groups include intravenous (IV) drug users who share needles or other equipment, persons with hemophilia, others who have had transfusions of blood products before 1985, and children born to HIV-infected women.

Over the next several years, nearly all of us in the United States will be affected in some way by AIDS. We may be infected ourselves or may have to watch the suffering and death of a loved one. This has already been true for many of us.

Recognize that AIDS is not just statistics and preventive measures. Although these points are important, statistics and preventive measures may cause us to overlook the tragedy of the condition. It is the loneliness, the too-frequent ostracizing by society, and the subsequent suffering that we must remember if, as nurses, we are going to make a difference for these people. Additionally, information about HIV and AIDS can be found by contacting infection control programs at major hospitals, local public health departments, and national AIDS information centers and hot lines.

One positive change for some persons with AIDS is the improvement in family relationships. Families are often more accepting now than they were, even just a few years ago, of homosexuality—one contributing factor to contracting AIDS. Some persons, estranged from families because of lifestyle, have been able to return to the fold and to find caring and concern there. Powell-Cope (1994), in her study on family caregivers of people with AIDS, found that caregivers appreciated being able to negotiate partnerships with health care providers. She indicated that these families are especially protective of their loved ones, and watch health care providers closely for signs of homophobia or fear of infection. As they learn to trust the care provider, they function well in a partnership where everyone works for the common good of the patient.

Health Problems Across the Life Span

Several health problems may occur across the life span (Table 7-2). Interestingly, injury is the leading cause of premature death in the United States (National Center for Health Statistics, 1988, p. 11). That many of these deaths are the result of homicide and suicide is noted by the U.S. Public Health Service Office of Disease Prevention and Health Promotion (1988, p. 40) and is more than ever true today.

Solutions

Many solutions for these problems have been proposed, and, indeed, a variety of health promotion policies and activities are already in place. Table 7-3 lists some currently available programs.

The aim of health-related programs is to increase society's awareness of existing needs. It is an attempt to help persons realize their options and take better care of themselves, thereby retaining control over their lives. However, Fitzgerald (1994) cautions us. She states, "Is there indeed a risk that we will establish a tyranny of health in which those who are unwell are assumed to have misbehaved (with certain areas of misbehavior forgiven and others condemned)?" (p. 197). While she encourages us to think about the meaning of health and the role of health care providers in working for health promotion, she continues in her cautious platform, "We must beware of developing a zealotry about health, in which we take ourselves too seriously and believe that we know enough to dictate human behavior, penalize people for disagreeing with us, and even deny people charity, empathy, and understanding because they act in a way of which we disapprove" (p. 197).

Management of Health Care Delivery

Over the years, we have used various strategies to manage the health care delivery industry. These strategies have involved the government, the private sector, or both. The following discussion presents several key points in the history of health care management. A review of these ideas may suggest new solutions for the future.

Government Structures

Currently, within the federal government, we have the Department of Health and Human Services. One of its branches, the Public Health Service (PHS) is of major concern to nursing. It was established by a congressional act in 1798 and
(*text continues on page 209*)

TABLE 7-2 *Health Problems Across the Life Span*

Age	Health Problems	Rank as a Cause of Death
Infants	Congenital anomalies	1
	Sudden infant death syndrome	2
	Respiratory distress syndrome	3
	Low birth-weight	
	Accidents	
	Influenza and pneumonia	
	Unfavorable resolution of trust versus mistrust	
Children, 1–14 years	Accidents	1
	Malignant neoplasms	2
	Congenital anomalies	3
	Abuse and neglect	
	Dental caries	
	Inadequate school functioning	
	Lead poisoning among inner-city children	
	Learning disorders	
	Problems begun in childhood as precursors for adult problems	

	Unfavorable resolution of
	    Autonomy versus shame and doubt
	    Industry versus inferiority
	    Initiative versus guilt	

Adolescents and young adults, 15–24 years	Accidents	1
	Homicide	2
	Alcohol and drug abuse	3
	AIDS	
	Gun shot wounds	
	Injuries	
	Life-style and behavior pattern as precursors for chronic disease	
	Mental illness	
	Risk-taking behavior	
	STDs	
	Smoking	

	Unfavorable resolution of
	    Identity versus role confusion
	    Intimacy versus isolation	

	Unwanted pregnancy	

(continued)

TABLE 7-2 (Continued)

Age	Health Problems	Rank as a Cause of Death
Adults, 25–44 years	Accidents	1
	Malignant neoplasms	2
	Heart disease	3
	AIDS	
	Gun shot wounds	
	Alcohol abuse	
	Cirrhosis	
	Diabetes	
	Feelings of stagnation and self-absorption	
	Homicide	
	Hypertension	
	Mental illness	
	Obesity	
	Peridontal disease	
	Unfavorable resolution of generativity versus stagnation	
Adults, 45–64 years	Malignant neoplasms	1
	Heart disease	2
	Cerebrovascular disease	3
	Other problems similar to those in the age group 26–44 years	
Older adults, 65 years and older	Heart disease	1
	Malignant neoplasms	2
	Cerebral vascular disease	3
	Arteriosclerosis	
	Decreased ability to care for self	
	Dependency	
	Depression	
	Diabetes	
	Fluid, electrolyte, and metabolic disturbances	
	Influenza and pneumonia	
	Injuries	
	Insufficient finances to meet basic needs	
	Neglect, loneliness	
	Nutritional deficiencies	
	Overmedication	
	Preventable and reversible mental deterioration and behavioral changes	
	Stress of loss and grief	
	Unfavorable resolution of Ego integrity versus despair Visual and hearing alterations	

National Center for Health Statistics. [1988]. Advanced report of final mortality statistics, 1986.

TABLE 7-3 *Possible Solutions for Health Problems*

Solution	Examples
Community support systems	Abuse prevention
	Parent counseling
	Runaway centers
	Stress control
	Suicide prevention
	Safe Houses
	Counseling centers for family violence and abuse
Counseling programs	Family planning
	Genetic counseling
	Nutritional counseling
Educational programs	Cardiopulmonary resuscitation (CPR) classes
	Health education throughout the school year
	Nutritional education
	Physical fitness activities and programs
	Information about signs of cancer
	Unemployment programs, teaching youths how to be employable
Health and safety protection	Automobiles designed for safety
	Changes in fabric (not inflammable)
	Childhood immunizations
	Control of firearms
	Control of disease (i.e., STDs, hypertension)
	Floridation of community water supply
	Lowering speed limits
	Occupational health and safety programs
	Poison control centers
	Proper reporting of disease, institution of regulations, and use of statistics
	Seat belts in moving vehicles
	Toxic-substance control
	Toy manufacturing safety regulations
Prevention programs	Dental hygiene
	Papanicolaou (Pap) smear
	Prenatal care and mental health
	Self breast examination
	Regular mammography
	Self testicular examination
	Regular prostate examination
	PSA blood level and rectal examination
Screening programs	Screening and diagnosis for high-risk factors across age groups
	Screening programs for diseases such as diabetes and hypertension

TABLE 7-4 *Agencies of the U.S. Public Health Service*

Agency	Mission
National Institutes of Health (NIH)	Research
Food and Drug Administration	Regulation related to consumer protection
Health Services Administration	Establishment of responsibility related to the delivery of health care and quality of care
Centers for Disease Control	Responsibility for preventive medicine and public health
Health Resources Administration	Development of health service resources and improvement of their use
Alcohol, Drug Abuse and Mental Health Administration	Development of strategies to deal with medical problems

is intended as a vehicle for health professionals and scientists to discover and apply knowledge to cure disease and improve health.

The Public Health Service comprises six major agencies (Table 7-4), the combined purpose of which is to provide better health services for Americans. Activities of PHS include the following:

- ❑ Review of health care—quality and appropriateness of medical care provided to Medicare and Medicaid subscribers
- ❑ Provision of grants to study widespread health problems such as venereal disease and hypertension
- ❑ Assistance with plans to raise public awareness of serious health problems
- ❑ Operation of hospitals for national health concerns such as narcotics addiction, TB, and mental illness
- ❑ Research on health problems
- ❑ Provision of training grants to educational institutions in the health services
- ❑ Publication of vital statistics pertinent to public health programs

Particular emphases associated with different presidential administrations, such as increased or decreased expenditures for health care, will alter the philosophy and functions of PHS. A flurry of activity on health care issues and designs for reform occurred in the early years of the Clinton Administration. However, Americans generally distrusted the plan that they were led to believe would nationalize health care and force those with insurance to pay the price for those who had none. Congress defeated the plan, and while much of this was political in nature, there were many who saw the Clinton plan as further damaging to health, and to the economy of the country. In August of 1996, President Clinton signed into law the Kassebaum-Kennedy Bill, an insurance reform bill that allows workers who have lost their jobs to keep their health care insurance coverage. This bill and law evolved through bipartisan efforts. President Clinton and his administration have indicated that health care is still heavily on their minds in this second term. Americans can expect continuing activity in governmental as well as private arenas on the issues of providing and financing health care.

The Center for Nursing Research, established in April 1986, has been renamed a National Institute of Health (NIH). This research center provides the first visible national governmental center devoted to nursing research—research about the human responses to persons' actual or potential health problems, and also the nursing interventions to promote, maintain, and restore health.

Financing Health Care Delivery

Health care costs have mounted alarmingly since 1900. Accordingly, many agencies can no longer be supported by fee for service alone, and must rely on voluntary contributions or tax dollars. Many Americans belong to a variety of health care insurance plans, or receive governmental assistance. However, as mentioned earlier, there are still those with inadequate or no coverage.

Funding Health Care Agencies

Agencies are funded from two basic sources: tax support and private support. Tax-supported agencies receive public aid through city, county, state, or federal agency funds. Often, several levels of government combine to provide assistance. These agencies are not necessarily free to those whom they serve; they usually charge a fee for service to offset operating costs.

Most tax-supported agencies are nonprofit. Those agencies that make a profit return monies to the agency for expansion of services and the purchase of new equipment. Examples of tax-supported agencies include health departments from all levels of government; many hospitals; the Bethesda, Maryland hospital complex; other Army, Navy, and veterans' hospitals; state mental hospitals; and neighborhood health clinics.

Non–tax-supported agencies include private profit-oriented agencies such as pharmacies, some hospitals, nursing homes, and private practices that are run on a fee-for-service basis.

Private, nonprofit agencies are supported by fees for service and voluntary contributions. Examples of this kind of agency include certain hospitals, VNA, and programs such as Motor Meals or Meals on Wheels. Another fast-growing nonprofit agency is the **hospice.** This agency is devoted to providing care to persons with life-limiting illnesses such as cancer, obstructive pulmonary disease, progressive neurologic deficits, or AIDS. Care, offered in residential facilities or the person's own home, centers around the total family.

Most voluntary agencies are also private and nonprofit oriented. They usually concern themselves with a single problem. The American Cancer Society, American Heart Association, and the National Foundation (March of Dimes) are exam-

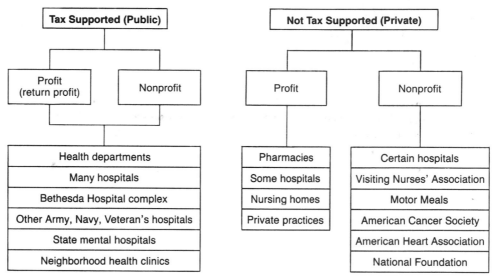

FIGURE 7-1 Funding of health care agencies.

ples of voluntary agencies. Figure 7-1 indicates the funding structure of health care agencies.

Financing Personal Health Care

PRIVATE INSURANCE

Private insurance is one way of financing personal health care. Nonprofit, tax-exempt organizations such as Blue Cross–Blue Shield provide payment for the health care needs of many Americans. Private, profit-oriented insurance companies also deal with the payment of health care needs. To become insured, members pay monthly premiums either individually or in combination with an employer. The best method of buying insurance is as a member of a contracting group through a union, an employer, or a club. This approach reduces the cost of insurance, because the pooled risks of all group members determine charges. These plans commonly pay about 80% of health care costs; the client pays the remainder.

Many other insurance plans are available that offer varying coverage. Many do not cover preventive health, health promotional care costs, or screening procedures such as routine chest x-rays. Some include benefits for psychiatric care and cancer follow-up care, but often coverage is limited for long-term disease. A certain amount of time must elapse between hospitalizations for a given disease before benefits resume. It should also be noted that the trend to increase copays and decrease benefits is on the rise. This is especially problematic for people on fixed incomes—in particular, for retirees.

Although nurses will not know specifics of each insurance program, we assist our clients to learn about their coverage and to plan their health care through the insurance agency resources. Most agencies today employ persons whose jobs are to understand payment plans and to seek authorization for payment for their clients' needs. As nurses, we can direct clients to these resource people and assist clients to make sound decisions.

MEDICARE

Medicare (Title XVIII of the Social Security Act of 1966), has existed since 1966. It is administered by the federal government and thus is uniform from state to state. Medicare serves persons aged 65 years or older, regardless of financial resources. It also covers disabled persons younger than age 65 years who have been entitled to Social Security benefits for 2 consecutive years, and certain other persons with renal failure. These persons are insured through a monthly premium deducted from their Social Security benefits, with additional amounts being paid by the federal government. These monies are placed in trust funds that pay medical expenses for insured persons. Medical expenses covered include costs of physician services, home health care, and outpatient services such as rehabilitation therapy. Hospital insurance under Medicare is financed by workers' payroll deductions.

Services sometimes cover certain hospital and home health care agencies, independent laboratories and x-ray services, some ambulance firms, chiropractors, and a variety of independent practitioners. Agencies and independent practitioners can decide not to accept persons insured by Medicare if they find administrative costs too high. In addition, Medicare often will not pay the fee charged by independent practitioners for a particular visit or procedure.

To be covered, care must be considered reasonable and necessary. Care provided by home health aides is not covered; drugs or meals delivered to the home are also not covered except in instances in which hospice care is provided by the Medicare hospice insurance rider. Nurses who provide care for persons receiving Medicare inform their clients to

- ❑ Carry their Medicare cards and present them whenever seeking services.
- ❑ Write their claim number on any bills or correspondence sent to the claims offices.
- ❑ Check agencies and services the person is seeking beforehand to determine that they are approved for reimbursement by Medicare and that they accept Medicare.
- ❑ Clarify services covered within a given agency before the agency is used.
- ❑ Exercise their right to appeal when disagreeing with the coverage by Medicare in a specific instance.
- ❑ Obtain a copy of *Your Medicare Handbook,* distributed by HEW (1996).

Medicare does not address certain common needs of persons aged 65 years or older, and preventive and promotional health care coverage is inadequate.

MEDICAID

Medicaid (Title XIX of the Social Security Act of 1966), another way of financing personal health care, also has existed since 1966. It is administered by both federal and state governments in a partnership arrangement. The states develop their

TABLE 7-5 *Services Covered by Medicaid*

Covered	Covered in Some States
Inpatient services	Dental care
Outpatient services	Prescribed drugs
Skilled nursing home care	Eye glasses
Physician's services	Intermediate-care facilities' services
Laboratory services	Diagnostic
X-ray procedures	Screening
Diagnosis and treatment of children under 21	Preventive
Home health care services	Rehabilitative
Family planning services	
Rural health-clinic services	

own programs within federal government guidelines, so benefits vary from state to state. The program provides benefits for certain eligible needy and low-income persons who are younger than age 65 years. In addition, it pays for certain expenses for persons older than age 65 years who are below a certain income level, including services that Medicare does not cover. Medicaid pays for medical expenses incurred by persons with complete visual loss and those classified as disabled, as well as by members of families with low income and with dependent children. The program is funded by federal, state, and local taxes. Table 7-5 lists services covered by Medicaid.

As with Medicare, nurses can assist clients who are eligible for Medicaid by providing them with information concerning the program, ensuring that they understand the necessity of always carrying their Medicaid cards, and checking agencies to determine whether they accept Medicaid clients and which services are covered. As the administration of all levels of government changes, programs and their rules, regulations, and benefits also will change. For example, in 1988, the largest expansion of Medicare instituted assistance for catastrophic illness. Similarly, at that time, Medicaid underwent significant change to prevent financial disaster of a spouse caused by nursing home care of a mate.

Both programs expect high standards of care and careful attention to cost containment. They encourage innovations in medical care delivery and require a review of the care provided. An amendment to the Social Security Act, called the Professional Standards Review Organization Act (PSRO), was enacted in 1972. This amendment mandated that physicians develop a mechanism for monitoring care and ensuring quality care to beneficiaries of Medicare and Medicaid. Physicians were the first target group of this law. However, nursing is now included, and nurses are involved in peer review and quality assurance programs. Agencies have learned that regardless of the quality of their programs and the care provided, if proper documentation and quality assurance reviews are not in place, reimbursement can be seriously affected.

National Health Insurance

A major proposed solution for the financing of health care delivery in the United States is **national health insurance,** which would provide guaranteed health care coverage to everyone. The Advisory Committee on National Health Insurance, charged by President Jimmy Carter (1977–1981), was instructed to develop a plan that would address the problems of availability of treatment, health promotion, and distribution of resources.

The Reagan and Bush administrations halted most discussions on this proposal; Americans will continue to see activity regarding the issue as we progress through the Clinton years.

Overall, the proponents of a national health insurance program seek to reflect the generally agreed-on notion that everyone is entitled to health care that is financially equitable, accessible, available, comprehensive, and uniform in quality of care. Although clearly impoverished people receive inadequate health care, this problem affects the middle class as well.

It behooves nurses to be aware of these concerns. Federal legislators have asked nurses to testify during hearings on national health insurance. Proposed nursing solutions could make a difference in the overall effectiveness of health care delivery.

For example, early testimony was provided by Barbara Nichols, president of the American Nurses Association (ANA; 1978–1982), before the Senator Edward Kennedy hearing in Denver on November 29, 1978 (Brewer, 1979). Nurses are being included as President Clinton continues to study the issues related to health care reform.

Politically active nurses can shape legislation that will delineate appropriate nursing services; in this way, we may be able to protect our clients from exorbitant expenses and ensure that preventive health care becomes a priority.

Nurses will want to consider the following questions concerning the plans for health care reform:

How will the government ensure both quality and cost containment?
Can we expect a change from illness-oriented care to preventive health care and health promotion?
Will national health insurance provide reimbursement of nursing services?
Does the federal government understand the difference between medical insurance and health insurance?

Nursing's Agenda for Health Care Reform

The National League for Nursing, in 1990, wrote a position statement called *Nursing's Agenda for Health Care Reform.* Although many organizations in both the private and public sectors are working on such statements, the uniqueness of the nursing proposal is within the set of values it portrays. The Executive Summary of the statement says:

Nursing has long supported the nation's efforts to create a health care system that assures access, quality, and services at affordable costs. [In this document] we call for a basic "core" of essential health care services to be available to everyone. We call for a restructured health care system that will focus on the consumers and their health, with services to be delivered in familiar, convenient sites, such as schools, workplaces, and homes. We call for a shift from the predominant focus on illness and cure, to an orientation toward wellness and care (p. 2).

Nursing does not, for example, look at just facilities or staffing or environment—rather, it views all aspects of the fiscal and human arenas that make up the realm of health. It is this holistic perspective that, as a profession, we have to offer in our contribution to health care reform.

Nursing's agenda emphasizes primary health care services and promotion, restoration, and maintenance of health. It calls for increasing consumer responsibility and focuses on partnerships between clients and providers. Moreover, nursing believes that the health care system has lost touch with individuals, and with community life. Most health care is not available within the communities that we actually serve. The agenda also indicates that with certain groups such as children and pregnant women, there is an even greater need to "catch up" than with health care in general, and that programs here need a special enrichment. Other considerations addressed by the Agenda focus on more interdisciplinary collaboration and improved research utilization.

The agenda suggests several possibilities to obtain revenue for needed reform. For example, it indicates that our tax structure will be one source, and that higher taxes on such items as alcohol and tobacco may be necessary. The main source suggested, however, is that monies gained from efficiencies realized after reform should be reallocated to necessary programs. In addition, the Agenda calls for making full use of the range of health care providers, which could have implications for both cost and quality. For example, there would be new opportunities for nurses to function as primary health providers and to be reimbursed in their own right rather than through other professionals such as physicians.

The Nursing Agenda clearly states that when there is a proper balance between individual health needs and self-care responsibilities with provider capabilities, care can be offered in a more efficient and coordinated manner, as well as be directed at health promotion activities that will ultimately improve outcomes and reduce costs. Nursing's plan is designed to achieve such a balance (p. 15).

Diagnostic Related Groups

The **diagnostic related groups** (DRG) system represents a major thrust by the federal government to contain health care costs. The system was devised by a group of Yale University researchers and is based on the International Classification of Diseases drawn up by the World Health Organization in the 1920s. The code letters ICD-9-CM, which stand for International Classification of Diseases, 9th revision, Clinical Modification, now appear on hospital records of Medicare clients to indicate in which category of the DRG system they have been placed for payment. The system officially went into effect on April 20, 1983, when President Ronald W. Reagan signed Public Law 98–21 (the Social Security Amendments of 1983). Title VI of this law deals with Medicare payments for hospital inpatient services under the DRG system. Private insurance companies, which do not specifically use the DRG system, have developed similar criteria for reimbursement.

Simply described, the DRG system works as follows. Mr. Jones enters a local hospital emergency room with severe lower abdominal pain. After appropriate studies, the diagnosis of appendicitis with a need for surgery is made. Mr. Jones is assigned the DRG number covering this condition that indicates that clients undergoing an uncomplicated appendectomy may stay in the hospital for 3 days. If his postoperative course is smooth and he indeed leaves in 3 days, the hospital is reimbursed accordingly. If the client is able to leave in just 2 days, the hospital will receive the same reimbursement as if the client had stayed for 3 days and, consequently, will make money. On the other hand, if the client remains more than 3 days and the hospital could not justify the necessity, such as a demonstrated complication from surgery, reimbursement would be paid for 3 days and the hospital would assume the rest of the cost. If the client develops a complication, such as a wound infection, the original DRG code number is changed to ensure proper reimbursement to the hospital. The code number also can be changed for other reasons, such as if the client is diagnosed with an additional disease while in the hospital.

Under the DRG system, clients are admitted to the hospital later in an illness and discharged earlier in convalescence than ever before. For example, in the past, clients about to undergo planned surgery usually were admitted one day or more ahead of the scheduled date. This time was spent in diagnostic studies and general preparation for the surgery. This work currently is done more often in ambulatory-care clinics, and clients enter the hospital on the day of surgery. Postoperatively, clients proceed through a planned program and are discharged as soon as possible, often leaving with a need for nursing care in the home.

The implications for nursing under the DRG system are many. The client acuity (severity of illness) in the hospital is greater than ever before, because only the sickest or those who need surgery are admitted. Joel (1987) stated, "Increased volume under DRG's equals more admissions. And new admissions demand significantly more nurse time and energy"(p. 794). Although we can often note examples from the very ill population, another group to consider in this dilemma is the less ill population. For example, there has been an increasing emphasis on the **23-hour admission.** An admission less than one full day (24 hours) is reimbursed differently, and to the advantage of both the agency and the insurer. Patients having oral, otologic, and ophthalmic surgeries provide common examples of the 23-hour admission. Although these persons may not be as ill, in the sense of critical illness or extensive surgery, their procedures and subsequent needs may still be intense. This type of admission requires all nursing interventions involving management of respiratory, bleeding, and pain issues, as well as preparation for discharge and home instruction, to be compressed into 23 hours. In the past, we might have had several days for these activities. Moreover, even the 23-hour admission is often reduced to ambulatory surgery, and patients are not admitted but sent home from ambulatory recovery rooms. This is true even though many have had general anesthesia.

Although administrators may indicate they are employing more nurses than ever before, the nursing profession has stated that the number of nurses is still inadequate to meet this increased need. Moreover, nurses nationwide have been the subject of concern regarding rising health care costs. Many have been released from their employment and replaced by less costly assistive personnel. This situation creates tension between nursing and administration because nurses are frequently required to justify their demands for more positions by proving their productivity. While we ought to be able to justify our worth, nursing is not an easily quantifiable profession.

In addition to the sicker client issue, implications exist for nursing regarding the surgical client who arrives on a nursing unit only after surgery. Time-honored nursing research has clearly indicated that postoperative complications are reduced when clients are given preoperative education and taught coping skills regarding the surgical experience. During the preoperative period, the nurse develops rapport with the client and assesses the client for baseline data with which to compare his or her postoperative response. Although assessment and education are being handled in some ambulatory clinics, the programs are in the developmental phase and clients may not receive adequate preparation. However, as nurses, we must be cost as well as quality conscious, and it behooves us to develop new economical ways of providing for our clients' needs.

Depending on the hospital, the DRG system can negatively affect nursing job security. Although tertiary care hospitals generally will not experience a decrease in client populations, some community hospitals already have, requiring the closure of sections or even entire hospitals. In these instances, nurses may want to consider a new setting. Although there may be more nurses than necessary in some places, there are shortages in others. In any event, clearly nurses and all other health care providers are expected to maintain quality and increase productivity while using fewer resources.

Nursing in the community also has been affected by the DRG system. Although hospital acuity is higher, acuity also is high in the community. Because clients remain at home longer and return home sooner, a need exists for more acute nursing care in this setting as well, which often involves sophisticated equipment. It is not unusual to find clients at home with oxygen, IV therapy, open wounds, or various drainage tubes. Even clients on ventilators (breathing machines) can sometimes be cared for at home.

*N*ursing Solutions for Cost-Containment in Health Care Delivery

Continuity of Care

Nurses have long known that continuity of care, that is, discharge planning, starts with admission to the agency. While we typically think of admission and discharge as referring to the hospital, nurses in community agencies, depending on the mission of the agency, also admit and discharge their clients. The concept of discharge planning has become even more critical with the advent of the DRG system. Many hospital and community agencies have nurses, often called home-care coordinators or discharge planners, who assist the general staff nurse in continuity of care activities. In other systems, the primary nurse or other staff nurses are responsible for this planning.

Planning for discharge as soon as the person is admitted requires nursing expertise in anticipating the usual needs of a particular client population, as well as expertise in assessing individual clients and their families for special needs. It also requires general knowledge of issues such as the operations of other departments within the agency that affect the client (e.g., physical therapy or social work); how to help with transportation; pharmacies where medications and supplies can be obtained; and how much nursing care need will continue after discharge.

Fagin (1982), in her article on ways in which nursing can be an alternative to the high cost of health care, referred to the research of Georgopoulus and Mann (1962): "Research data accumulated over the past twenty years indicate the importance of nursing and nursing care in affecting patient outcomes in and out of hospitals and show that nursing services can contribute immeasurably to the goals of a competitive delivery system"(p. 59). Fagin suggested that specialization in nursing is one solution to burgeoning costs, and mentioned such specialties as nurse–midwifery; nurse–practitioner (pediatric, psychiatric, cardiovascular, and so forth).

Primary Nursing

Marie Manthey (1980) is recognized as the first person to describe the concept of **primary nursing.** She indicated that it is a system of nursing care delivery that renders the nurse responsible and accountable, although not necessarily present or available, on a 24-hour basis. This accountability is possible through coordination, management, and communication of care so that others can provide that care in the absence of the primary nurse.

Joel (1987) spoke harshly of those who would not see the value of professional nursing care: "Faced with patients who are less functionally able and more acutely ill, the fool's answer to economic constraints is to dilute staffing: the foolish will sacrifice two professional positions to hire three ancillary workers. This reasoning proves disastrous"(p. 794).

At this juncture, primary nursing is considered too expensive a system to continue. Although it remains intact in some agencies, many have turned away from the concept, which suggests a need for redesign of the system. However, it is our basic premise that it has been nursing care that has decreased admissions, acuity, and length of stay in both hospital and community agencies. Nursing care is a major reason why many clients can stay within the limits of the DRG system. Consider the following example:

Paul, a 21-year-old man, had been through a rugged experience with kidney stones, pain, hemorrhage, and infection. Because he was otherwise healthy, everyone expected that following appropriate treatment he would get well and be discharged. Instead, he became weak and depressed. Finally, the primary nurse uncovered the problem. Paul said that he was exhausted but could not sleep because he was afraid of suddenly hemorrhaging during the night. He thought that if his sister could spend the night with him he would not be afraid. The primary nurse was criticized by some for encouraging dependence when she permitted his sister to stay. However, the nurse recognized that his unmet need for safety was contributing to the dependency. Criticism evaporated when Paul slept through the night for the first time in several weeks, showed considerable improvement the next day, and was discharged the day after. He told the nurse, "It was because you let my sister stay that I got well." Although Joel's (1987) comments and the example of Paul present important points, the national movement of work redesign for nursing is also acknowledged here.

Work redesign is a restructuring of the system of nursing work, or a change in the actual structure of the jobs nurses perform. This restructuring is managed by measuring the work that is required to attain the outcomes expected and then reshaping jobs and adapting them to workers with varying levels of expertise. Nurses know that, in addition to providing care, they are involved in activities that do not require their particular skills. For example, they perform clerical tasks, arrange for transportation, run errands, and run interference with different departments within their settings. Identifying all tasks currently performed by nurses helps us to determine whether they are necessary and appropriate and who ought to be doing them. In this way, many tasks can be delegated to the appropriate level, freeing nurses to provide the expected quality of care. In addition, it is proper to use care extenders or nursing assistants to assist the primary nurse with direct patient care as long as the nurse and assistant work closely together. The following discussion on managed care incorporates work redesign initiatives that involve other professionals as well.

Managed Care: A Collaborative Solution

Health care providers have been mandated to define care specifically so that quality is maintained in a less resource-intensive environment. In order to accomplish this, **managed care** has become the system of our era. The essence of managed care is the organization of unit-based care so that specific patient outcomes can be achieved within fiscally responsible time frames. This means that hospital and community agency lengths of stay decrease and resources are used appropriately (in amount and sequence) to the specific case type and the individual patient (Etheredge, 1989). Managed care also means that ambulatory and clinic services are tailored to specific patient needs, and decisions are made as to the necessity and relevancy of certain diagnostic and treatment procedures. Ostensibly, the goals of managed care are to achieve the expected patient outcomes while facilitating early discharge and reducing the use of resources; to promote collaborative practice, coordination, and continuity of care; and to direct the contributions of all care providers toward the achievement of high-quality patient outcomes. Unfortunately, professionals (i.e., nurses and physicians) have indicated that they are not always consulted and that unilateral decisions are sometimes made by the payor that reflect the health care industry's needs rather than the patient's needs.

An example of the payor's attempt to make decisions is described by one client. She said, "I had several problems during my pregnancy, necessitating that a diagnostic test be done twice within a few months. Again, about two months later, I had an additional problem requiring that same procedure a third time. I was told that the care manager for our insurance company would not agree to pay for it. She did not understand why I would need the test yet again. Fortunately we were delayed only briefly while my doctor explained her decision to the care manager." While this situation seems harsh for the client, the fact that care providers are having to justify their decisions does require the use of critical thinking, and serves to make us more careful.

One important concept relevant to the managed care system is that of **capitation.** This is a system of reimbursement in which providers receive a fixed amount of income per enrollee, regardless of the services they perform. Thus it is up to providers to keep their clients healthy and to work at health promotion and illness prevention. Health care consumers are also expected to manage care within their capabilities so that they stay as healthy as possible.

Health Maintenance Organizations

Health maintenance organizations (HMOs) are group health practices whose major distinguishing feature is prepayment and whose existence suggests one major solution to the problems of health care costs. Thus they are examples of a managed care system. Members pay a fixed fee on a yearly basis and receive health care whenever they need it, either for a nominal additional charge or for no charge, depending on the plan. The HMO provides comprehensive health care services that include both wellness care and illness care. The program is arranged so that a broad group of specialists participate in care and are available for referral. Most HMOs have participating hospitals as well.

The emphasis on preventive health services and wellness care encourages persons to seek care early in a disease process, thereby avoiding hospitalization or costly diagnostic and treatment procedures; the healthier the clients are, the more financially stable the HMO remains. The traditional approach to health care has been to pay doctors and hospitals to provide care to the sick, thus giving incentives for illness care. The HMO has sought to change that by providing incentives for health care.

One of the most successful HMOs is the Kaiser-Permanente prepaid care plan, which provides medical and hospital and clinic services to more than 3 million persons. Agencies and physicians throughout a large portion of the western United States, as well as Ohio and Hawaii, participate in this program. Kaiser-Permanente has developed six basic principles from which it operates:

1. Group practice
2. Integration of facilities (combining both hospital and outpatient facilities)
3. Prepayment
4. Preventive health care (emphasis on keeping the person well, in addition to treating the sick)

5. Voluntary enrollment
6. Physician responsibility (for client care, financing, planning, and allocation of resources)

Central to the operation of Kaiser-Permanente is the principle that the program must be self-sustaining. Equipment and facilities are paid for by client fees and long-term loans. Less than 1% of Kaiser-Permanente costs have been supported by either private or government sources.

Using the Kaiser-Permanente plan as a model, the federal government enacted the Health Maintenance Organization Act of 1973. The act was developed to study various methods of health care delivery in the hope of generating a model for comprehensive health care. It was to deal with issues such as the distribution and availability of quality health care, cost-containment, and quality control. It provided for members of HEW (federal government) to collaborate with Professional Standards Review Organization (PSROs) to ensure quality of care.

"Between 1976 and 1986, the number of (HMOs) increased from 174 to 623 and enrollment rose from 6 million to 26 million" (National Center for Health Statistics, 1988, p. 4). Although the number of HMOs has burgeoned during the past 10 years, their future is uncertain. Much depends on what course the government takes with regard to national health care reform. A combination of the two concepts—HMOs and universal health care coverage—is a distinct possibility.

Case Management

Case management is a companion concept to managed care. Karen Zander and her nursing associates at the New England Medical Center are credited with the development of this concept in the mid 1980's. The National Case Management Task Force of 1995 focused on the collaborative nature of this system of care delivery. "Case management is a collaborative process that uses assessment, coordination, and evaluation to consider potential services for individual health care needs. The process considers resources, quality, and effective outcomes (Chapter 7, p. 221)."

Case management is nurse driven, family focused, and uses medical, nursing, and treatment protocols in its implementation. The protocols are planned to be outcome driven and multidisciplinary. That is, the system uses a variety of health professionals to provide cost effective, quality care. While managed care can be considered the umbrella concept and the aspect most closely associated with actual payment, case management focuses on seeing that reimbursement will occur relative to case types and individual clients.

Features of Case Management

Suppose that a person has been admitted to the hospital for a *radical nephrectomy* (kidney removal). Based on case type, the nurse knows approximately how long it will take this person to recover from the surgery, that is, to ambulate, void, eat, resolve pain and nausea, and become independent enough for discharge. As the patient becomes more independent and needs fewer nursing interventions, the nurse teaches the patient about care at home, and within a specified number of days, the patient is discharged. Nurses generally know the care plan and length of stay for persons who have had a radical nephrectomy. However, with managed care, this general knowledge is specified into a written critical pathway or care map. Consider the following discussion for a clearer understanding of the system.

Critical pathways are the key events in the hospitalization of a particular case type that must occur for the patient to reach the outcomes set by the DRG parameters. These events are planned in a collaborative manner between nurses and physicians and other professionals as needed to determine the interdisciplinary interventions necessary in the care of the patient. See Table 7-6 for an example of a critical pathway for a patient having a radical nephrectomy.

Care maps are broader than critical pathways and include statements from medicine, nursing, and other disciplines that address problems frequently related to specific DRGs. Care maps also include intermediate and long-term goals for resolution of these problems. The critical pathway portion of the care map shows the critical incidents that must occur to keep the patient's length of stay within the planned time frame.

Variances in Case Management

Incidents may occur, however, that delay a patient's discharge, increase cost, or alter the quality of care. These incidents or events are called *variances* and occur for many reasons. Variances are as follows.

NURSING OR PHYSICIAN VARIANCE

A *nursing or physician variance* is a variance due to an occurrence or omission in nursing or medical practice. The patient is required to spend another day in the hospital because a medication was not ordered or not given, or because the nurse did not report changes, or the physician did not assess the patient's condition in a timely manner.

SYSTEM VARIANCE

A *system variance* is a variance due to an occurrence or omission in the hospital system. For example, the patient has to wait too long in the admitting department for a bed, and thus certain diagnostic procedures are delayed for another day; the unit clerk does not schedule the ordered diagnostic procedure, delaying the patient's discharge; or the patient is scheduled for surgery on a particular day but accidentally receives and eats breakfast that morning.

PATIENT VARIANCE

A *patient variance* is a variance due to a patient's preexisting condition, such as diabetes, or a complication such as a deep vein thrombosis that occurs despite proper nursing and medical intervention.

The use of critical pathways may avoid many of these variances. Nurses and

TABLE 7-6 *Critical Pathway for a Patient Having Radical Nephrectomy*

DX ____ Date/Length of Surgery ____ Days Preop ____
Outcome—Discharged to Home ____ Transfer ____ Expired ____ LOS: ____

Date	Operative Day	POD 1	POD 2	POD 3	POD 4	POD 5	POD 6
Consults	Social services Cont. Care OT, PT, prn						
Test	CBC, A, B	CBC, A, B					
Activity	Bedrest	OOB with assist	B Ambulate with assist	A Ambulate with assist	Up ad lib	Up ad lib	Up ad lib
Self-care		Wash face	Self bath except back and legs	Self bath	Self bath	Self bath	Self bath
Diet	NPO	NPO	NPO	NPO	Clear liquids	Regular	Regular
Drains	NG–Sxn Foley–dd	NG–Sxn Foley–dd	NG–Sxn Foley–dd	NG–Sxn/dd Foley–d/c'd	NG–D/C'd		
Medications	Prophylactic IV ABX Analgesics prn	Prophylactic IV ABX Analgesics prn	IV D/C IV ABX Analgesics prn	IV Analgesics prn	IV D/C'd Colace Analgesics prn PO ABX	PO ABX Colace Analgesics prn PO ABX	PO ABX Colace Analgesics prn PO ABX
Treatment	IS, TEDS/SCD Mental care	IS, TEDS/SCD Mental care	IS, TEDS/SCD Mental care	IS, TEDS/SCD Discharge mental care	Discharge	TEDS, IS	
Teaching	IS, use of PCA	IS, mental care	IS, mental care	IS, mental care	Radical nephrectomy discharge sheet given	Review radical nephrectomy discharge for sheet, wound	Review discharge sheet phone nos., return visit
Discharge planning	Assess patient supports	Assess patient supports	Assess patient supports	Assess patient supports	Assess patient supports	Assess patient supports	Discharge to home with prescription medications

DX = Diagnosis
Preop = Preoperative
LOS = Length of stay
POD = Postoperative day
Cont. = Continuing
OT = Occupational therapy
PT = Physical therapy
PRN = Latin term meaning "whenever necessary"
CBC = Complete blood count
OOB = Out of bed
Up ad lib = Up whenever one wishes and without assistance
NPO = Latin term meaning "nothing by mouth"

NG–Sxn = Nasogastric tube to suction
NG–Sxn/dd = Nasogastric tube to suction and change to dependent drainage
Foley–d/c'd = Discontinue Foley
IV = Intravenous
PO = By mouth
ABX = Antibiotic
D/C IV = Discontinue IV
IS = Incentive spirometer
SCD = Antiembolic device
TEDS = Antiembolic stockings
PCA = Patient-controlled analgesia

Although this particular pathway has been updated recently (2/96), six days may be longer than most patients currently stay in the hospital. This table offers one possible pathway format. Recognize that there may be many variations among agencies.

223

physicians will know exactly when certain treatments or procedures are to occur and then professionals will collaborate to ensure that the treatment plan follows its course. Collaboration among departments such as admitting, clerical services, and dietetics also occurs, affecting professional practice.

SHIFT REPORT RELATED TO CRITICAL PATHWAYS

During *shift report,* the nursing staff reports the patient's diagnosis or surgery; anticipated length of stay; DRG number; the day number (e.g., day 3 of a 5-day stay); present condition; and how the individual patient compares with the critical pathway for his or her diagnosis. Variances are reported and plans are made for resolving variance issues.

The case management approach is meant to add efficiency to the value of quality espoused by our current approach to health care. The purpose of case management is to virtually eliminate glitches that can occur in patient care systems. As nursing students, for example, you may have experienced both nurses and physicians who have their own ideas about pain management. New ideas are critical and should be tried and researched. In the daily administration of health care, however, approaches with some uniformity will decrease our expenditures. Although some professionals worry that we will lose the uniqueness of the individual with such systems, this is unlikely. With approaches that decrease nursing time spent on unnecessary work such as dealing with variances, more energy can be devoted to person-centered care.

Consumerism and Preventive Health Care

A **consumer** is a person who uses a commodity or service. All of us are consumers of health commodities and services. Some of these services require the specialized knowledge and skills of health care professionals, whereas many of the commodities—such as antidandruff shampoos or aspirin—may be purchased according to our own choice. For a variety of reasons, consumers may settle for less than optimum value, especially when illness and financial considerations affect their ability to make rational choices. Moreover, sometimes we are hesitant to ask questions of or check the references of health care providers.

Characteristics of the Health Care Consumer

Consumers of health care, like all persons, have certain characteristics that have important implications for nursing.

Interrelated Biophysical and Psychosocial Concerns

Consider the following examples. Ms. Jones, the single mother of a teenage daughter, is hospitalized for surgery. The nurse is concerned with providing preoperative teaching, but Ms. Jones is worried about leaving her teenager with inadequate supervision and cannot focus on preoperative teaching. Clinical studies have indicated that preoperative teaching instruction shortens a hospital stay if barriers to the client's learning are removed. Helping Ms. Jones to plan for her daughter will ease her worries so that she can absorb important information. Ideally, a well-prepared client will have a smoother postoperative course and return home quickly, thus alleviating the family situation.

Next, consider a client who must convalesce for several weeks following a heart attack. The client is discharged and told to rest and relax. This may be difficult, because long illnesses usually compound preexisting job, financial, or family concerns. One home-care nurse observed a client writing checks to pay bills within hours after the client was discharged following major surgery (a laryngectomy with tracheostomy).

Such examples focus on physiologic problems and suggest that psychosocial needs increase the harmful effects of physical illness. Viewing these examples in another way, we note that preexisting psychosocial needs may precipitate physical problems. The interrelationship of these factors reinforces the need for nurses to treat clients from a holistic perspective.

Ill-Matched Concerns

The consumer of health care has a set of concerns that may differ from those of the health care providers. One woman with diabetes, during an assessment about this condition, stated that diabetes was not a problem, since she was only hospitalized for sugar control. However, she stated that the inability to do housework since her heart attack was a problem.

In her book *Heartsounds*, Martha Weinman Lear (1980) described her husband's attempts to cope with progressive heart disease. He discovered, to his horror, that his mental abilities had declined following heart surgery. His memory was poor and he often felt confused. His cardiologists told him to be patient, that his mind would recover. His concern, they said, should be his life-threatening heart condition.

Personal Priorities

Community nurses often consider immunizations a top priority. However, a mother with chronic fatigue and financial burdens may not have the time or energy required to take her children to even a free immunization clinic. The possibility of her children contracting a disease such as polio seems remote.

Self-Care Abilities and a Knowledge of Personal Needs

The philosophy of self-care purports that persons have knowledge and abilities regarding their health. However, because they sometimes cannot communicate their knowledge or mobilize their strengths, they become health care consumers.

Variables That Influence Health Behavior

Health behaviors are learned and develop from customs particular to one's social system, culture, and family. A person adopts a health behavior if he or she perceives it to have value, meaning, and relevance to his or her particular needs. There are often variances among care providers and receivers as to the importance of certain health behaviors.

Biophysical Variables

Health care is sought more quickly if a symptom interferes with the person's functioning. The following physical symptoms are those that most commonly motivate a person to seek health care:

- ❐ Pain
- ❐ Respiratory distress
- ❐ Insomnia
- ❐ Visual and auditory alterations
- ❐ Dizziness
- ❐ Malfunctions of a body part

Psychological Variables

HESITANCY TO CONSULT A PHYSICIAN OR TO ENTER A HEALTH CARE SYSTEM

Consumers prefer to seek health care from professionals they know or have previously consulted; they want affordable health care without the confusion of a large system. When their experience does not meet these expectations, they may put off seeking needed care. Some persons have grown up in families who used home or cultural remedies rather than traditional care, and these individuals may be suspicious of practices with which they are unfamiliar.

THE NEED TO KNOW AND THE FEAR OF KNOWING

Some persons who are fearful that they might have a serious illness seek medical care immediately, whereas others minimize symptoms hoping that they will go away. Those who put off obtaining health care usually seek help once they accept the idea of coping with serious illness.

KNOWLEDGE LEVELS

Our knowledge of health and disease frequently affects the way in which we seek health care. Some persons know that symptoms are serious and can seek appropriate help. Those who know about health services and systems can pursue health care with less difficulty than those who know little.

SELF-ESTEEM

Our sense of self-worth affects when and how we seek health care services. Although feelings of self-esteem may not be conscious, some persons may not believe that they will receive attention unless they are ill. This may motivate them to seek health care repeatedly for the secondary gain it provides.

Sociocultural Variables

AVAILABILITY OF HEALTH CARE SERVICES

Persons generally desire health care services that are near their homes. Both healthy and ill persons may find distances or public transportation difficult.

FINANCIAL STATUS

For many years, persons with limited financial resources had difficulty obtaining care. They may have refused or have been denied health services because they were unable to pay. Today, insurance programs cover a large percentage of health care costs for those who can pay the program premiums, and government programs have been developed that assist needy persons to obtain health care. However, depending on the plan, certain necessary services may not be covered.

ALTERNATIVE HEALING SYSTEMS AND SPECIFIC RELIGIOUS PHILOSOPHIES

Some individuals trust the shaman or curandero, and practices such as acupuncture or astrology, more than the Western cultural practice of calling the physician. Others of the Judeo–Christian faith have been attracted by the laying on of hands and other faith-healing practices. Often, these alternative practices can be effective—remember that persons survived on this earth for centuries before the advent of modern health care. More recently, alternative practices have become more accepted by both nursing and medicine. Therapeutic touch, massage, art, music, and aroma therapies, relaxation training, and imagery are just a few of the many alternative practices that are currently being used.

MEDIA

Television and news publications have had a far-reaching effect on our lives, especially in the past 40 years. Through these sources, we receive health-related information that is not always accurate or useful. Nurses can assist clients to develop decision-making skills to judge the quality of information from the media. Computer sources of information, now widely available through the world wide web, make using such judgment ever more important.

In one instance, however, information from a television program about a hospital emergency unit helped a young girl save a young boy's life. When he accidentally electrocuted himself, his 11-year-old sister performed CPR that she had learned from watching the program.

All health care consumers have their own definitions of health and illness. Decisions about whether and when to seek health care and to engage in health practices are based on many variables. Although our health practices reflect our cultural and family customs, our uniqueness has an even greater influence on how we perceive health. As nurses, we believe persons are holistic, and we consider the interactions among all variables that influence perceptions of health.

Consumer Movement

Before World War II, there were few medicines or surgical techniques. Chemotherapy, dialysis, radiation, and other technologic advances to help persons manage disease were minimal. Sick persons often were kept at home, and families used private duty nurses for help, if they could afford them. Advances in medicine and science began to change this picture. In 1921, insulin was first used successfully in the treatment of diabetes mellitus. By the early to mid-1940s, antibiotics were introduced to combat bacterial infections. Miraculous drugs turned life-threatening diseases into treatable problems, and tranquilizers changed the whole concept of care for mentally ill persons. Throughout the 20th century, many new drugs became available, including medicines for hypertension and cancer, as well as drugs for infertility and birth control.

Eventually prescriptions, rather than the person's individual needs or self-care abilities, became the focus of treatment. Although drugs were often appropriate (as when antihypertensive drugs were prescribed for persons with high blood pressure), they were relied on completely, without giving much thought to other aspects of the person's life, which are emphasized in the holistic view. Examination of certain factors known to precipitate hypertension might teach us other ways to control blood pressure. Professional nurses possessed skills to assist clients in this regard, but the emphasis remained on the new miracle drugs and the easy solutions they provided for health problems.

As the age of science and technology progressed, consumers no longer remembered the effects of polio or strep throat. Doctors and nurses became more controlling with their advanced knowledge, and often indicated that they knew best, without consideration for the client's ideas—although care provided by large hospitals and clinics was not particularly individualized. Moreover, care providers were anxious to use the expensive new techniques and equipment, and often consumers came to expect this. As the costs of health care were being driven upward, persons began to voice other concerns:

Drugs and surgical procedures that were expected to cure sometimes made them sicker.
Return visits to doctors were expensive and often seemed unnecessary.
The cost of health care was escalating beyond reasonable levels.
Scandal was frequent: nursing home administrators pocketed money provided for client care, and physicians received percentages of prescription costs from pharmacists to whom they sent customers.
Nurses were often perceived as uncaring and unavailable.

The consumer movement in health care originated from these concerns. It probably began with Ralph Nader's (1965) book *Unsafe at Any Speed*. Nader berated car manufacturers for their failure to respond to the needs of the public and for their disregard for safety. Nader has continued his fight for consumer protection in a variety of products and services. Others have followed his lead, contributing to the growth of the movement.

As consumer pressure developed, consumer advocates were hired by hospitals and other health care organizations. The governing boards of health care agencies of hospitals and communities, and certain agency committees, were required to have consumer representation. Human subject protection committees were developed in institutions where research was being done, and these also are required to have consumer members.

The consumer movement has produced many positive effects, especially in promoting protective and educational functions. Committees have been formed to set standards for commodities and services, and quality assurance programs have been developed to ensure that these standards are followed. In the health care industry, the consumer movement has clearly established that persons have a right to receive information about their disease and treatment, to participate in the decision making, and to understand the charges for treatment. These rights have been outlined in the Patient's Bill of Rights developed in 1972 (revised in 1990 and 1992) by the American Hospital Association (AHA; see Display 7-1). Publications are available from government, private agencies, and individuals to increase health consumers' knowledge and decision-making abilities.

The consumer movement has helped create **responsible consumerism.** Responsibility is an obligation as we all learn the necessity of guarding our resources.

A negative effect of the consumer movement has been the proliferation of malpractice lawsuits. Consumers have recently discovered their rights and have taken to the courts. As a result, malpractice insurance premiums have become astronomical, particularly for physicians.

Some persons who merit payment due to physician error would prefer to settle quickly without litigation. One such situation involved a woman who was to have minor surgery for diagnosis of her infertility problem. Another woman was scheduled for a sterilization procedure on the same day. The physician confused the two women and tied the tubes of the one with the infertility problem. He stated, "As soon as I realized my mistake, I called a surgeon in another city who was known for his ability to repair tubes, and made arrangements for him to see this woman the next week. Then I called my attorney and prepared to make a settlement for my error." Attorneys for both parties were able to negotiate a reasonable settlement that included payment for future medical expenses as well as reimbursement for the emotional distress and pain incurred by the woman who was supposed to have had minor surgery. Such reasonable settlement of problems might prevent malpractice insurance premiums from becoming prohibitive.

Still, many consumer complaints reach the courts. Some professionals may be reluctant to admit mistakes. Sometimes persons are looking for a reason to file suit in the hope of gaining attention or money, and some attorneys encourage this practice for their own financial gain. Whatever the reason for litigation, the result is increased malpractice insurance premiums, which are then passed on to the consumer.

Although the increased incidence of malpractice suits is a problem, it has had positive effects. The health care professions have begun to review and evaluate their practices more carefully. Committees for standardizing diagnostic and therapeutic procedures are a part of most agencies that provide health care. Their purpose is to provide quality and safety in the care of the individual, as well as to protect the agency from litigation. These committees, concerned with both medical and nursing procedures, have attempted to set standards for the most common medical diagnostic tests and procedures and for most technical nursing procedures. Regulatory agencies such as state departments of public health and

DISPLAY 7-1 A Patient's Bill of Rights

1. The patient has the right to considerate and respectful care.
2. The patient has the right to and is encouraged to obtain from physicians and other direct caregivers relevant, current, and understandable information concerning diagnosis, treatment, and prognosis.

   Except in emergencies when the patient lacks decision-making capacity and the need for treatment is urgent, the patient is entitled to the opportunity to discuss and request information related to the specific procedures and/or treatments, the risks involved, the possible length of recuperation, and the medically reasonable alternatives and their accompanying risks and benefits.

   Patients have the right to know the identity of physicians, nurses, and others involved in their care, as well as when those involved are students, residents, or other trainees. The patient also has the right to know the immediate long-term financial implications of treatment choices, insofar as they are known.

3. The patient has the right to make decisions about the plan of care prior to and during the course of treatment and to refuse a recommended treatment or plan of care to the extent permitted by law and hospital policy and to be informed of the medical consequences of this action. In case of such refusal, the patient is entitled to other appropriate care and services that the hospital provides or transfer to another hospital. The hospital should notify patients of any policy that might affect patient choice with the institution.

4. The patient has the right to have an advance directive (such as living will, health care proxy, or durable power of attorney for health care) concerning treatment or designating a surrogate decision maker with the expectation that the hospital will honor the intent of that directive to the extent permitted by law and hospital policy.

   Health care institutions must advise patients of their rights under state law and hospital policy to make informed medical choices, ask if the patient has an advance directive, and include that information in patient records. The patient has the right to timely information about hospital policy that may limit its ability to implement fully a legally valid advance directive.

5. The patient has the right to every consideration of his privacy. Case discussion, consultation, examination, and treatment should be conducted so as to protect each patient's privacy.

6. The patient has the right to expect that all communications and records pertaining to his/her care will be treated as confidential by the hospital, except in cases such as suspected abuse and public health hazards when reporting is permitted or required by law. The patient has the right to expect that the hospital will emphasize the confidentiality of this information when it releases it to any other parties entitled to review information in these records.

7. The patient has the right to review the records pertaining to his/her medical care and to have the information explained or interpreted as necessary, except when restricted by law.

(continued)

8. The patient has the right to expect that, within its capacity and policies, a hospital will make reasonable response to the request of a patient for appropriate and medically indicated care and services. The hospital must provide evaluation, service and/or referral as indicated by the urgency of the case. When medically appropriate and legally permissible, or when a patient has so requested, a patient may be transferred to another facility. The institution to which the patient is to be transferred must first have accepted the patient for transfer. The patient must also have the benefit of complete information and explanation concerning the need for, risks, benefits, and alternative to such a transfer.

9. The patient has the right to ask for and be informed of the existence of business relationships among the hospital, educational institutions, other health care providers, or payers that may influence the patient's treatment and care.

10. The patient has the right to consent to or decline to participate in proposed research studies or human experimentation affecting care and treatment or requiring direct patient involvement, and to have those studies fully explained prior to consent. A patient who declines to participate in research or experimentation is entitled to the most effective care that the hospital can otherwise provide.

11. The patient has the right to expect reasonable continuity of care when appropriate and to be informed by physicians and other caregivers of available and realistic patient care options when hospital care is no longer appropriate.

12. The patient has the right to be informed of hospital policies and practices that relate to patient care, treatment, and responsibilities. The patient has the right to be informed of available resources for resolving disputes, grievances, and conflicts, such as ethics committees, patient representatives, or other mechanisms available in the institution. The patient has the right to be informed of the hospital's charges for services and available payment methods.

Reproduced by permission of the American Hospital Association. *A Patient's Bill of Rights* was first adopted in 1973. This revision was approved by the AHA Board of Trustees in 1992.

the Joint Commission on Accreditation of Healthcare Organizations perform periodic inspections of hospitals and home-care agencies. Their role is to determine that both governmental and professional standards and regulations are being met and that agencies adhere to their own standards and policies.

Nurses as Client Advocates

An *advocate* is a person who supports, upholds, defends, or intercedes on behalf of another person. Nurses perform this function when they assist and support clients. The following details ways nurses can function as client advocates:

❐ Uphold the Patient's Bill of Rights.
❐ Respond to the social and ethnic uniqueness of the person.
❐ Provide scientifically current nursing care.
❐ Establish continuity of care.
❐ Empower your clients by providing for their participation and decision making in all aspects of health care.

❏ Serve on a committee for standardizing agency procedures.
❏ Become involved in community-level health care.
❏ Become involved in governmental programs that affect health care.
❏ Intervene on behalf of a person with any other health care provider involved in that person's care.
❏ Coordinate all services used by the client in the attempt to restore, maintain, or promote health.

The following example occurred a number of years ago. It demonstrates how a nurse acting as a client advocate, while she served on a standardizing committee at a large medical center, paved the way for improved quality of care. The nurse manager in a nursery ICU became concerned because of the large amount of blood that was being removed from babies for diagnostic tests. She pointed out that the amount of blood taken from the babies was often as much as that taken from adults for the same test. She stated that, although 5 mL or 6 mL of blood was not a great deal for an adult to lose, it was too much for a baby, especially true when more than one test was to be conducted on a given day. On occasions when this subject was before the committee, laboratory personnel were consulted. Often they indicated that the amount of blood specified was necessary. On each of these occasions, the nurse persisted in the following way: she remained composed; she came to the committee with data about her tiny clients; she elicited support from other members of the committee (often before the meeting); and she was willing to compromise. She stated, "I know this is difficult for the labs, but we must try to reach a better solution because these little ones cannot tolerate the loss of so much blood." In this way, she attained the respect of her colleagues and paved the way for protection of her clients. Her work from several years ago brought about major changes now clearly evident in the policies and procedures of the agency.

Nurses can become involved in the community by serving on the governing board of directors for agencies whose activities are designed to meet consumers' needs. Because of their unique skills in understanding the biopsychosocial aspects of persons, nurses can identify consumers' needs and how these needs can be met. For example, one nurse sitting on a board of a community clinic that serves persons with special socioeconomic needs is able to identify these needs for funding agencies. Using knowledge about perceptions of health and health behavior, the nurse is able to inform others more clearly of her clients' special needs.

Nurses can be advocates for individual consumers by assisting them to deal with the process of entering a health care agency, by helping them to find information they need, and by encouraging them to solve problems and identify solutions for their health care needs. Nurses, with their knowledge of biologic, psychologic, and sociocultural functioning, are well-suited to this role. Because nurses spend more direct time with clients than do other health care providers, they are in an ideal position to listen to their problems, identify their needs, and assist them to find solutions. When the hospital nurse helps a client contact a dietitian for concerns about the client's low-sodium diet, and when a community-health nurse

---

DISPLAY 7-2 **Person-Centered Health Care Goals**

1. To receive care that subscribes to the philosophy of the whole integrated person with spiritual, psychological, physiologic, and sociologic components.
2. To collaborate with health care providers and direct the planning and implementation of one's own care
3. To receive information from health care providers about the person's health concerns or disease to assist him or her in making appropriate decisions about the care
4. To receive care that considers the person's unique needs when he or she has a diminished ability to participate
5. To communicate the person's knowledge about his or her unique needs and expect that health care providers will incorporate these into the care plan
6. To have the person's strengths assessed by health care providers and mobilized toward supporting, maintaining, or promoting health status
7. To have the person's unique characteristics (biopsychosocial–spiritual) assessed and care provided that is safe and relevant, given those characteristics
8. To expect confidentiality concerning the person as a person and the care he or she is receiving
9. To be provided with the most modern and scientifically sound medical and nursing care available
10. To be advised of the rules, regulations, policies, and procedures of the agency or persons from whom he or she is seeking care
11. To receive continuity of care
12. To receive a full explanation of the expected costs of the health care for which the person is contracting and the actual costs of it after completion
13. To have consideration given to the person as a member of a family
14. To have family included where possible and appropriate

---

helps a client identify an agency that provides needed financial assistance, both are acting as consumer advocates.

To cite a challenging example, reflect on the recent publicity involving physician-assisted suicide. This intervention has generally been associated with the suffering incurred from life-limiting illnesses. Although space does not allow for a major discussion of this issue, client advocacy by nurses offers effective alternatives to such measures. The mission of the hospice movement, for example, is to assist clients to die with grace, comfort, and dignity. Although this includes facilitating the grieving process for both client and family, the pursuit of aggressive symptom control by both nurses and physicians, and particularly pain control, constitute the major focus—thus omitting the need for suicide.

Our challenge is clearly marked: as professional nurses, we have the knowledge, skills, and numbers necessary to make a difference to the health of both individuals and groups. Display 7-2 presents a list of person-centered health care goals. These goals reflect the philosophy of person-centered health care.

The Globalization of Health Care

Our world today has decreased in size. Growth in the travel industry, information systems technology, importing and exporting, and the transfer of knowledge among nations have all contributed. Opportunities to share experiences and gain new insights in many arenas are unlimited. Donald Berwick, MD (1996) from the Institute of Healthcare Improvement describes the "globalization of health care." He believes that health care can emulate the globalization of enterprises such as the automobile and food industries. From the study of other countries, Dr. Berwick recognizes that quality health care for a reasonable cost is also possible. He laments the fact that health care providers in the United States often believe there is little to learn from other countries who are "different" than we are. He states, "When our awareness of our differences impedes our learning, we pay a high price in missed opportunity. Improvement thrives everywhere and good ideas do not end at any border. Health care delivery may not yet be international, but health care improvement can be if only we let it"(p. 2).

Nursing has been aware for a long time that we can both share and gain from others around the world. Nursing leaders in years past, particularly in the early years of this century, took part in international nursing affairs. Several examples are as follows:

❑ Annie Warburton Goodrich (1966–1954): always active in national and international nursing affairs, was at various times president of the American Federation of Nurses, The American Nurses Association, and the International Council of Nurses (ICN) (Christy, 1970).

❑ Lavinia Lloyd Dock (1858–1956): Possibly our most colorful early leader, she was an ardent pacifist and did not hesitate (in fact some of her colleagues thought she enjoyed it) to serve time in the local jails for demonstrating against the government, war, and for women's suffrage. She served as secretary for ICN upon its founding in 1899, traveled extensively visiting hospitals in Europe and Asia, was editor of the American Journal of Nursing's Foreign Department (1900-1923), and was a member of the International Almshouses Committee (Christy, 1969).

❑ Lillian D. Wald (1867–1940): founder of the Henry Street Settlement in New York City often said, "the whole world is my neighborhood." She traveled throughout Europe and Asia, attending conferences and representing such organizations as the International Red Cross, and the League of Nations Child Welfare division. Passionate and far reaching in her pleadings for peace and child welfare, she was called "That Damned Nurse Troublemaker" by New York City officials and referred to as "That Woman" by President Woodrow Wilson. She was often an international consultant on issues of Public Health and nursing education (Coss, 1989).

In the years before World War II, it was not unusual for groups of nurses to travel to the ICN meetings throughout the world. Although the war may have dampened this enthusiasm for a while, international sharing is now clearly a prominent issue once more. Current nurse leaders and many schools of nursing participate in international activities to "globalize" nursing and to strive for professional recognition, as well as quality improvement, of health care world wide. Visiting scholar and professor programs, and more open doors for international graduate students, are just two ways this is happening. In addition, calls have come from many countries to the United States asking for textbooks, even older editions, because they are not plentiful in certain areas. This particular text, for example, has been translated into Italian and Japanese, as have many others. The point is that nursing as well as medicine, and health care in general, are challenged to make this a better, healthier world for all peoples.

KEY CONCEPTS

✔ Health care delivery has changed markedly during this century and will change even more rapidly as we approach the new millennium.

✔ Health care delivery, while often called a system, frequently does not provide adequate care or coverage for the people of the United States.

✔ The many changes in our society during the past 100 years are reflected in the development, the health problems, the changes and the solutions, in health care delivery.

✔ Attempts at solutions for our problems in health care delivery are more reflective of economics than overall program planning (e.g., Medicare and Medicaid, insurance plans, managed care and national/universal health insurance).

✔ With the advent of consumerism, the public has achieved more empowerment toward affecting its own destiny.

✔ Nurses become advocates for their clients by supporting, upholding, defending, and interceding on behalf of these clients.

✔ Historically, nurses have long supported the private and public efforts for health care reform. Moreover, nurses have been forerunners in these efforts through their holistic perspectives, health promotional activities, advanced practice, research, and the globalization of nursing and health care.

✔ We have much to learn from each other, and those advocating the globalization of health care encourage us to share across international borders.

CRITICAL THINKING QUESTIONS

1. Consider a health care agency with which you are familiar (i.e., hospital unit, pharmacy, physician's office or crisis center).

   a. Identify the professionals and nonprofessionals in the agency. Consider how geographically accessible it is to a broad spectrum of people.

   b. Identify the philosophy and standards of care in the agency.

   c. Identify the larger system of which it is a subsystem.

2. Considering the problems of health and health care delivery, suggest some ways nursing could advance health in the United States.

3. Examine the ideas behind national health insurance and HMOs. Describe how these two concepts might work together toward a health care delivery system for all Americans.

4. Assess and describe the biologic, psychologic, and sociocultural variables that influence your personal health behavior.

5. How have health care delivery systems changed in your community in the past decade? Have they increased or decreased in number? Changed in focus? Consolidated?

REFERENCES

American Hospital Association. (1992). *A patient's bill of rights*. Chicago: Author.

Berwick, D. (1996). The globalization of health care. *Quality connection: News from the Institute for Healthcare Improvement, 5*(2), 1–2.

Brewer, K. (1979). Inclusion of nursing services vital to any national health insurance program. *American Nurse, 11*(1) January 20, *31.*

Christy, T.E. (1970). Portrait of a leader: Annie Warburton Goodrich. *Nursing Outlook, 18*(8), 46–50.

Christy, T.E. (1969). Portrait of a leader: Lavinia Lloyd Dock, *Nursing Outlook, 17*(6), 72–75.

Coss, C. (Ed.). (1989). *Lillian D. Wald: Progressive activist.* New York: The Feminist Press.

Etheredge, M.L. (Ed.). (1989). *Collaborative care: Nursing case management.* Chicago: American Hospital Association—AHPI.

Fagin, C. (1982). Nursing as an alternative to high-cost care. *American Journal of Nursing, 82,* 56–60.

Fitzgerald, F. (1994). The tyranny of health. The New England Journal of Medicine, *331*(3), 196–198.

Georgopoulus, B.S., & Mann, F.C. (1962). *The community general hospital.* New York: Macmillan.

Hess, M.R. (1993). Preparing a nurse workforce appropriate for current and future health care delivery. In *U.S. Department of Health and Human Services, Public Health Service, Health Resource Administration, Bureau of Health Professions. Ninth report to the President and Congress on the status of health personnel in the United States,* Rockville, MD: Author.

Joel, L.A. (1987). Reshaping nursing practice. *American Journal of Nursing, 87,* 793–795.

Lear, M.W. (1980). *Heartsounds.* New York: Simon & Schuster.

Manthey, M. (1980). *The practice of primary nursing.* Boston: Blackwell Scientific Publications.

Munson, R. (1996). *Intervention and reflection: Basic issues in medical ethics.* (5th ed.). Belmont, CA: Wadsworth Publishing Co.

Nader, R. (1965). *Unsafe at any speed.* New York: Grossman Publishers.

National Center for Health Statistics. (1988). Health, United States, 1987 (U.S. Department of Health and Human Services Publication No. PHS 88-1232). Hyattsville, MD: Author.

Norling, R. (1996). Talk shows. *Hospitals and Health Networks, 70*(14) 66–76.

Powell-Cope, G.M. (1994). Family caregivers of people with AIDS: Negotiating partnerships with professional health Care providers. *Nursing Research, 43*(6), 324–329.

U.S. Department of Health and Human Services (1993) *Health Personnel in the United States, Ninth Report to Congress.* Hyattsville, Maryland: Public Health Service.

U.S. Department of Health, and Human Services (1995) *Healthy People 2000.* Hyattsville, Maryland: Public Health Service.

U.S. Department of Health and Human Services. (1996). *Your Medicare Handbook* (Publication No. HCFA-10050). Baltimore, MD: Health Care Financing Administration.

U.S. Department of Health and Human Services (1996-96). *Healthy people: 2000 Review: National health promotion and disease prevention objectives.* (DHHS Publication No. [PHS] 96-1256).

U.S. Public Health Service, Office of Disease Prevention and Health Promotion. (1988). *Disease Prevention/Health Promotion: The Facts.* Palo Alto, CA: Bull Publishing.

8

The Nursing Process

Key Words

Aggregation	Evaluating	Nursing	Nursing process
Assessing	Implementing	diagnosis	Planning
Defining	Intuition	Nursing	Problems
characteristics	North American	Intervention	Quality assurance
Diagnosing	Nursing Diagnosis	Classification	Standard
Diagnosis	Association	(NIC)	Strengths
	(NANDA)	Nursing Outcome	
		Classification	
		(NOC)	

Objectives

After completing this chapter, students will be able to:

State the purpose of the nursing process.

Describe how the nursing process has developed over time as the problem-solving process of nursing science.

Describe how the nurse collects data about the person to individualize care.

Describe how the nurse plans and implements individualized nursing care.

Discuss how evaluation and revision enhance the nursing process and improve nursing care.

The nursing process provides a way to identify the health, strengths, and needs of clients. This problem-solving process emphasizes the responses of persons to various situations and experiences, thus offering a means to plan effective and individualized nursing care. After years of development and testing, the nursing process has become the framework of professional nursing practice. Its importance is reflected in the standards of nursing practice, which were developed by the American Nurses Association (ANA, 1973, 1991) and incorporate the phases of the nursing process. The nursing behaviors that are tested on the licensing examination for registered nurses are grouped under the five parts or phases of the nursing process.

Before the Nursing Process

Historically, nursing focused more on health problems or specific disease conditions than on persons receiving care. Often, nursing care was based on the intuition of individual nurses or on orders written by physicians. Such care suggested that nurses were extensions of physicians rather than health professionals who provided a different service called nursing. As the knowledge base of nursing expanded, it became clear that this approach to planning care did not view persons as holistic beings with unique strengths and needs. Schedules of activities or procedures, so common to this traditional method of planning care, omitted the purpose of nursing—caring. As nursing developed into both a science and an art, the problem-solving method of science—that is, the scientific method—was adopted as a systematic approach to nursing practice.

The Nursing Process Defined

The **nursing process** is a series of scientific steps that assist the nurse in using theoretical knowledge to diagnose the strengths and nursing care needs of persons and to implement therapeutic actions for the purpose of attaining, maintaining, and promoting optimal biopsychosocial functioning. The nursing process proceeds logically through this series of scientific steps or phases from data collection to evaluation of care. Most nurse–scholars suggest that five distinct phases—(1) assessing, (2) diagnosing, (3) planning, (4) implementing, and (5) evaluating—comprise the nursing process. Additionally, diagnosing and the actual nursing diagnosis component of this phase are discussed extensively because of the current national and international focus on these areas. Figure 8-1 depicts the sequence of phases in the nursing process.

Phases

Phase 1 in the nursing process, assessing, consists of collecting information, data, or facts about the client so that the nurse may better understand the individual's feelings, ideas, values, and biophysical responses. With this information, the nurse and the client work together to identify the client's strengths and needs, and to develop an effective nursing care plan.

Phase 2 in the nursing process is diagnosing. Nursing diagnoses generated during this phase represent conclusions drawn by the nurse and the client from data collected and analyzed. Thus, analyzing follows assessing and precedes the actual care planning. Nursing diagnoses, the outcome of analysis, summarize the

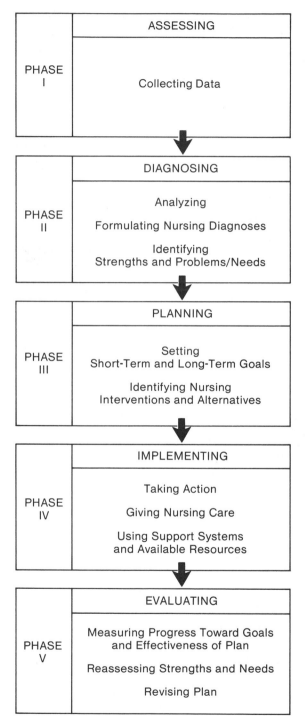

FIGURE 8-1 Five phases of the nursing process.

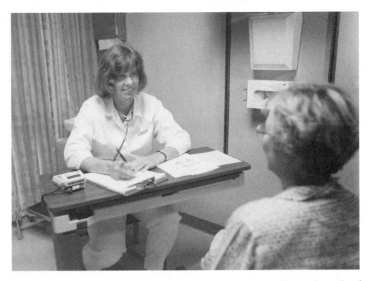

The nursing process is a way to identify the health, strengths, and needs of our clients.

client's strengths and needs within those specific functional areas for which nurses are qualified and licensed to provide support and care.

Phase 3 in the nursing process is planning. During this phase, the nurse and the client plan achievable outcomes and actions that both will take. The client participates in this step as well as he or she is able and is assisted by the nurse as needed.

Phase 4 in the nursing process, implementing, is the activation of the care plan. The nurse and the client work to achieve mutually planned objectives using actual nursing interventions.

Phase 5 in the nursing process, evaluating, is the act of determining the client's progress toward outcomes planned in phase 3. As before, the nurse and the client evaluate and revise the plan as needed to make continued progress toward the goals or to maintain identified strengths.

Aggregation: A Basis for Theory Development

These scientific steps form the accepted standard for basic professional care by aspiring nurses and mature professionals. Guides for particular components of the process (e.g., assessment guides and standard diagnoses) evolved as nurses collectively gained experience in their use. As individual nurses progress from novice to expert status, the additional potential of such a scientific approach becomes apparent. For example, as nurses mature, they accumulate a wealth of experience while caring for many persons with similar needs, problems, and concerns (Benner, 1984). An extension of the nursing process that provides an added potential is an activity called "aggregation." *To aggregate* is "to compile or gather together individual pieces of information'' (Erickson, Tomlin, & Swain, 1983, p. 252).

Although not usually identified as a phase in the nursing process, **aggregation** is defined as the process of collecting and summarizing many nursing interventions and their outcomes. The five steps in aggregation are as follows:

1. Collect and summarize clinical interventions.
2. Establish relationships.
3. Synthesize nursing principles.
4. Conduct nursing research.
5. Develop nursing theory.

From such summaries, nurses determine relationships among outcomes to predict the most effective interventions for a given age, gender, culture, health concern, life-style, and so forth. The idea of aggregation was first suggested by Swain (1973), and has since evolved as one method for developing a theory base for nursing practice.

Aggregation is a natural result of the many observations nurses make during the course of their practice, and it demonstrates how persons are unique, yet similar. Based on this information, nursing can develop interventions that are useful for certain common needs, such as altered mobility, pain control, unmet basic needs, experiences of loss, or feelings of hopelessness. Interventions developed through aggregation can be researched in actual clinical practice. Informal hunches can be tried and formal hypotheses tested. It was from just such informal hunches that Dumas and Leonard's (1963) pioneering research arose concerning preoperative interventions to stem postoperative nausea and vomiting. Thus, aggregation, the process of synthesizing data collected from many persons, contributes to nursing principles, nursing theories, and general nursing knowledge. Ultimately, aggregation can expand the knowledge base of nursing and stimulate theory-based practice.

For assistance in applying the concept of aggregation, consider the following discussion. In a course for RNs studying for a baccalaureate degree, the nurses had an opportunity to think about aggregation with regard to three clients. They were immersed in a project that included nine assignments over the course of the term (the idea for the project originally developed in a course by Erickson & Swain, 1983). In the beginning, they chose three clients for whom they had provided care sometime during their student or career days. They were encouraged to choose clients that just came into their head, and not to look for those obviously alike. Thus they chose clients of different ages, settings, cultures, diagnoses, and so forth. To begin with, they briefly told the ''story'' of each client, and then, as the term progressed, applied ideas from concepts such as person, family, sexuality, and culture to each. At the end of the project, they applied the process of aggregation to their three clients by considering the similarities and differences—among all three clients as a group, and among their own nursing interventions. They also identified three ''informal hunches'' that occurred to them as they thought about their clients. Consider the following examples:

"My clients were three unique individuals with three distinct life stories. At first it seemed that their only similarity was residence in an extended care facility. However, as I looked at these clients over the term, based on the course concepts, I saw them more broadly than I had at first. For example, Marianne barely ate for days, until Tim came and took her to the diner across the street, where she ate ravenously. When Tim was with her, she felt whole. Mr. Murray, following a failed marriage, and retirement from the job where he had felt complete, had a wound that would not heal, and Dr. Roget, still active professionally, died a few weeks after his wife died because he felt that he was nothing without her. Thus one hunch I formed is that a person's love and belonging needs often override basic physiological needs"(Contributed by Maricar Uy, RN).

"When we started this project I would have said that all three of my clients were unique with absolutely no similarities. As I studied them in greater depth, I gained a new understanding of each one and of the group as a whole. For example, all three were female. Marian and Karen were in their twenties and Caucasian, and Julie was African-American. Marian was married, Karen engaged, and Julie was single. Although Marian was pregnant, none had children. All lacked family support and all had ill health. Each had significant stressors that could be considered causative or contributory factors in their illnesses. Marian became pregnant to please her husband and then developed hyperemesis (severe nausea and vomiting) and eventually miscarried. Julie had little friend or family support, and after retirement felt worthless and without direction. At this point she developed osteomyelitis (a bone infection) that would not resolve. Karen was estranged from her mother and felt abandoned. Although she tried hard to overcome this loss, even turning to her fiance as if he were a parent, her health began to fail. Eventually she developed lung cancer and died at age twenty-six. Thus I began to realize that there may well be a correlation between the physical symptoms or manifestations of a person's illness, and stress or loss preceding the illness"(Contributed by Ashling Farelly).

These nurses and their classmates experienced a beginning step in the thinking process that moves us from clinical practice and informal hunches to hypotheses, research, and the development of new knowledge for nursing.

The Nursing Process as a Problem-Solving Process

The nursing process can be compared with the problem-solving approach and the scientific method as shown in Table 8-1. All of these processes follow a logical sequence of steps, beginning with the gathering of information and concluding with an evaluation of the outcome. Use of the scientific method is common to all professions, but each profession alters the method to suit its particular focus. For example, two characteristics of the problem-solving method—interaction and goal direction—are particularly well-suited to the nursing process.

Interaction and Goal Direction

The interaction between client and nurse is the nursing profession's unique use of the scientific problem-solving process. The nursing process guides nursing practice and is essential for effective, safe, quality care. Interaction is emphasized in

TABLE 8-1 *Comparison of Nursing Process With Scientific Method and Problem-Solving Method*

Scientific Method	Problem-Solving Method	Nursing Process
Define the problem	Gather information in a situation	Assess the situation, collect data
Collect data from observation and experimentation	Analyze information and identify the problem	Make a nursing diagnosis after analyzing data
Devise and execute a solution	Plan a course of action	Plan care, set goals or expected outcomes, establish nursing interventions
Evaluate the solution	Carry out the plan	Implement interventions
	Evaluate the plan and its outcomes	Evaluate and revise the process

the nursing process: the nurse interacts while working with the client to set goals and devise a plan directed at the client's strengths and needs. The patient is both the recipient of and a participant in the nursing care. The goal direction is a process and an outcome of the interaction. Thus, the professional work of nursing is approached in a scientific manner, as suggested in the discussion of the criteria for a profession in Chapter 2.

The interactive components of the nursing process (listening, observing, and responding purposefully) result in meaningful nursing care. Clients have described interacting with the nurse as helpful in identifying their health needs. Professional nurses have developed the knowledge and skills necessary for this helping role. Purposeful use of that knowledge and those skills will help clients understand their needs and identify and attain their goals. Gaining independence and self-awareness helps clients assume more control over their own care. Those who are more dependent and have complex needs may require more active involvement from the nurse. Achieving a balance between taking and returning control can be difficult for the nurse. However, it is the aim of nursing to promote self-care abilities through appropriate use of the nursing process. Nurse–client interaction is basic to the achievement of this end.

Now that the nursing process is the accepted professional practice method, nurses are becoming more sophisticated in its use. For example, initially, as the nursing process method came into vogue, most of the attention was focused on assessing—the data-gathering phase. The pioneering McCain (1965) article reflects the era when general assessment skills predominated. Taking a history and performing a physical examination, much as a physician would do, received major emphasis. Gradually, however, assessment skills both deepened and broadened to include psychosocial issues and data that would enhance nurses' diagnostic skills in specialty areas of nursing practice. With the continuing development of nursing as a profession, the growth of an assessment data base is recognized.

The creation of nursing diagnoses also indicates an increased sophistication in the use of the nursing process. The current emphasis on nursing diagnosis, including the development and continued work on standard nursing diagnoses, can be compared with nursing's earlier emphasis on assessment. Currently there is advanced work being done on the development of a nursing intervention classification system to be used with particular standard diagnoses. The next developmental wave, that of a nursing outcome classification, is in the early stages. Moreover, as nurses have recognized and acknowledged the importance of scientifically testing nursing interventions and outcomes in actual practice, classification systems have been developed by research teams. The University of Iowa has provided much leadership in this endeavor. Nursing's scientific development provides a legitimate scientific rationale for the care nurses give. This scientific development is also a necessary step toward aggregation, the important theory development phase that will expand the science of nursing.

The Nursing Process and Promotion of Self-Care

The nursing process as depicted in this chapter represents full client participation with the nurse in planning care. However, many variations exist in nurse–client approaches and responses. Ours, though perhaps an ideal, envisions clients as active participants and nurses as facilitators in the achievement of health promotion goals. In principle, this ideal is appropriate to all settings where professional nursing care is given, and can be practiced even when nurses modify the process to meet certain reality situations (refer to the discussion of self-care in Chapter 6). Further development of these ideas occurs throughout this chapter.

Standards of Nursing Practice

A *standard* is a specification set up and established by authority as a rule for the measure of quantity, weight, extent, value, or quality. A standard may be considered a criterion by which individuals or actions are compared and judged. The practice of nursing involves various settings, specialty areas, and levels of care. Nursing practice also reflects varying individual perspectives (both nurse and client) regarding the process of effective care. Therefore, the use of standards for practice has become necessary for professional functioning. Standards provide a common base or unifying force in this diverse profession. Although nurses may function in different ways, they still provide services from a shared understanding of the essence of nursing.

The American Nurses Association (1991) states, "Standards reflect the values and priorities of the profession. Standards provide direction for professional nursing practice and a framework for the evaluation of practice"(p. 1). The American Nurses Association reminds us that, as nurses, we are accountable to the public and to our clients for the outcomes of the nursing care we provide. The association sets professional standards for the purpose of maintaining a high level of quality in the practice of nursing. Because there is a close relationship among the defining characteristics of nursing practice—that is, the development and application of theory through nursing action, the nursing process, and the standards of nursing practice—the standards are identified in this section. Students will note that the standards are stated with consideration for the phases of the nursing process (see Fig. 8-2).

The American Nurses Association first introduced the document *Standards of Nursing Practice* in 1973. This document focused primarily on the nursing process and standards for practice related to this problem-solving method. In 1991, the document was revised and is called *Standards of Clinical Nursing Practice*. In this revision, ANA focused on two areas:

> Standards of Care consist of assessment, diagnosis, outcome identification, planning, implementation, and evaluation, and describe the competent level of nursing care as demonstrated by the nursing process (pp. 2–3).

> Standards of Professional Performance consist of quality of care, performance appraisal, education, collegiality, ethics, collaboration, research, and resource utilization, and describe a competent level of behavior in the professional role (pp. 2–3).

Thus, ANA has set professional standards for the purpose of defining a high level of quality in the practice of nursing and a means by which to measure it. The association has dealt with the level of client care and the growth of both individual nurses and the profession as a whole.

Standards are defined at several levels. The standards as developed by ANA provide the profession with a broad conceptual foundation for practice that is expected from all nurses, regardless of setting or type of care delivery. Using these standards as a base, organizations such as the American Association of Critical Care Nurses or the National Gerontologic Nursing Association, and institutions such as hospitals and home-care agencies have developed another more specific level of standards particularly directed to their practice. Nurses practicing at the bedside or in the home define standards suited to the daily operations of nursing care.

For example, consider the issue of client education. One ANA standard directed at this aspect of practice states, "The nurse develops a plan of care that prescribes interventions to attain expected outcomes"(ANA, 1991, p. 10). For institutional practice, another level of the standard for client education might read, "The nurse provides clients and families with health care education using appropriate principles of learning and in accordance with their specific assessed needs and abilities." Standards regarding many other specific interventions, such as those indicated for pain management and discharge planning, would also emanate from this same ANA standard.

At the bedside, the level of standards for patient education might read, "Patient education includes:

❏ An explanation of rationale for procedures and medications
❏ Written material and instructions applicable to test and surgical procedures
❏ Observation of client's demonstration of care activities for home"

Even more specifically—on a urology unit, for example, nurses develop stan-

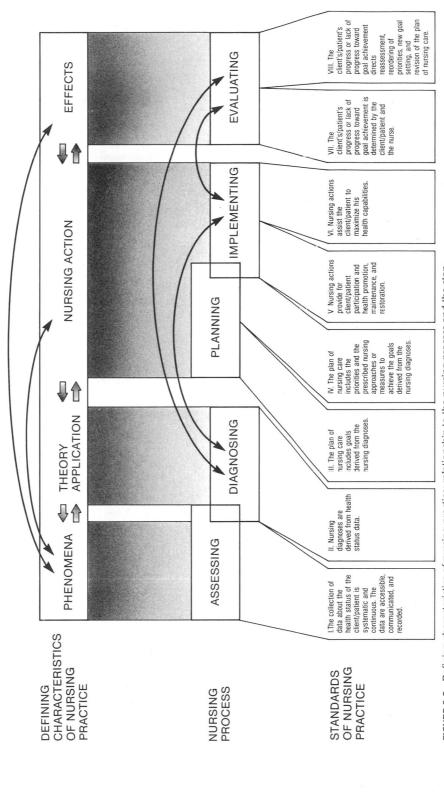

FIGURE 8-2 Defining characteristics of nursing practice: relationship to the nursing process and the standards of nursing practice.

247

dards that include step-by-step instructions for performing self-catheterization at home. This level of standard development flows nicely into the standard nursing care plan. Although it is acknowledged that care plans are developed to suit the individual client, the standard plan can be altered as necessary. However, a standard plan that describes general needs of all clients with a certain condition or problem provides the nurse with a basic direction for care. Carpenito (1990) offered what she termed "Generic Care Plans." These plans "present nursing diagnoses and collaborative problems that commonly apply to clients (and their significant others) undergoing hospitalization or out-patient treatment for any medical disorder or surgical procedure"(pp. 629, 641, 657). In addition, she presented more specific, yet still generic, care plans for certain nursing diagnoses and nursing plans for response to medical or surgical disorders. In this way, she provided direction for nurses using a standardized and quality-oriented approach that can be altered according to individual client and family needs.

Standard statements prescribe the expectations of nurses for client care or professional practice. Included in these statements are criteria for measurement. Using these criteria, nurses can determine that expectations have been met and with quality. For example, the aforementioned ANA standard includes the following five measurement criteria:

1. The plan is individualized to the client's condition or needs.
2. The plan is developed with the client, significant others, and health care providers as appropriate.
3. The plan reflects current nursing practice.
4. The plan is documented.
5. The plan provides for continuity of care.

Each level of practice develops measurement criteria that become more specific and provide a means for evaluation of whether the standard has been met. Determination that expectations have been met can be found through review of the following:

❐ Documentation on the client record
❐ Methods of peer review
❐ Nursing care conferences
❐ Statements of client satisfaction
❐ Decrease in a client's need for certain interventions, such as pain medication and assistance with daily activities
❐ Decrease in unnecessary complications (i.e., client is assisted with hourly coughing and deep breathing, resulting in clear lungs)
❐ Maintenance or decrease in the expected length of stay for clients with certain needs.

Quality Assurance

The discussion of standards prefaces the importance of a concept called **quality assurance (QA).** Quality assurance programs were first defined as such in the 1970s, and were developed to assure that products or services provided met certain standards of quality. These programs are found throughout the industrial as well as the professional world. *Quality assurance* can be defined as the establishment of professional standards and the monitoring of performance by colleagues. Essential to this concept is that quality control and self-regulation remain in the hands of professionals within their own practice. Thus, nursing will monitor itself and be reviewed, rather than monitored, by other professionals and government or regulatory agencies. Note that the "new generation" of QA programs that have developed over the last twenty years have been given more descriptive names, such as Quality Circles, and Continuous Quality Improvement.

The purpose of nursing quality programs is to improve and maintain the quality of nursing care and to determine how well nursing meets its stated objectives. Essential to this idea is the determination that the caregiver's knowledge and skills are at a level to ensure safe, effective client care. A quality program, like the nursing process, uses the problem-solving method. Quality programs are formal and systematic processes whereby problems are identified, activities or corrective actions are planned to resolve problems, and follow-up steps are performed to ensure that corrective actions have been effective. This process incorporates major issues confronting nursing today, such as accessibility to care, effectiveness and continuity of care, and cost-containment. Consider the example of a nursing quality activity on pages 280–281.

This text will not provide a comprehensive discussion on the issue of major quality programs. However, the comments provided introduce students to the concept, and demonstrate that nursing care can affect client outcomes and that nursing recognizes its accountability to society. In addition, note that regulatory agencies such as JCAHO (Joint Commission on Accreditation of Health Care Organizations), and our own professional organizations such as the ANA (American Nurses' Association) have definite Quality Assurance/Improvement programs.

Assessing (Collecting Data): Phase 1

The **assessing** phase of the nursing process consists of collecting data about the client and his or her family. Data are information, facts, or findings that the nurse gathers to understand feelings, ideas, values, and biophysical responses of persons and their families. These data are also used to identify client strengths and needs.

Purposes of Collecting Data

The nurse collects data during the assessing phase to obtain relevant information about the strengths and needs of both clients and their families. The nurse uses this data to plan effective care collaboratively with clients, families, and other professionals. The collected data provide a basis for expected outcomes and for planning interventions to maintain strengths or to cope with particular problems. Table 8-2 describes purposes for collecting data as discussed by nurse–scholars. Additional important priorities of data collection include the following:

The nurse communicates with the client rather than secondary or tertiary

TABLE 8-2 *Purposes of Collecting Data*

Nurse–Scholar	Quotation
Yura & Walsh (1978b)	"The purpose of this phase [assessment] is to identify and obtain data about the client that will enable the nurse and/or client or his family to designate problems relating to wellness and illness." (p. 95).
LaMonica (1979)	"Data collection is the continuous process of obtaining information needed in providing care." (p. 2).
Jones (1982)	"Assessment is defined as an interactive process through which the nurse gathers information about the client and the client's responses and interprets the information to derive an understanding of the level of wellness and the pattern and level of coping." (p. 196).
Marriner (1983)	"To deal with a problem one must first determine what the problem is. Therefore assessment is the first phase of the problem-solving process. It begins with the collection of patient data that have implications for nursing actions and ends with the nursing diagnosis, a statement of the patient's problems" (p. 27).
Carpenito (1993)	Data collection focuses on identifying the client's: ❏ Present and past health status ❏ Present and past coping patterns (strengths and limitations) ❏ Present and past functional status ❏ Response to therapy (nursing, medical) ❏ Risk for potential problems ❏ Desire for a higher level of wellness Nurses collect data to determine the need for nursing service and to assist other professionals (e.g., pharmacists, nutritionists, social workers, physicians) in determining their activities. (p. 46–47)
Erickson et al. (1983)	"—To develop an overview of the client's situation from the client's perspective —To develop an understanding of the client's personal orientation in terms of the client's expectations for the present and future —To determine the nature of the external support system —To determine the client's strengths and virtues —To determine the client's currently available internal resources —To determine the current developmental status in order to understand the client's personal model [view of the world] and to utilize maximum communication skills. The purpose for data collection within each of these major categories is to be able to interpret the data and specify nursing diagnoses." (p. 118).

sources to gather a major portion of the data. Family members are included in data collection if the nurse and client view this as important. The nurse uses judgment and data from the client to determine the proper approach.

Data collection includes information about both strengths and needs.

Data collection includes the client's and family's responses to current alterations in health and to past biopsychosocial stressors that may have pre-cipitated the current alterations.

Classifying Data

Data can be classified as subjective or objective. The literature describes these two types of data as follows:

1. *Subjective data* (symptoms) represent the person's description of his or her strengths, needs, perceptions, feelings, and experiences, that is, data that cannot be seen or felt by the observer. Examples include the client's statements "I feel warm" or "I am very tired."
2. *Objective data* (signs) consist of information obtained from clinical obser-vation, examination, and diagnostic studies. Examples include skin le-sions, blood pressure readings, and swelling associated with a bone fracture.

Both types of data are essential for accurate data analysis. Although these definitions of subjective and objective data are generally accepted, some would suggest they ought to be reversed in keeping with the emphasis on person; that is, the client's own observations may be more objective than those of the nurse (D. A. Finch, personal communication, September 1984). In research terminol-ogy, this would be using a phenomenologic approach. The term suggests that it is the client's perceptions of or the meanings he or she attaches to his or her experience that provide the most objective data about the phenomenon.

Sources of Data

Data about a client can be obtained from primary, secondary, or tertiary sources.

❏ The *primary source* is always the client.
❏ *Secondary sources* include the nurse's own observations and data from fam-ily and friends.
❏ *Tertiary sources* are the client's record and other health care providers, such as other nurses, physicians, and dietitians.

When evaluating data sources, the nurse considers the client as the first point of observation, hence the word *primary*. When collecting data from one whose communication abilities are limited (e.g., from an infant or from a comatose or confused person), the primary source is obviously limited. Therefore, the nurse uses data from secondary and tertiary sources as well to develop a more complete understanding of the client.

Tools for Collecting Data

Several tools can be used for collecting data. These tools are helpful in the exami-nation or testing of a phenomenon against established norms to make compari-sons. Table 8-3 describes the most common tools. Figure 8-3 illustrates physical assessment tools.

TABLE 8-3 *Tools for Collecting Data*

Assessment	Definition	Tools Needed	Examples
Observation	The art of seeing or sensing	Senses: sight, hearing, smell, touch, taste	Severe pallor Respiratory wheezing Cold, clammy skin Verbal and nonverbal behavior
Interview	A conference held in a face-to-face situation for the purpose of discussing and exploring a particular point	Conducive environment: comfortable, private Communication skills	Informal or unstructured (i.e., when bathing client) Formal or structured (i.e., planned conference for initial assessment data)
Listening	The act of purposefully attending to hear another person express his or her feelings, beliefs, strengths, and needs	All senses Conducive environment: comfortable, private Communication skills	Recognition of a person's underlying grief statement, "I don't really care."
Consultation	The use of additional resources to supplement data	Expert knowledge Literature Agency records Family, friends, and others who know client Client	Read literature or speak with expert regarding a subject or technique Discuss with client, family how to arrange house for disabled person
Inspection	A close and purposeful observation involving the visual and auditory examination of a client to obtain qualitative and quantitative data	Vision, hearing Tools such as scale, otoscope, stethoscope, thermometer, and so forth Standard charts for comparison	More focused than observation Color and integrity of skin Height and weight Blood pressure Body temperature, and so forth
Palpation	The use of the hands or fingers to examine the external surface of the body to determine surface or underlying characteristics	Hands Senses: touch, vision	Location of pain, tenderness, hardness Degree of edema Location, rate, quality, and strength of peripheral pulses
Percussion	Light but sharp tapping on an area of the body to produce vibration, resonance, and pitch of sound or resistance	Hands Senses: touch, hearing Reflex hammer tool	Determine position, size, and density of the underlying structure Presence of fluid in a cavity (e.g., normal: urine in bladder or abnormal: fluid in the lungs)
Auscultation	The act of listening with a stethoscope or other similar instrument for sounds in organs or body cavities	Stethoscope Senses: hearing Doppler, ultrasonic probe Sphygmomanometer Fetoscope	Heart, lung, and bowel sounds: duration, frequency, relative intensity, quality of pitch as well as adventitious sounds, i.e., rubbing, rumbling, gurgling Apical and brachial pulses Fetal heart tones

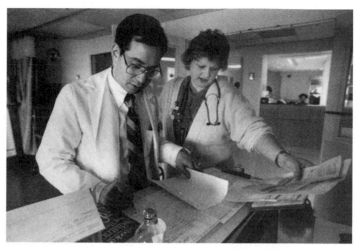

Data collection from tertiary sources is an interdisciplinary activity.

The Environment for Collecting Data

Selecting a Time and Place

Data collection occurs whenever a person is under the care of an agency such as a hospital, clinic, or nursing organization. Peace, quiet, and privacy are essential elements of the environment in which nurses and their clients talk. Difficulty in finding this environment is a common frustration. In the home, family members, phone calls, and the television provide distraction. In health care settings, interruptions occur frequently. In hospital ward settings, others may hear the client's responses. Despite these difficulties, nurses usually create a comfortable atmosphere so that clients can share private thoughts and information.

Establishing Trust

In addition to having a peaceful, private environment, clients need a sense of trust in the interviewer. Trust is developed as people work together. The nurse can begin to build trust by establishing a harmonious atmosphere of honest acceptance and empathy. Display 8-1 suggests interventions that encourage the development of trust.

Issues of Confidentiality

During interactions with the nurse, clients often share personal information. The nurse must decide which data to report. The key is to protect the client from exposure and yet provide enough data so that others may give consistent care. Nurses must decide whether information has been revealed to them in confidence or can be generally known. How one conveys data is often more important than

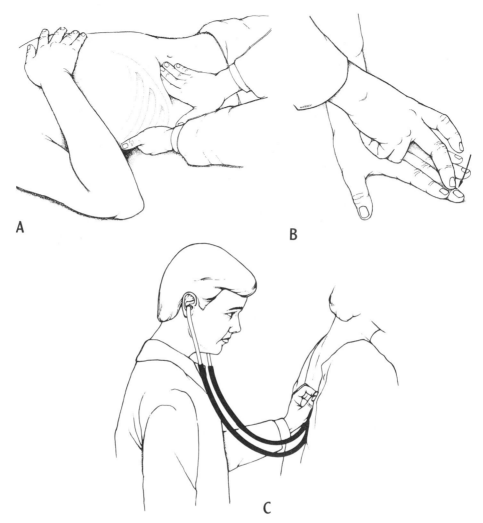

FIGURE 8-3 Physical assessment tools. (A) A Light palpation. (B) Percussion. (C) Stethoscopic examination.

the actual information given. Consider the following clinical example illustrating this point.

One nursing instructor relates,

The students and I were listening to morning report. The night nurse, addressing the entire day staff, reported on a patient who had not slept. She then disclosed, in great detail, a disturbing incident about the woman's alcoholic son. Later I asked the students for their response to the nurse's report. They believed that the client had been exposed and the report had seemed like gossip. When I asked how data should be passed on so that relevant care could be given, the students came to the following conclusion: the nurse could have recorded some general statements and

DISPLAY 8-1   **Interventions to Develop Trust**

Develop rapport
  Demonstrate
    Concern
    Belief in the intrinsic value of the person
    Unconditional acceptance of the person with his or her strengths and limitations
    Empathy
    Compassion
Develop trust
  Demonstrate
    Consistency in behaviors exhibited toward the person
    Willingness to clarify communications
    Genuine interest
    Truthfulness
  Remember that trust is not spontaneous but must be earned
    Spend time with the person.
    Use a relaxed and unhurried manner.
    Visit when there is nothing specific to do.
    Address the person by name.
    Do not invade privacy; hesitate at the door; ask the person if he or she feels like talking; ask if you may sit down.
    Do not interrupt.
  Do not issue direct commands, such as "you should."
  Ask for clarification of statements you do not understand.
  Let the person know you remember what he or she has told you on another occasion.
      For example, ask how the situation is now; say, "I remember when you told me. . . ."
  Communicate that you wish to understand what the client is experiencing.
  Offer touch; assess the person's comfort level with touch, and start slowly and gently.
  Move your body toward the person as he or she speaks.
  Allow the person to tell his or her complete story, even when it is uncomfortable for you, or explain your discomfort honestly and find someone else to listen.
  Inform the person early of your time limitations.
  Be reliable. It is all right to forget or change your plans, but be honest about what you did and why.
  Be consistent in behavior.
  Facilitate the person to regain control over his or her care and life.
  Help the person plan and carry out goals.

(B. Kennison, personal communication, January 1980.)

then talked privately to the day nurse. She might have explained the situation in some, but not total, detail. They reasoned that if the day nurse were aware of the problem, she could make herself available should the woman choose to talk. Further, if this nurse approached the client with care, the woman would not feel that everyone knew her troubles.

Many nurses find the confidential nature of client–nurse interactions to be both challenging and satisfying. However, in this day of the computer, confidentiality becomes more critical. Professionals who access information about others on their computer systems, unless needed for client care, can be subject to dismissal. In one instance, nurses wanted to know their manager's birthday so that they could plan a special party. They were able to access this via her records on the computer. While well meaning, this was clearly an improper use of the computer. In another instance, Carol, age 25 and single, decided to seek an abortion. Later she became ill and had to be hospitalized. She told the nursing staff that her family did not know about her pregnancy. Carol's sister, however, was a nurse in the same institution and accessed Carol's records on the computer. This created major problems for Carol and her family. While the nurses in these two examples were not reported, they would have been disciplined had their actions been known. No matter how tempting it is to seek information about family, friends, or others via computer records, it is always inappropriate unless professionally necessary. It is also correct to ask for a reassignment when given a client whose privacy might be violated by your knowledge of his or her needs. Moreover, do not assume that you know whether privacy would be violated or not, assume that it would be. One nurse reported that whenever there is a client whom she knows on her unit, she informs the person that she will not be caring for him or her, or reviewing the records.

*A*pproaches to Collecting Data

Frameworks

Several specific frameworks or guides have been created to help nurses collect and organize data. Displays 8-2 through 8-4 provide details of the following nurse–scholars' frameworks:

- ❐ Virginia Henderson (1966), Activities of daily living
- ❐ Faye Abdellah (Abdellah, Beland, Martin & Matheney, 1960), 21 Nursing Problems
- ❐ Marjory Gordon (1982, 1989, 1994), 11 functional health patterns

Although the first two references are comparatively old, they are generally acknowledged as classics. Furthermore, they have withstood the test of time, and present several enriching perspectives that contribute to a basic understanding of collecting data.

Even though Abdellah referred to her framework as problems, and the others used more health-oriented titles, all of these frameworks emanate from a health perspective. Abdellah has developed her framework around nursing goals to be

---

DISPLAY 8-2   Henderson's Activities of Daily Living

1. Breathe normally.
2. Eat and drink adequately.
3. Eliminate by all avenues of elimination.
4. Move and maintain a desirable posture (walking, sitting, lying, and changing from one position to another).
5. Sleep and rest.
6. Select suitable clothing; dress and undress.
7. Maintain body temperature within normal range by adjusting clothing and modifying the environment.
8. Keep the body clean and well-groomed and protect the integument.
9. Avoid dangers in the environment and avoid injuring others.
10. Communicate with others in expressing emotional needs, fears, and so forth.
11. Worship according to faith.
12. Work at something that provides a sense of accomplishment.
13. Play or participate in various forms of recreation.
14. Learn, discover, or satisfy the curiosity that leads to "normal" development and health.

(Henderson, V. [1966]. The nature of nursing. *New York: Macmillan, pp. 16–17.*)

DISPLAY 8-3   Abdellah's 21 Problems

1. To maintain good hygiene and physical comfort
2. To promote optimal activity, exercise, rest and sleep
3. To promote safety by preventing accident, injury, or other trauma and by preventing the spread of infection
4. To maintain good body mechanics and prevent and correct deformities
5. To facilitate the maintenance of a supply of oxygen to all body cells
6. To facilitate the maintenance of nutrition of all body cells
7. To facilitate the maintenance of elimination
8. To facilitate the maintenance of fluid and electrolyte balance
9. To recognize the physiologic responses of the body to disease conditions—pathologic, physiologic, and compensatory
10. To facilitate the maintenance of regulatory mechanisms and functions
11. To facilitate the maintenance of sensory function
12. To identify and accept positive and negative expressions, feelings, and reactions
13. To identify and accept the interrelatedness of emotions and organic illness
14. To facilitate the maintenance of effective verbal and nonverbal communication
15. To promote the development of productive interpersonal relationships
16. To facilitate progress toward achievement of personal spiritual goals
17. To create or maintain a therapeutic environment
18. To facilitate awareness of self as an individual with varying physical, emotional, and developmental needs

(continued)

DISPLAY 8-3 (*Continued*)

19. To accept the optimum possible goals in the light of physical and emotional limitations
20. To use community resources as an aid in resolving problems arising from illness
21. To understand the role of social problems as influencing factors in the cause of illness

(*Abdellah, F. G., Beland, I. L., Martin, A., & Matheney, R. V. [1960]. Patient-centered approaches to nursing. New York: Macmillan, pp. 16–17.*)

DISPLAY 8-4 Gordon's Typology of 11 Functional Health Patterns

1. *Health perception–health management pattern*–Describes client's perceived pattern of health and well-being and how health is managed
2. *Nutritional–metabolic pattern*–Describes pattern of food and fluid consumption relative to metabolic need and pattern indicators of local nutrient supply
3. *Elimination pattern*–Describes patterns of excretory function (bowel, bladder, and skin)
4. *Activity–exercise pattern*–Describes pattern of exercise, activity, leisure, and recreation
5. *Cognitive–perceptual pattern*–Describes sensory–perceptual and cognitive pattern
6. *Sleep–rest pattern*–Describes patterns of sleep, rest, and relaxation
7. *Self-perception–self-concept pattern*–Describes self-concept pattern and perceptions of self (e.g., body comfort, body image, feeling state)
8. *Role–relationship pattern*–Describes pattern of role engagements and relationships
9. *Sexuality–reproductive pattern*–Describes client's patterns of satisfaction and dissatisfaction with sexuality pattern; describes reproductive patterns
10. *Coping–stress-tolerance pattern*–Describes general coping pattern and effectiveness of the pattern in terms of stress tolerance
11. *Value–belief pattern*–Describes patterns of values, beliefs (including spiritual), or goals that guide choices or decisions

(*Gordon, M. [1989]. Manual of nursing diagnosis. St. Louis, MO: C. V. Mosby, p. 302–305*).

accomplished with each client. Henderson has used a person-focused approach, that is, the areas for collecting data are suggested from the person or client's perspective. Gordon's (1989) typology of functional health patterns provides groupings for the development of the nursing diagnoses currently accepted by the **North American Nursing Diagnosis Association (NANDA).**

In addition to these frameworks, nursing scholars have suggested theory bases from which nursing care may be practiced. A review of the discussion of the theorists in Chapter 3 will offer ideas in this realm. The use of a theoretical perspective for assessing and planning care, as well as for theory-based practice in general, provides the following essential elements for nursing:

❑ A common language
❑ A purpose and rationale for care planned
❑ An approach for communication with other professionals
❑ A base for the development of research
❑ An increase in nursing's body of knowledge
❑ Continued growth toward meeting the criteria for a profession (Chinn & Jacobs, 1987)

A General Approach

A person-centered approach is essential to this text's format for collecting data. Learning about the client's life experiences and understanding his or her particular view (model) of his or her life will provide a base for effective nursing care (Erickson et al., 1983).

Choosing some general-purpose tool that facilitates the comprehensive, orderly collection of data is most important at this point. Regardless of the particular theoretical perspective used, common areas exist across which data may be collected. The data obtained can be analyzed to yield diagnoses that conform to the evolving NANDA diagnoses. The work of NANDA is discussed in the ''Nursing Diagnosis'' section of this chapter. The essential point is that collecting data, that is, assessing, is an ongoing process that occurs wherever and whenever it is needed. Consider Display 8-5 for an example of data collection.

DISPLAY 8-5 Data Collection for Mrs. Carroll

Physical Signs and Symptoms
72-year-old woman admitted in wheelchair for a mitral valve repair
Height, 5'1"; weight, 160 lb
Very pale complexion
Lungs clear on auscultation
Respirations regular and unlabored but audible
Dyspnea on exertion beyond dressing self and ambulating a few steps
Heart rate strong and regular
Skin clear and intact
Shoulders hunched
Sad affect
Speech slow and barely audible
States: "I can change my clothes, but it will take me a long time."
Sighs frequently

(continued)

DISPLAY 8-5 (*Continued*)

Mental and Emotional Concerns

NURSE: You do look very tired to me. Have you been unable to rest or sleep well lately?"

CLIENT: "I've stayed up all night crying this past week. I'm so afraid of this surgery."

NURSE: "Can you tell me more about your fears?"

CLIENT: "I'm afraid because I know they are going to put that tube down my throat during surgery. Then when they take it out they will rip my trachea and I'll die. That's what happened to my sister-in-law, right here in this hospital. My father died here, too, from cancer."

NURSE: "Have you discussed some of these worries with your family?"

CLIENT: "It has been 8 years since my husband died but I still miss him. My daughter and her family try to help, but I still feel as if there is no one to turn to."

Diagnosing: Phase 2

Analyzing Data

Diagnosing is phase 2 of the nursing process. This phase includes analyzing data, an important mental activity that follows collecting data. *Analyzing* is the cognitive (thinking) process in which nurse and client form conclusions on which to base nursing care. Analyzing occurs whenever there are data, whether from a full assessment or a brief interaction. The focal points of the analysis are both the client's strengths and needs.

A classic and still helpful statement by Durand and Prince (1966) described data analysis as the thought process leading to the recognition of a pattern that precedes the nursing diagnosis. They indicated that this thought process is influenced by scientific knowledge applicable to nursing, by a definition of nursing, and by past experiences that lead to the recognition of a pattern and thus the nursing diagnosis (p. 55). LaMonica (1979) presented the data processing, or data analysis, segment of the nursing process as the bridge connecting rote nursing responsibilities with individualized client considerations (see Fig. 8-4).

Carnevali (1983) suggested a strategy for analyzing data and thus developing nursing diagnoses. She stated, "The actual organization, storage, and creation of accessing pathways must be done by the individual clinician"(p. 38). Three basic activities are involved:

1. Accumulating knowledge from reading, listening, observing, and analyzing experience
2. Storing facts, cues, variations, contexts, and experiences in a purposeful and systematic way in one's long-term memory
3. Engaging in ongoing critiqued clinical practice of using "accessing routes" to the stored knowledge and testing the effectiveness of recognition features and treatment options (pp. 38–39)

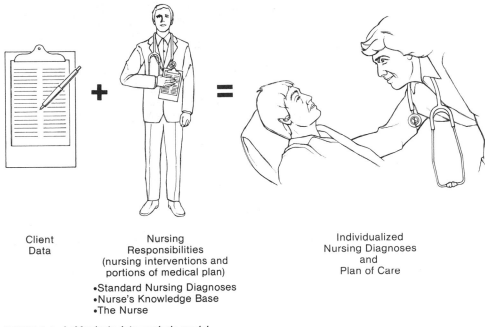

Client
Data

Nursing
Responsibilities
(nursing interventions and
portions of medical plan)
•Standard Nursing Diagnoses
•Nurse's Knowledge Base
•The Nurse

Individualized
Nursing Diagnoses
and
Plan of Care

FIGURE 8-4 LaMonica's data analysis model.

Thus, when analyzing data, the nurse compares facts gathered from the client with a number of accepted norms: anatomic, physiologic, psychologic, and developmental. At the same time, the nurse draws on accepted nursing knowledge and personal nursing experiences to recognize patterns in, or relationships among, the data. The nurse then discusses his or her conclusions or checks with the client to determine the validity or soundness of those conclusions.

Analyzing data occurs in an ongoing way when working with a client. The nurse constantly considers, sifts, and sorts the facts presented. Often, conclusions are drawn quickly with little chance for discussion with the client or others. However, many interactions with a client may be required before the nurse has data suitable for planning comprehensive care. Frequently during interactions between nurse and client, both form perceptions and begin analysis. In one research study (Kennison, 1983), clients described the nurse's questions as helpful because, in answering them, the client was able to do his or her own sorting, which assisted the client in attaching more meaning to his or her experiences. See Table 8-4 for details of the thinking process followed by the nurse in analyzing data and formulating nursing diagnoses for a specific client.

Nursing Diagnosis

Establishing a **nursing diagnosis** is the outcome of analyzing in the diagnosing phase. Diagnosing has long been considered the prerogative of the medical profession. Indeed, dictionaries frequently list the first definition of the term as the art

TABLE 8-4   *Analyzing Data for Scenario With Mrs. Carroll*

Summary of Nurse's Observation	Rationale
Communicates readily with the nurse and talks about feelings and experiences	Strengths identified using both psychosocial and physical data (nurse's observations, past experiences, anatomy and physiology sources)
Can take care of self and activities of daily living	
Lungs clear on auscultation	
Breathing unlabored with limited exertion	
Heart rate strong	
Skin clear and intact	
Demonstrates feelings of extreme fatigue, fear, grief, and abandonment	Affect: slow, quiet speech; statement that she has no one to turn to (Engel's [1964] theory of grief and loss, Piaget's [1973] theory on object permanence)

Demonstrates unmet needs in following areas:
Physiologic
Safety and security
Love and belonging
Esteem
	Rest, sleep, cardiac output, circulation
	  Statements about what will happen to her
	  Statements that she misses husband and has no one to turn to
	  Statements suggest that she does not feel in control but that others will cause things to happen (Maslow's [1970] basic needs theory)

Distrustful of caregivers	Statements about what will happen to her during and after surgery (Erikson's [1963] psychosocial development theory)
Perceives little control over destiny	Statements regarding what others will do to her (Maslow [1970] and Erikson [1963])
Unsure of boundaries between self and sister-in-law, self and father	Comments suggest that it happened to them so it will happen to me (Piaget's [1973] cognitive development theory—preoperational thinking)

or act of identifying a disease from its signs and symptoms. Nursing diagnoses, however, summarize the client's strengths and problems within those specific functional areas for which nurses are qualified and licensed to provide support or care. In differentiating the nursing diagnosis from other clinical problems, that is, medical problems, Carpenito (1987) suggested the following questions:

> Can the nurse identify the problem legally and educationally?
> Can the nurse legally order the necessary interventions to treat or prevent the problem?
> Can the nurse legally treat the problem? (p. 17)

Nursing diagnosis emphasizes the unique contribution nurses can make to the health of individuals and the community. Gordon (1994) suggests the following helpful ideas:

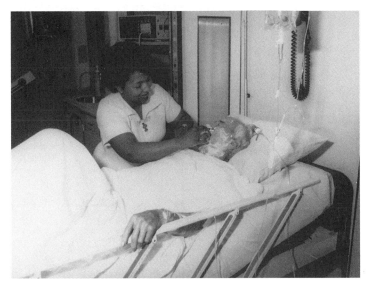

The client and the nurse plan care together.

Characteristics of Conditions Labeled Nursing Diagnoses

1. Nurses can obtain the critical assessment data necessary for making the diagnosis independently.
2. The condition can be resolved primarily by nursing interventions.
3. Nurses assume responsibility for patient/client outcomes related to the condition.
4. Nurses assume responsibility for research on the condition—including its prevention, diagnosis, and treatment (p. 23).

Definition of Nursing Diagnosis

A *nursing diagnosis* represents a nursing judgment drawn from data concerning client strengths and needs that guides decisions for care. The following are five essential elements of the nursing diagnosis:

1. Represents a statement, judgment, or conclusion
2. Focuses on the client's responses (either strengths or problems)
3. Comes from and follows data collection
4. Labels conclusions
5. Suggests interventions

At the ninth conference of NANDA, the following definition was adopted: "A nursing diagnosis is a clinical judgment about individual, family, or community response to actual or potential health problems/life processes. Nursing diagnoses provide the basis for selection of nursing interventions for which the nurse is accountable"(Carroll-Johnson, 1991, p. 373). Just as there are many tools for collecting data, there are numerous definitions of nursing diagnosis. See Table 8-5 for several early definitions of nursing diagnosis.

STRENGTHS

The following definition of strengths describes this component of nursing diagnosis:

> **Strengths,** also called internal resources, are biologic, psychologic, social, or spiritual qualities that contribute to a person's character, integrity, and uniqueness, and that can be mobilized to cope with a problem or to attain a goal. Strengths are an inherent part of each individual, but may not be maintained or mobilized in an adaptive manner without nursing interventions.

Strengths represent inner health that promotes greater wellness. Strengths are important considerations when planning nursing care. See Display 8-6 for examples of strengths. Popkess-Vawter (1984) stated,

> Without a strengths list, nursing care is planned in isolation; there is no recycling of patient energy back into his or her system to revitalize the person's recovery process. Without assessing the patient's strengths, the nurse is second-guessing what would be a therapeutic approach to care for the patient's problems (p. 435).

The client's external resources also assist the nurse when planning care and can be included in the individual client's diagnosis list because they provide important sources of support in coping with health problems. Consider the following categories:

- ❏ Support systems—Family, friends, health care professionals
- ❏ Financial resources—Income, insurances
- ❏ Environmental resources—Health care, recreation, shopping, transportation, education
- ❏ Education—Level, training, and occupational experience

TABLE 8-5 *Definitions of Nursing Diagnosis*

Author	Definition
Mundinger & Jauron (1975)	"The statement of a patient's response which is actually or potentially unhealthful and which nursing intervention can help to change in the direction of health. It should also identify essential factors related to the unhealthful response" (p. 97).
Gordon (1976)	"Actual or potential health problems which nurses, by virtue of their education and experience, are capable and licensed to treat" (p. 1299).
Kim & Moritz (1982)	"The judgment or conclusion that occurs as a result of nursing assessment" (p. 107).
Marriner (1979)	"A statement of the patient's problems, including his strengths, limitations, and methods of adapting to that problem" (p. 2).
Thomas & Coombs (1966)	"A statement of a conclusion resulting from a recognition of a pattern derived from a nursing investigation of the patient" (p. 66).

DISPLAY 8-6   **Examples of Strengths**

Has resolved developmental tasks favorably
   Trust versus mistrust
   Autonomy versus shame and doubt
   Initiative versus guilt, and so forth
Meets own basic needs
   Physiologic
   Safety and security
   Love and belonging
   Esteem
   Growth
Values independence
Relates warmly with spouse, children, and others
Expresses spirituality and faith
Expresses a comfortable philosophy of life
Verbalizes knowledge about health problems
Displays a sense of humor
Uses pain control methods effectively
Displays unique talents and interests (music, art, languages, cooking, woodworking, needle-
   work, gardening, extensive reading, athletic endeavors, and so forth)
Demonstrates effective problem solving
Accepts help from the nurse and others
Gives and receives warmth, affection, friendship
Expresses readiness to learn about health concerns
Expresses readiness to start coping with health concerns
Has insight into personal situations and responses
Has progressed through stages of grief and loss appropriately
Sleeps well
Absorbs and digests food effectively
Maintains a stable blood pressure
Maintains effective breathing patterns
Moves about with ease
Maintains skin integrity

PROBLEMS/NEEDS

Another element of nursing diagnosis is the problem or need category. **Problems** can be classified into three areas: (1) actual problems, (2) potential problems, and (3) possible problems.

Actual problems or needs are those that can be identified from the current data. Examples include:

- ❏ Decreased endurance
- ❏ Respiratory distress with minimal exertion
- ❏ Anxiety related to forthcoming surgery
- ❏ Chronic nausea

Potential problems or needs are those that the person is at high risk to develop, given his or her particular situation. Examples include:

❏ Skin breakdown related to decreased mobility
❏ Increased respiratory secretions related to postoperative state
❏ Diminished self-esteem related to alteration in usual functioning.

Possible problems or needs are those for which the nurse has obtained enough data to suggest a hunch, but not enough to identify an actual problem. An example might be possible financial problems. The client may indicate that he or she is not worried about finances, yet the nurse notes that the client wrings his or her hands when questions of finances arise.

Purposes of Nursing Diagnoses

In 1973, a group of nurses from the United States and Canada met to identify nursing functions and to establish a classification system of nursing diagnoses. These nurses represented all specialties and roles within the nursing profession. Foreseeing future needs, they envisioned a classification system suitable for the age of computerization. These and other nurses interested in nursing diagnoses have continued to meet at intervals to develop and establish the classification system further. The most recent convention, the 12th, was in 1996, and the most recent list of accepted nursing diagnoses can be found in Display 8-7.

This international group, NANDA, has identified several purposes for the establishment of a classification system for nursing diagnoses:

❏ Identifying nursing's independent practice domain
❏ Providing a common reference system to assist in the growth of clinical knowledge through research
❏ Assisting in computerization of the nursing process

Other nurse–scholars concur and have given additional purposes such as the following:

❏ Meeting record-keeping requirements
❏ Evaluating quality of care
❏ Assessing charges for reimbursement.

Nursing diagnoses will continue to evolve over time; two recent modifications deserve special mention. In 1987, Taxonomy I was organized according to the nine human response patterns that prevail today:

1. Choosing
2. Communicating
3. Exchanging
4. Feeling
5. Knowing
6. Moving
7. Perceiving
8. Relating
9. Valuing (Fitzpatrick, 1991)

DISPLAY 8-7 Approved Nursing Diagnosis Labels of North American Nursing Diagnosis Association

Activity intolerance
Activity intolerance, risk for
Adjustment, impaired
Airway clearance, ineffective
Anxiety
Aspiration, risk for
Body image disturbance
Body temperature, risk for altered
Breastfeeding, effective (potential for enhanced)
Breastfeeding, ineffective
Breastfeeding, interrupted
Breathing pattern, ineffective
Cardiac output, decreased
Caregiver role strain
Caregiver role strain, risk for
Communication, impaired verbal
Constipation
Constipation, colonic
Constipation, perceived
Coping, defensive
Coping (family), ineffective: Compromised
Coping (family), ineffective: Disabling
Coping (family), potential for growth
Coping (individual), ineffective
Decisional conflict (specify)
Denial, ineffective
Diarrhea
Disuse syndrome, risk for
Diversional activity deficit
Dysreflexia
Family processes, altered
Fatigue
Fear
Fluid volume deficit
Fluid volume deficit, risk for
Fluid volume excess
Gas exchange, impaired
Grieving, anticipatory
Grieving, dysfunctional
Growth and development, altered
Health maintenance, altered

Health-seeking behaviors (specify)
Home maintenance management, impaired
Hopelessness
Hyperthermia
Hypothermia
Incontinence, bowel
Incontinence, functional (urinary)
Incontinence, reflex (urinary)
Incontinence, stress (urinary)
Incontinence, total (urinary)
Incontinence, urge (urinary)
Infant feeding pattern, ineffective
Infection, risk for
Injury, risk for
Knowledge deficit (specify)
Management of therapeutic regimen, ineffective
Mobility, impaired physical
Noncompliance (specify)
Nutrition, altered: less than body requirements
Nutrition, altered: more than body requirements
Nutrition, altered: potential for more than body requirements
Oral mucous membrane, altered
Pain
Pain, chronic
Parental role conflict
Parenting, altered
Parenting, risk for altered
Peripheral neurovascular dysfunction, risk for
Personal identity disturbance
Poisoning, risk for
Post-trauma response
Powerlessness
Protection, altered
Rape-trauma syndrome
Rape-trauma syndrome: compound reaction
Rape-trauma syndrome: silent reaction
Relocation stress syndrome

Role performance, altered
Self-care deficit, bathing/hygiene (specify level)
Self-care deficit, dressing/grooming (specify level)
Self-care deficit, feeding (specify level)
Self-care deficit, toileting (specify level)
Self-esteem, chronic low
Self-esteem, disturbance
Self-esteem, situational low
Self-mutilation, risk for
Sensory/perceptual alterations (specify): auditory, kinesthetic, gustatory, tactile, olfactory, visual
Sexual dysfunction
Sexuality patterns, altered
Skin integrity, impaired
Skin integrity, risk for impaired
Sleep-pattern disturbance
Social interaction, impaired
Social isolation
Spiritual distress (distress of the human spirit)
Suffocation, risk for
Swallowing, impaired
Therapeutic regimen (individuals), ineffective management of
Thermoregulation, ineffective
Thought processes, altered
Tissue integrity, impaired
Tissue perfusion, altered (specify type): cerebral, cardiopulmonary, gastrointestinal, peripheral, renal
Trauma, risk for
Unilateral neglect
Urinary elimination, altered
Urinary retention
Ventilation, inability to sustain spontaneous
Ventilatory weaning response (dysfunctional)
Violence, risk for: self-directed or directed at others

(*SOURCE:* North American Nursing Diagnosis Association, *Nursing Diagnoses: Definitions and Classification, 1995–1996.* Philadelphia: NANDA. Used by permission.

In 1989, Taxonomy I-Revised was translated into the International Classification of Disease code as a step toward international acceptance of nursing's diagnostic and therapeutic domains in anticipation of Taxonomy II (Carroll-Johnson, 1991).

Let us consider writing nursing diagnoses or diagnostic statements in the forms suggested by Gordon (1989, 1994) and Carpenito (1987, 1995). As an illustration, consider the actual problems listed previously in an informal format as

❐ Decreased endurance
❐ Respiratory distress with minimal exertion
❐ Anxiety related to forthcoming surgery
❐ Chronic nausea.

Now, using the more formal three-part wording, they are transformed to a format of

PROBLEM—related to—ETIOLOGY—as evidenced by—SYMPTOM

ACTIVITY INTOLERANCE related to ALTERATION IN OXYGEN TRANSPORT SYSTEM as evidenced by DECREASED ENDURANCE and RESPIRATORY DISTRESS WITH MINIMAL EXERTION.
ANXIETY related to FORTHCOMING SURGERY as evidenced by FEELINGS OF LOSING CONTROL.
NAUSEA related to STRESS as evidenced by CLIENT COMPLAINTS OF FEELING "SICK TO MY STOMACH."

No single correct way exists to write such diagnoses. In part, the decision about how to write is based on the emphasis desired. For example, is nausea primarily a comfort problem or a long-standing manifestation of a nutrition problem? If a long-standing manifestation of a nutrition problem, the nursing diagnosis might have been written as follows: ALTERED NUTRITION: LESS THAN BODY REQUIREMENTS related to ANOREXIA as manifested by COMPLAINTS OF NAUSEA.

Or, if the client can verbalize his or her concerns about surgery, the problem might be written, FEAR related to FORTHCOMING SURGERY as manifested by patient statement, "I KNOW I WON'T COME THROUGH THIS OPERATION." When a standard diagnosis does not cover the specific situation, the nurse describes or creates a diagnosis as necessary to plan care, and validates the statement with professional nurse colleagues.

As you grow in an understanding of the nursing process, and nursing diagnosis in particular, consult both Gordon's and Carpenito's work over the years. These books and manuals will offer you the current generation of thinking, and will provide an historical perspective as well. This history helps us understand the progress of the problem-solving method called nursing process, and also demonstrates the development of the nursing profession.

Analyzing and Diagnosing: An Illustration

Analyzing and diagnosing have now been presented from several specific viewpoints. Using the analysis of data for Ms. Carroll (see Table 8-4), nursing diagnoses can now be formulated for this client from a general person-centered approach.

This approach incorporates the various theoretical frameworks introduced in the conceptual discussion of person in Chapter 4; however, the data presented are incomplete in the sense of a total person assessment. The facts, however, are considered accurate because the client's actual statements and the nurse's objective observations are provided. In addition, the nurse has validated some of his or her observations with the client through the questions the nurse asked.

In analyzing these data, the nurse notes that the client can communicate her fears and express at least some of her feelings. Ms. Carroll can also perform certain activities of daily living, for example, changing her clothes. Using knowledge from physiology and pathophysiology, the nurse understands that the faulty mitral valve has compromised cardiac output and thus circulation throughout the body, which in turn contributes to the extreme fatigue. The nurse also recognizes from nursing theory and past experiences that fear and unresolved issues of loss and grief may contribute to fatigue. The frameworks of Maslow, Erikson, and Piaget are helpful in understanding Ms. Carroll's statements and her personal model of the world. The following list may be considered the nursing diagnoses or conclusions drawn from this data base. The first list uses the NANDA standardized diagnoses, and the second list individualizes or expands on these standard diagnoses, using the client's data base (Table 8-6).

Nursing diagnoses according to the NANDA list of standard nursing diagnoses are as follows:

❑ Activity Intolerance
❑ Sleep Pattern Disturbance
❑ Grieving, Dysfunctional
❑ Anxiety
❑ Thought Processes, Altered

Nursing diagnoses expanded according to the individualized data set are as follows:

Strengths
❑ Able to express feelings
❑ Can establish rapport with a helpful person (nurse)
❑ Self-care asset: can dress self.

TABLE 8-6 *Examples of Strengths Derived from NANDA List*

Accepted Diagnoses	Strengths
Breathing Pattern, Ineffective	Breathing pattern, effective
Communication, Impaired Verbal	Communication, effective
Fluid Volume Deficit	Hydration, adequate
Grieving, Dysfunctional	Grieving, appropriate
Powerlessness	Control, ability to maintain
Skin Integrity, Impaired	Skin integrity, maintained
Sleep Pattern Disturbance	Sleep pattern, restful

Problems

❏ Activity Intolerance related to decreased cardiac output and decreased circulation feelings of fear, abandonment, grief
❏ Sleep Pattern Disturbance, insomnia related to fear of surgery
❏ Grieving, unresolved issues related to death of husband, father, sister-in-
law
❏ Deficit in ability to meet basic needs physiologic safety and security love
and belonging esteem growth (Maslow)
❏ Unresolved issues of trust versus mistrust autonomy versus shame and
doubt (Erikson, 1963)
❏ Preoperational thinking mode related to death of father, sister-in-law (Piaget, 1973)

Note that the nurse has identified both strengths and problems derived from
the available data. In this way, he or she can use the strengths to assist with
problem solving. For example, Ms. Carroll can express her fears and concerns.
Therefore, the nurse knows that listening carefully and providing time for verbalization will help the client begin to work through her feelings. Ms. Carroll's
exhaustion does not prevent her from being somewhat independent. This fact
indicates that the nurse can support Ms. Carroll's independence and help the
client maintain the abilities she still has. Further data collection will help the
nurse determine how to promote the client's independence optimally. If this
process seems confusing, remember that nursing students have many opportunities for clinical practice under the guiding assistance of a clinical instructor.

Establishing Priorities Among Nursing Diagnoses

After determining the nursing diagnoses, the nurse will rank them in a particular
order to plan the most effective approach for the delivery of nursing care. When
establishing priorities, the nurse considers the following questions:

What strengths does the person have, and how can they best be used?
Are there acute or life-threatening problems?
What is the client's most pressing stated concern?
Which problems, not acute or pressing, does the client prefer to work on
first?
Which problems can the client work on by himself or herself, and with
which ones will the client need nursing assistance?
Which strengths can the client mobilize at the present time to facilitate his
or her problem solving?
Are there several problems that are acute or pressing? If so, how can the
approach to care accommodate the client's needs in several areas?

The nurse will often note that a client has many pressing needs that cannot
be met at once. When this occurs, it is best to consider urgent safety issues first,

and then comfort. Returning to the client and determining with him or her how to order nursing care uses both the client's model of the world and his or her strengths. Usually when life-threatening problems are involved, several persons are available to assist. In this way, emergency needs can be attended to by some personnel while others consider safety, security, and comfort needs. Maslow's hierarchy of basic needs may be helpful if used with the client to explore his or her needs. If the client is unconscious or is otherwise unable to make his or her needs known, the nurse reviews the physiologic needs using a head-to-toe assessment process. At the same time, the nurse attends to psychological needs by talking to the client and providing comfort. During this time, it is useful and comforting to remind the client of strengths the nurse has identified—for example, a strong heart rate, regular breathing, and positive responses to care. Additionally, secondary and tertiary data sources are consulted as necessary. The nurse attempts to determine this particular client's perspective, as well as interventions that have been helpful in the past.

When writing a list of the client's nursing diagnoses, strengths are often listed first so that the nurse and the client are clearly aware of them. Strengths, as an integral part of the person's holism, are used to assist the client generally. Strengths may be correlated with specific problems, however, if suitable.

Guidelines for Using Standardized Lists of Nursing Diagnoses

The standardization of nursing diagnosis has provided a way for the nursing profession to define and articulate practice. When the movement was relatively young, and particularly in the early 1980's, some nurse–scholars cautioned us to use this standardization format with care. In general, they advised nurses not to let a standard format substitute for individualized and holistic care. They worried that standard diagnoses could become labels that would stereotype our clients. In particular, Shamansky and Yanni (1983, p. 48) stated, "It is therefore inappropriate to be constrained by a predigested set of labels into which one must force bits of information. Rather, it is incumbent upon us to describe carefully and thoughtfully and fully the phenomena we see." We are well advised to consider these points today. In addition, we offer the following three suggestions:

1. Develop nursing diagnoses from a theoretical foundation rather than from disease or pathology.
2. Develop a format for describing the phenomena observed in the individual client's data base, including both strengths and problems (e.g., maintains a stable blood pressure, unresolved trust versus mistrust).
3. Avoid using the standardized nursing diagnoses as labels or value judgments, and develop a procedure for describing the individual client's perspective and experiences.

Nurses are encouraged to expand on or enlarge the standard diagnoses to describe the individual client's responses and to develop new diagnoses as a situation warrants. Although a standard diagnosis assists the nurse by providing a general category, it should be made specific enough to give others an understanding of the problem. For example, "Ineffective coping" is a standard diagnosis used in instances in which the client is unable to participate in his or her care. This diagnosis provides us with the concern. However, the nurse also explores—with the client—whether plans are irrelevant or too overwhelming to follow. Nursing care can then be expanded to deal with the client's perceived needs, thus changing the diagnosis and the nursing care as clients and their responses change.

Currently, nurse–scholars are continuing their work to further classify standard diagnoses as they further develop and refine lists of defining characteristics for each diagnosis. For example, the NANDA diagnosis of "Pain," according to Gordon (1989), includes the following defining characteristics:

❑ Communication (verbal or coded) of pain description
❑ Narrowed focus (altered time perception, withdrawal from social contact, impaired thought process)
❑ Distraction behavior (moaning, crying, pacing, seeking out other people or activities, restlessness)
❑ Facial mask of pain (eyes lack luster,"beaten look," fixed or scattered movement, grimace)
❑ Alteration in muscle tone (may span from listless to rigid)
❑ Physiologic responses (excessive perspiration, blood pressure and pulse rate change, pupillary dilatation, increased or decreased respiratory rate) (p. 154)

Panels of nurses with defined expert knowledge are polled to determine whether, in their judgment, certain defining characteristics are generally present with a given diagnosis. This process will further clarify the actual diagnosis and, when used with an individual client's experience and perspective, can provide a basis for planning nursing care. For easy access to the up-to-the-minute nursing diagnoses, consult Doenges and Moorhouse (1996) (listed in the references).

Legal Implications of Nursing Diagnoses

When nurses collect and analyze data and develop nursing diagnoses, they have a professional obligation to communicate and record these items; moreover, it is expected that the professional nurse will develop and implement a care plan relative to the diagnoses. Accurate record keeping that reflects the nursing care plan and the client's response to the plan is essential. Documentation on the legal record, that is, the client's agency chart, is required for several reasons, which will be discussed in Chapter 11. However, one important reason for documentation is to have available, in the event of legal questions or litigation, an account of the client's care while associated with a particular agency.

In 1991, Iyer identified a trend involving a shift from narrative charting to focus charting, which offered a way to structure a progress note more concisely by targeting the "focus" of the note—for example, a sign or symptom or nursing diagnosis. In 1995, Iyer again notes that focus charting documentation is continuing (pp. 256–257). This trend demonstrates progress toward safer as well as more effective care.

Client Participation in Establishing a Nursing Diagnosis

A major challenge for nurses is determining how best to facilitate the client who disagrees with the nurse regarding a nursing diagnosis. Consider the following situation: based on physiologic principles and nursing knowledge, the nurse knows that ambulation (walking) following surgery facilitates the return to former functioning. Moreover, the nurse can identify problems that may occur if a regular ambulation regimen is not followed. However, because of postoperative fatigue and pain, the client may prefer to rest rather than ambulate.

Standards of care developed through research indicate that nurses would be negligent if they did not intervene at this point. The client's participation usually can be gained if the nurse first addresses his or her concerns and finds mechanisms to help the client cope. For example, establishing a pain management plan and regular rest periods may help relieve pain and fatigue. This relief facilitates ambulation, a necessary part of postoperative care. The person who is still unable to become involved in his or her own care may be expressing a deeper unmet need that requires further data collection.

Respecting a client's right to ignore or deny an obvious health problem is difficult, particularly if doing so has serious implications. If nurses assess the meaning behind the avoidance behavior and consider the client's perception of his or her real needs, they are more likely to intervene effectively. For example, imagine a man who has high blood pressure and does not take his medications as prescribed. The nurse might identify the problem as noncompliance with the health care regimen. The man, however, may feel that the pills cause unpleasant side effects, or he may not remember to take them. The nurse who respects his right to make decisions about health care will spend time talking with him and concentrate on the client's perception of the situation. For instance, the client may tell the nurse that his family is struggling with complex problems. Working to solve some of these problems may seem more relevant to the client than trying to cope with the nurse's main concern. If he is assisted to improve his family relationships, the client may decide to take the medications as scheduled. Moreover, if the client is happier in his family life, his high blood pressure may return to a more normal level.

Nursing Diagnosis Versus Collaborative Problems

The discussion of nursing as a science and a profession described nursing as having independent, interdependent, and dependent functions. The discussion of nursing diagnosis has focused primarily on those problems that are within the domain of nursing's independent function. These are problems for which nurses can legally determine the actions to avert, solve, or relieve the problems.

Nursing as a science and profession also is primarily concerned with persons' health generally and clients' specific responses to their particular health problems.

However, many of nursing's clients also have diagnosed medical problems (disease). In addition, these same clients have a likelihood of developing difficulties or potential complications related to a disease or to medical or surgical interventions used to treat the disease. Other clients are at risk for developing medical complications from diagnostic tests, whether or not they have actual disease. These actual or potential problems, which are outside the realm of nursing's independent function, are designated as *collaborative problems.* Carpenito (1990) defined collaborative problems as "potential physiological complications," and the corresponding nursing goals as "determin(ing) onset or status, (and) management of change in status"(p. 8). "Nurses collaborate with medicine for definitive treatment"(Carpenito, 1987, p. 24).

Collaborative problems require nurses to collaborate with other health professionals for their resolution. This collaboration usually involves physicians but may involve health professionals other than physicians. For example, nutritionists, physical therapists, and dentists may be some of the professionals with whom nurses collaborate. This collaboration often involves nurses' interdependent and dependent functions. However, just as the greater part of professional nursing's functioning should be independent, the greater share of professional nurses' activities should be focused on resolving problems for which nursing has prime responsibility.

For example, Mr. Jones, 75 years old, is at high risk for increased respiratory secretions related to his recent surgery performed under general anesthesia. The nurse may initiate teaching and positioning as well as coughing and deep breathing to assist the client's return to health. If, however, Mr. Jones develops pneumonia, a medical postoperative complication of surgery, the nurse and physician will work together to solve the resulting collaborative problem of respiratory insufficiency. The physician may prescribe antibiotics and oxygen as specific medical treatments. The usual supportive care of the nurse, that is, regarding positioning, coughing, and deep breathing, may be supplemented by additional nursing measures to conserve energy and maintain comfort. The nurse will also continue to perform the monitoring interventions that are within nursing's independent function and will administer the prescribed medication, a dependent nursing function.

As a postscript to the discussion of nursing diagnoses versus collaborative problems, another point should be clarified. In its most general meaning, the word collaborate denotes working together. Because health care encompasses the care by nurses, physicians, and other health professionals (e.g., dentists or social workers), all professional health care workers "collaborate" in the general sense of the word. They do this to provide a broad spectrum of efficient and effective care for their clients, even when they are functioning in their independent professional practice modes.

Planning: Phase 3

Phase 3 in the nursing process is **planning.** As this discussion begins, consider general notions about the nursing process. The assessing, analyzing, and diagnosing aspects, as described earlier, may sound laborious. In actuality, nurses perform and record a fairly complete assessment and care plan when the client enters an agency.

In most instances, however, they perform the nursing process briefly. For example, while listening to the client, the nurse is assessing, analyzing, and diagnosing. Likewise, planning, implementing, and evaluating may take only moments. This approach to the nursing process occurs many times through the course of providing care to a client. Often, the data and care plan are not written down immediately. Although certain aspects are recorded later, even these will be a synopsis of the actual interaction. Thus, the nursing process becomes primarily a way of thinking.

Planning, implementing, and evaluating are sometimes grouped together as the therapeutic or action portion of the nursing process. One aspect of planning is projecting the realization of achievement. Together, the nurse and the client identify outcomes that are reasonable and relevant, choose among alternative interventions, and implement the plan.

Iyer et al. (1986) stated, "Planning involves the development of strategies designed to prevent, minimize, or correct the problems identified in the nursing diagnosis"(p. 114). This component consists of four stages:

1. Setting priorities
2. Developing outcomes
3. Developing nursing orders (measures or interventions)
4. Providing documentation

Bower (1982) stated, "Planning nursing care for people in a constantly changing milieu (environment) demands that the nurse be able to analyze, and organize an incredible amount of data. . . . Nursing care planning . . . is a process that requires a systematic and comprehensive approach" (p. 10). She stated also that nurses must "preserve the individuality of the person or family, assess health needs, establish priorities in nursing care, determine nursing interventions, and refer persons to appropriate resources" (p. 10).

In addition to this description of the planning phase, several thoughts can be included. First, planning occurs as the result of systematic data collection and nursing diagnosis and follows naturally from these primary activities. Second, in keeping with this text's philosophy, the notion of health and strengths will also be added to the planning phase in the following discussion. Third, both the Iyer et al. and Bower definitions suggest that the nurse does the planning. Although this may happen in certain instances, the goal is client participation in the planning phase according to his or her ability. The notion of the client's active role may be confusing at first. For clarification, consider that the nurse does not necessarily stop the thinking process to consult the client. Moreover, the nurse, coming from a knowledge and experience base, does planning that the client could not be expected to do. Essentially, there are a variety of ways to plan with clients, the most important of which is to listen when developing a plan. A clinical illustration at the end of this chapter demonstrates these ideas.

Goals and Expected Outcomes

Goals or *expected outcomes* are predictions of what the client hopes to attain given his or her strengths and needs. Goals are developed to maintain and promote strengths and move toward problem solving and decision making.

The client's particular wishes are considered equally with the knowledge base of the nurse. As goals are developed, expectations of how the client will look, act, or feel are stated for the purpose of evaluating the outcome. Goals can be adjusted to meet changing needs. The following criteria provide guidelines for constructing goals.

Goals are written in behavioral terms and individualized to suit the person who expects to attain the result, in other words, the client.

Goals are constructed to reflect the person's rather than the nurse's behavior. For example, stating a goal, "The client will maintain . . ." or "The client will demonstrate . . ." clearly identifies the person as the one who will achieve the result. Thus, the client goal becomes person-centered. The nurse's goal is to facilitate the client in that venture.

Goals are written using measurable terms with outcome criteria.

Use of action verbs will demonstrate for both client and nurse that outcomes have been attained. Examples include state, verbalize, demonstrate, recite, gain, lose, smile, or exercise. Consider the goal, "The person will state his or her new low-sodium diet from memory." This is a start, but does not include the time-frame criterion. If the client is hospitalized, the goal might be ". . . state his or her diet by discharge." However, if there are other goals to attain that go beyond this one, such as the client learning to choose the correct foods from the daily menu, then the time frame may be different. For example, "The client will state his or her new diet from memory within 1 week after instruction begins." Then, "The client will choose the correct foods for a low-sodium diet from the daily menu by discharge." In this day of shortened hospitalization periods, goals may be stated in days or even hours, rather than weeks. This will necessitate communication between the nurse and family members, as well as nurses in clinics where the client might return for followup, and nurses who visit the client at home.

Other examples of criteria-referenced goals include the following:

❏ The client will state that his or her pain has decreased within 2 days after beginning relaxation techniques.
❏ The client will demonstrate the ability to take his or her own blood pressure by discharge.
❏ The client will maintain his or her blood pressure within the current range (150/90 to 130/80).
❏ The client will maintain his or her ability to achieve a restful sleep.
❏ The client will smile three or four times a day.
❏ The client will walk in the hall 2 days after surgery.

Some goals cannot be structured easily within a time frame. For example, "The client will verbalize feelings of increased safety and security" provides one means of measurement with the action word "verbalize." The time frame, however, is missing. Nursing interventions are planned—avoiding a time frame for the present—to help the client feel safer, and eventually to verbalize those feelings. When the goal is affective, or feeling related, the nurse begins where the client is. Then, following some success, a time frame for further achievement is planned.

Goals are written to reflect plans for a short time or for a more extended period. *Long-term goals* often refer to a broader accomplishment that, although eventually realistic, can only be attained through a series of smaller steps—for example, "The client will lose 50 pounds over the next 12 months." *Short-term goals* reflect smaller steps that can be pursued one at a time. They demonstrate achievement, provide encouragement, and suggest ways to attain the long-term goal.

Consider the following short-term goals suggested to meet the long-term goal of a 50-pound weight loss:

The client will

❒ Identify his or her weight as a problem
❒ State his or her wish to lose weight
❒ Verbalize knowledge of good basic nutrition
❒ Plan with the nurse a diet relevant to his or her needs
❒ Lose 1 pound a week beginning in 2 weeks

To make these goals clearer, a time frame could be added, particularly after the first two goals have been achieved; thus, note the time frame suggestion of 2 weeks to attain the other goals before the client begins to lose weight. Perhaps after assessment, 2 weeks seems to be a realistic time period for the overall plan to begin. Specific time frames for the first few goals are omitted, however, to provide some freedom, but further evaluation may suggest a need for readjustment of the goals and the addition of a time frame. Continued plans for weight loss also can be developed.

Consider the following goals for Ms. Carroll, the client discussed earlier:

The client will

❒ Continue to express her feelings regarding fear, abandonment, and grief
❒ Maintain a positive client–nurse relationship
❒ Perform own basic hygiene by 3 days after surgery
❒ Establish a plan to decrease fatigue
❒ State that she feels safe when asked by the nurse
❒ State differences between herself and family members who have died from a similar disease

To summarize, goals are planned with the client and reflect both his or her ability and readiness to work toward attaining his or her plans. Goals are written in measurable terms according to the behavior of the client. Goals may be long- and short-term, and are evaluated and revised as necessary.

Nursing-Sensitive Outcomes Classification (NOC) (Johnson & Maas, 1995) refers to the most recent movement in nursing process development. Note first the term classification: the act of classifying is arranging ideas, facts, or objects into groups or categories based on their relationships, and so that they can be identified and recognized in an orderly fashion. When one orders ideas, one achieves a classification.

Since August 1991, a research team at the University of Iowa has been working on an outcomes classification for patient care. For the purposes of their work, the research team has defined a nursing-sensitive patient outcome as a variable patient or family caregiver state, condition, or perception responsive to nursing interventions. In other words, the researchers hope to study outcomes for both patients and family that nurses can effect through nursing care. One purpose of this research is to identify, label, validate, and classify nursing-sensitive outcomes. Eventually through this project, these outcomes and their indicators will be evaluated and their usefulness tested.

The outcomes are stated as concepts, such as mobility or self-esteem, that can be measured along a continuum, rather than as goals. Each outcome has an associated group of indicators that can be used to determine the level of outcome achieved. The research will provide the first standardized language and measurement for nursing-sensitive patient outcomes. Nurses can use this language to compare outcomes for large numbers of patients across settings, diagnoses, age groups, cultural expressions, and other aggregates being considered. Note that this plan fits well with the earlier discussion of the aggregation phase of the nursing process. Outcomes given as neutral statements can then be measured, and nursing care evaluated, over a continuum of care rather than at one point in time.

Note the following two examples of outcome concepts, their indicators, and an evaluation measurement for each (see Table 8-7 and Table 8-8).

TABLE 8-7 *Mobility Level: Ability to Move Purposefully*

Indicators	Dependent, Does Not Participate	Requires Assistive Person & Device	Requires Assistive Person	Independent With Assistive Device	Completely Independent
Balance performance	1	2	3	4	5
Body positioning performance	1	2	3	4	5
Muscle function	1	2	3	4	5
Joint movement	1	2	3	4	5
Transfer performance	1	2	3	4	5
Ambulation: walking	1	2	3	4	5
Ambulation: wheelchair	1	2	3	4	5
Other_____ (Specify)	1	2	3	4	5
	Dependent, Does Not Participate	Requires Assistive Person & Device	Requires Assistive Person	Independent With Assistive Device	Completely Independent
Mobility Level	1	2	3	4	5

Maas, M. (1991). Impaired physical mobility. In M. Maas, K. Buckwalter, & M. Hardy, (Eds.), *Nursing Diagnosis and Interventions for the Elderly* (pp. 263–284). Redwood City, CA: Addison-Wesley Nursing.

TABLE 8-8 *Self-Esteem: Perception of Self Worth*

Indicators	Never	Rarely	Sometimes	Often	Consistently
Verbalizes self acceptance	1	2	3	4	5
Accepts self-limitations	1	2	3	4	5
Maintains erect posture	1	2	3	4	5
Maintains eye contact	1	2	3	4	5
Describes self in positive terms	1	2	3	4	5
Demonstrates minimal embarrassment	1	2	3	4	5
Demonstrates minimal shame	1	2	3	4	5
Demonstrates regard for others	1	2	3	4	5
Communicates honestly & openly	1	2	3	4	5
Fulfills personally significant roles	1	2	3	4	5
Maintains grooming/hygiene	1	2	3	4	5
Manages anxiety effectively	1	2	3	4	5
Balances participation & listening in groups	1	2	3	4	5
Displays confidence	1	2	3	4	5
Accepts compliments from others	1	2	3	4	5
Expects to be received well	1	2	3	4	5
Accepts constructive criticism	1	2	3	4	5
Reports no somatic problems	1	2	3	4	5
Expresses opinions in spite of possible disagreements	1	2	3	4	5
Expresses success in work or school	1	2	3	4	5
Expresses success in social groups	1	2	3	4	5
Expresses pride in self	1	2	3	4	5
Other _____ (Specify)	1	2	3	4	5

	Extremely Poor	Poor	Fair	Good	Extremely Good
Self-Esteem	1	2	3	4	5

Maas, Johnson, and Moorhead (1996) of the Iowa Intervention Project state,

"The benefits of standardized languages and their contributions to quality care open exciting possibilities for nursing science, education, and practice. Data from standardized nursing diagnoses, interventions, and outcomes will provide nurses with information only imagined in the past, make nursing a visible and influential science and practice discipline, and benefit clients through more informed health care policy and data-based practice (p. 300)."

Implementing: Phase 4

Implementing refers to accomplishing or fulfilling. Implicit in this notion is the attainment of certain planned goals or outcomes, making implementation the active rather than the mental portion of the nursing process. Implementation may otherwise be known as nursing measures, nursing actions, or nursing interventions.

Nursing Interventions

Nursing interventions, nursing actions, or nursing measures are the steps taken to help the client attain the stated goals or outcomes, and are directed toward promoting or maintaining health. They are planned using the person's strengths and are implemented to mobilize those strengths toward self-care capabilities. Nursing interventions are derived from

- ❏ Scientific knowledge associated with the biophysical and behavioral sciences
- ❏ Nursing theory based on research
- ❏ Past nursing experience

Interventions can be categorized as diagnostic and therapeutic as indicated in the following examples.

Diagnostic Interventions

Diagnostic interventions are nursing actions that help the nurse and the client better determine the needs and the course of events in a given situation. They are also interventions in the sense that they help maintain the safety of the client during the observation or monitoring that must occur. Examples of diagnostic interventions include the following:

- ❏ Observe—Consider such aspects as nonverbal behavior, skin-color changes, progress in ambulation, and response to medication.
- ❏ Inspect—Examine a wound for signs of infection.
- ❏ Monitor—Check vital signs on a regular schedule, test blood glucose level four times a day, weigh the client daily.
- ❏ Percuss—Determine changes in condition.
- ❏ Listen—Obtain data to detect changes in voice tones, either for cues to respond in a specific way or for clues to a person's needs, concerns, or wishes; auscultate (listen with a stethoscope) to determine changes in condition (see Fig. 8-3).

Therapeutic Interventions

Therapeutic interventions are nursing actions planned to maintain strengths and treat problems. Examples of therapeutic interventions include the following:

- ❏ Listen—Provide opportunities for the person to verbalize; sit with and talk to the person; use touch and acknowledge strengths.

❐ Problem solve.
❐ Support physiologic needs—Assist persons with activities of daily living as needed; irrigate wounds and change dressings; encourage fluids to prevent dehydration; provide interventions for pain relief.
❐ Educate—Provide specific health information as needed and appropriate.
❐ Plan—Plan a diet with the client, a stop-smoking regimen, or a program of family discussions to improve relationships.
❐ Refer—Assist the person to find other professionals, services, or facilities to help with his or her needs.
❐ Meet basic needs (see Figure 4-2).
❐ Support developmental task resolutions (see Table 4-2).

Effective Interventions

Although assessing and planning represent formal phases within the structure of the nursing process, they require approaches that are suited to the needs of the individual person. As mentioned in our discussion of the holistic person in Chapter 4, all of a person's subsystems are interrelated, with the healthier parts contributing to overall coping efforts. When coping becomes ineffective, energy may be borrowed from stronger subsystems, causing them to become weaker. If too much energy is drained away, feelings of hopelessness may occur. The result may be a perceived loss of control and a diminished sense of self-esteem.

The use of a framework on which to base interventions often will increase their effectiveness. The concept of caring, as described in Table 8-9, is one such framework. When using this approach, the nurse first works toward a trusting relationship with the client, and then gradually assists the person to maintain or recover control over his or her life. Suggested interventions for achieving control within this trusting relationship are listed in Display 8-8. As the client experiences more control, the nurse helps the client establish goals, using a conscious effort to support and promote the client's strengths, thus elevating his or her self-esteem. Gradually, the client develops a more positive orientation, that is, an ability to project himself or herself into the future. As the client feels more hopeful, the cycle of trust, control, goal development, self-esteem, positive expectations, and hope repeats itself, resulting in greater control and less dependence on others. The following display exemplifies the QA intervention efforts of one hospital:

The nurses on one particular hospital unit offer primary nursing as a method of care delivery for their clients. One value of this system is that clients are able to name, or at least describe, their primary nurse. Nurses must clearly introduce and identify themselves to clients as the primary nurse. To determine that this standard was being met, the nurses decided to survey the clients. In the first survey, clients were able to name or describe their primary nurse 50% of the time. The nurses considered this response problematic. After discussion at a staff meeting, they decided to continue the surveys, unannounced, on a quarterly basis and to inform individual nurses whether their clients could name or describe them. It was

(continued)

TABLE 8-9 *The Concept of Caring*

Interventions	Definitions
Develop a trusting relationship.	*Trust*—The assumption that another is responsible and honest and has integrity; the belief that we are safe with another; the ability to take risks concerning another person, a pet, or an inanimate object such as a car; the ability to act without fear of the outcome; a mode of positive expectation and hope
Assist the person to maintain or recover control over his or her life.	*Control*—The act of exercising restraint or direction over some thing or person
Assist the person to establish goals.	*Goal*—The aim or end toward which effort is directed
Assist the person to develop higher self-esteem.	*Self-esteem*—The individual's personal judgment of his or her own worth obtained by analyzing how well his or her behavior conforms to the person's self-ideal; the frequency with which the person's goals are achieved will directly result in feelings of increased self-esteem
Assist the person to develop a sense of positive expectations and hope.	*Hope*—Expectation of something desired; confidence (trust) in another person, event, or outcome; promoting the promise of advantage or success
	Hopelessness—Despondency, despair, abandonment of self to one's "fate"; inability to mobilize resources to cope; the sense that nothing can help, that the situation will never improve
	Despair—The state of believing that one has no further control over a situation, an event, or even of one's life
	Helplessness—Weakness, dependence, ineffectiveness; inability to mobilize resources; being without hope
	Impoverishment—The state of feeling, in some measure, helpless—hopeless, sad, and fatigued, and often hostile and bitter; one's self-esteem is low and problem-solving skills are minimal

(*M. A. Swain, H. Erickson, E. Tomlin, personal communications*)

expected that the surveys and subsequent feedback would increase the nurses' awareness of the need to introduce themselves properly. After two additional surveys, the clients' positive responses had increased to 85%. This level of response was considered more satisfactory, and the surveys were decreased to twice yearly for the purpose of maintaining the standard.

Iyer et al. (1986) stated, "Implementation is the initiation of the nursing care plan to achieve specific outcomes" (p. 177). Implementation indicates that the nurse and the client together have put the plan into action. "Implementation is the actual giving of nursing care. It is nursing therapy or nursing treatment, each of which is the giving of nursing care. . . . Implementation of the nursing care plan

DISPLAY 8-8   **Interventions to Assist the Client in Regaining Control**

❏ Help the person recognize and recall his or her strengths.
❏ Respect the person's ability and right to make decisions about his or her care.
❏ Support the decisions the person makes and gear your interventions toward helping the person carry out his or her plans.
❏ Explain all nursing actions to the person and ask for his or her suggestions on how to proceed.
❏ Use the person's ideas about his or her care and provide the person with appropriate information to make safe decisions.
❏ Acknowledge the person's accomplishments and express your respect. Remind the person of other successful problem solving he or she has done.
❏ Listen to the person's statements of how he or she feels. The person knows better than anyone else what those feelings—both physical and psychological—mean.
❏ Provide opportunities for the person to perform activities as he or she is capable.
❏ Use a positive approach that indicates your expectation that the person will become increasingly able to take care of himself or herself.

contributes to comprehensive care because the plan considers the biopsychosocial aspects of the client'' (Marriner, 1979, p. 127).

Implementation is a complex undertaking. Certain activities, such as providing oral hygiene or teaching the side effects of particular drugs, are obvious interventions, whereas other nursing actions, such as providing support, are less clear. The notion of giving support is a conglomerate of many interventions that must be identified individually so that the nurse has specific direction. Encouraging verbalization, identifying strengths, and assisting with problem solving are some examples of giving support. Using a theoretical framework will assist the nurse to develop interventions with a conscious and purposeful approach to decision making. Maslow's basic need theory and the concept of caring that is derived from the linkages of several theorists are just two examples of such frameworks.

Consider the following interventions for Ms. Carroll:

❏ Use interventions from Display 8-1, Table 8-9 (concept of caring), and Display 8-8 (interventions to assist the client to regain control).
❏ Provide opportunities throughout the day for the client to explore thoughts and feelings.
❏ Suggest how the client is different from father and sister-in-law.
❏ Help the client reminisce about past with her husband.
❏ Plan a daily program with periods for rest and activity.
❏ Monitor blood pressure, pulse, and respiration after periods of activity or when the client expresses fatigue.
❏ Help the client determine which activities tire her, and suggest ways to conserve energy.

Nursing Intervention Classification (NIC)

To continue the discussion regarding further expansion of the nursing process, a research team, again at the University of Iowa, has also developed a Nursing Information Classification system known as NIC. This system is linked with the NANDA nursing diagnoses, and was actually created prior to the outcome work (NOC) described in the outcome section above. McClosky and Bulechek (1996) have written extensively on the purposes of a classification of nursing interventions. They have indicated that the development of the system is an ongoing process as interventions are identified and tested in the clinical arena. They point out that NIC has many features and uses as follows:

❏ Helps demonstrate the impact that nurses have on the health care delivery system
❏ Standardizes and defines the knowledge base for nursing curricula and practice
❏ Facilitates the appropriate selection of a nursing intervention
❏ Facilitates communication of nursing treatments to other nurses and other providers
❏ Enables researchers to examine the effectiveness and cost of nursing care
❏ Assists educators to develop curricula that better articulate with clinical practice
❏ Facilitates the teaching of clinical decision making to novice nurses
❏ Assists administrators in planning more effectively for staff and equipment needs
❏ Promotes the development of a reimbursement system for nursing services
❏ Facilitates the development and use of nursing information systems
❏ Communicates the nature of nursing to the public (1996).

Note in the following example of an intervention according to NIC, that the intervention is stated (Weight Management), then defined, and that the activities or nursing interventions to assist the client are stated (McClosky and Bulechek, 1996).

Weight Management

Definition: Facilitating the maintenance of optimal body weight and percentage of body fat.

   Activities:

1. Discuss with the patient the relationships among food intake, exercise, weight gain, and weight loss.
2. Discuss with the patient the medical conditions which may affect weight.
3. Discuss with the patient the habits, customs, and cultural and hereditary factors that influence weight.

4. Discuss risks associated with being over- and underweight.
5. Determine patient motivation for changing eating habits.
6. Determine patient's ideal body weight.
7. Determine patient's ideal percentage of body fat.
8. Develop with the patient a method for keeping a daily record of intake.
9. Encourage the patient to write down realistic weekly goals for food intake and exercise, and to display them in a location where they can be reviewed daily.
10. Encourage patient to chart weekly weights as appropriate.
11. Inform patient if support groups are available for assistance.
12. Assist in developing well-balanced meal plans consistent with level of energy expenditure.

The NIC taxonomy is arranged in six domains as follows:

Domain 1, Physiological: Basic care that supports physical functioning
Domain 2, Physiological: Complex care that supports homeostatic regulation
Domain 3, Behavioral: Care that supports psychosocial functioning and facilitates lifestyle changes
Domain 4, Safety: Care that supports protection against harm
Domain 5, Family: Care that supports the family unit
Domain 6, Health System: Care that supports effective use of the health care delivery system

In each domain, general interventions are identified with the specifics to be found under each general intervention as indicated above in weight management (McCloskey & Bulechek, 1996, pp. 56–57).

Evaluating: Phase 5

Evaluating is, in part, appraising by an authority. The nurse may be viewed as the authority in a given situation because of theory base, past experience, and assessment skill. The client, however, is the authority on his or her particular strengths and needs. Therefore, implicit in this interpretation of evaluating is the collaboration of the nurse and client, each using his or her particular authority to decide together on future directions of care.

Evaluating and revising represent that phase of the nursing process in which the person's strengths, needs, and goals, along with the planned interventions, are reassessed and revised as necessary. Iyer et al. (1986) stated, "Evaluation is defined as the planned, systematic comparison of the client's health status with the outcomes" (p. 237). The stated goals or expected outcomes are used as a standard for evaluating the degree to which the person has improved his or her health status.

Evaluation begins with the implementation of the nursing care plan.

Throughout the delivery of care, the nurse considers the effectiveness of the plan in helping the client achieve his or her goals. If, for example, the client is working on a weight reduction plan but continues to overeat, the nurse reassesses the situation and a more relevant plan is developed. Interventions may be better suited to the client's resolution of trust and control issues than to diet planning. Or, if the client is ready to move through a care regimen more quickly than usual, for example, is able to ambulate, do daily self-care activities, or begin fluids, the nurse adjusts the usual plan to accommodate the client's adaptation.

Although evaluation as a phase in the nursing process has focused on the individual person and on his or her attainment of health-directed goals, evaluation can also be applied in a broader sense. Evaluation can be used to determine the quality of health care delivered in an agency, or to judge the performance of health care personnel, either through self-evaluation or through the peer-review process.

Another important aspect of the nursing process is its interactive nature. Erickson et al. (1983) "view the nursing process predominantly as an ongoing, interactive, interpersonal relationship that includes use of the formal scientific mode of thought" (p. 105). These authors indicate that a formal step-by-step process is not necessarily followed, but rather, forms the moment of contact between nurse and client: the nurse is "analyzing while listening, intervening, and evaluating; evaluating while intervening, analyzing and listening—in short, doing the nursing process (as general problem solving) in her head while simultaneously giving [implementing] care" (p. 105).

Little and Carnevali (1976) helped with this notion by stating "The concept of the nursing process has several general properties. This pattern of thinking and behaving:

- ❏ Is cyclic and recurring
- ❏ May be carried on with awareness, or almost automatically
- ❏ Can be learned in terms of skill and speed
- ❏ May be carried out with varying speed ranging from almost instantaneous thinking to protracted deliberation
- ❏ Integrates priority setting and feedback mechanisms into every step
- ❏ Is dependent upon the effective use of a body of knowledge
- ❏ Involves verbal symbols (words)" (p. 11)

The clinical illustration in the display is offered as an example of the planning, implementing, and evaluating phases of the nursing process.

At midnight, the hospital telephone operator phoned the nursing unit stating that our patient, Betty Drayton, had called the switchboard. Betty said that she needed help but the nurses would not answer her light. I thanked the operator and went to Betty, whom I knew well. I approached her and said, "Betty, how can I help?" She brightened momentarily when she saw me but then began to cry. "Those nurses, they were so awful tonight. They would never come when I called. They're mad at me; everyone is mad at me because I wouldn't go to exercise class today and I wouldn't walk. But I don't want to do anything

(continued)

but go home." I responded, "The nurses feel that these activities will help you get home faster. They worry about you and get frustrated when you don't follow the plan."

I had sat down on her bed rather than in a chair, putting my hand on her arm, because I knew that Betty needed the closeness and acceptance this movement would indicate. Listening to her, I remembered that she had raised many children and had been extremely tired and psychologically impoverished before her surgery. She had stayed in intensive care longer than usual and had relied on having her own nurse. I had worked with her occasionally and knew that her special need was to be cared for. If she had perceived that she was being ignored, she would experience a deficit in her love and safety needs. I also thought she was struggling with issues of trust and autonomy (Erikson, 1963). For example, because she mentioned going home, I asked her how she might help herself get ready. She thought a moment and then said, "Well I suppose I could do all those things they wanted me to do today, but I want to decide that for myself instead of always being told what to do." I asked her how she might do that. Again she thought and then stated that she would get up in the morning without being told and start her own care. She was hesitant about being independent but her need to go home was becoming greater than her need to be taken care of in the hospital. I affirmed her strengths by supporting her statements and telling her I thought she was planning well for herself. I also assessed her blood pressure, pulse, and respirations to be certain that her restlessness was not related to a physiologic change. I told her that I was not assigned to her during the night, but would be across the hall, and she should call me if her nurse was busy.

The whole interaction took about 7 minutes. Using the nursing process, I moved back and forth among the five phases as we talked. From a theory base linking physiology with Maslow, Erikson, and nursing knowledge, I considered her physiologic, belonging, safety, and esteem needs. I used her health-oriented statement that she wanted to go home to help her deal with her need for autonomy, or more control over her own activities. I let her know that I would be available if she needed me so that she would feel safe and have some of her sense of trust restored. I followed this up by smiling and waving as I passed her room for awhile until she fell asleep. I was able to evaluate my plan and nursing interventions because I saw that she had stopped crying, began smiling a little, and announced that she would take a walk before she tried to sleep. In addition, I observed that she arose early and began her care. I believe that this transformation occurred in a short time because I focused on her rather than on her disease or annoying behaviors.

KEY CONCEPTS

The **nursing process** is a scientific problem-solving method with the goal of promoting the client's self-care abilities.

The nursing process is divided into five phases: **assessing, diagnosing, planning, implementation** and **evaluation.**

Data analysis is the first portion of the diagnostic phase, and can be described as the cognitive process the nurse uses to recognize patterns and relationships among the data.

Aggregation can be thought of as an extension of the nursing process that involves synthesizing the results of nursing interventions to make predictions about the most effective approach for a group of clients or for a given situation.

✓The nursing process is **person-centered** in that it is used as a collaborative process between the nurse and the client.

✓The use and continued reinforcement of the nursing process stimulates the development of **nursing research and theory** and thus promotes nursing's growth as a profession.

CRITICAL QUESTIONS

1. Describe a health care situation from your experience in which identifying a person's strengths would have assisted the problem-solving process.

2. Suppose your friend, a medical student, asks you what nursing diagnosis is all about. Using the ideas from this chapter about purposes of nursing diagnoses and client strengths as a component of nursing diagnoses, outline the points you would list to answer this question.

3. Suppose your friend who is majoring in business asks you what nursing is all about. Using the ideas from this chapter about the nursing process, outline the main points you would use to answer this question.

REFERENCES

Abdellah, F.G., Beland, I.L., Martin, A. and Matheney, R.V. (1960). *Patient-centered approaches to nursing.* New York: Macmillan.

American Nurses Association. (1991). *Standards of clinical nursing practice.* Kansas City, MO: Author.

American Nurses Association. (1973). *Standards of clinical nursing practice.* Kansas City, MO: Author.

Benner, P. (1984). *From novice to expert: Excellence and power in clinical nursing practice.* Menlo Park, CA: Addison-Wesley.

Bower, F.L. (1982). *The process of planning nursing care: Nursing practice models* (3rd ed.). St. Louis, MO: C.V. Mosby.

Carnevali, D.L. (1983). *Nursing care planning: Diagnosis and management* (3rd ed.). Philadelphia: J.B. Lippincott.

Carpenito, L.J. (1995). *Nursing care plans and documentation: nursing diagnoses and collaborative problems* (2nd ed.). Philadelphia: J.B. Lippincott.

Carpenito, L. J. (1993). *Nursing diagnosis: Application to clinical practice* (5th ed.). Philadelphia: J.B. Lippincott.

Carpenito, L.J. (1990). *Nursing care plans and documentation: nursing diagnoses and collaborative problems.* Philadelphia: J.B. Lippincott.

Carroll-Johnson, R.M. (ed). (1991) Classification of nursing diagnoses proceedings of the ninth conference. North American Nursing Association. Philadelphia: J.B. Lippincott.

Carpenito, L.J. (1987). Nursing diagnosis (2nd ed.). Philadelphia: J.B. Lippincott.

Chinn, P.L., & Jacobs, M.K. (1987). Theory and nursing: A systematic approach (2nd ed.) St. Louis, MO: C.V. Mosby.

Doenges, M.E. & Moorhouse, M.F. (1996). *Nurses' pocket guide: Nursing diagnosis with interventions* (5th ed.). Philadelphia: F.A. Davis.

Dumas, R.G., & Leonard, R.C. (1963). The effect of nursing on the incidence of postoperative vomiting. *Nursing Research, 12*(1), 12–15.

Durand, M., & Prince, R. (1966). Nursing diagnosis: Process and decision. *Nursing Forum, 5,* 50–64.

Engel, G. (1964). Grief and grieving. *American Journal of Nursing, 64*(9), 93–98.

Erickson, H.C., Tomlin, E.M., & Swain, M.A. (1983). *Modeling and role-modeling: A theory and paradigm for nursing.* Englewood Cliffs, NJ: Prentice-Hall.

Erikson, E.H. (1963). *Childhood and society* (2nd ed.). New York: W.W. Norton.

Fitzpatrick, J.J. (1991). *Taxonomy II: Definitions and development.* In: Carroll-Johnson, R.M. (Ed.). *Classifications of nursing diagnosis: Proceedings of the Ninth Conference.* North American Nursing Diagnosis Association. Philadelphia: J. B. Lippincott.

Gordon, M. (1994) *Nursing diagnosis: Process and application.* New York: McGraw-Hill.

Gordon, M. (1989). *Manual of nursing diagnosis* (3rd ed.). St. Louis, MO: C.V. Mosby.

Gordon, M. (1985). *Manual of nursing diagnosis.* New York: McGraw-Hill.

Gordon, M. (1982). *Nursing diagnosis: Process and application.* New York: McGraw-Hill.

Gordon, M. (1976). Nursing diagnoses and the diagnostic process. *American Journal of Nursing, 76,* 1276 1300.

Henderson, V. (1966). *The nature of nursing.* New York: Macmillan.

Iyer, P.W. (1995). Nursing process and nursing diagnosis (3rd ed.). Philadelphia: W.B. Saunders.

Iyer, P.W. (1991). New trends in charting. *Nursing '91, 91, 21,* 48–50.

Iyer, P.W., Taptich, B.J., Bernocchi–Losey, D. (1986). *Nursing process and nursing diagnosis.* Philadelphia: W.B. Saunders.

Johnson, M., & Maas, M. (1995). *Classification of nursing-sensitive patient outcomes.* In ANA, Nursing data systems: The emerging framework (pp. 177–183). Washington, DC: American Nurses Association.

Jones, P.E. (1982). The revision in nursing diagnosis terms. In M.J. Kim & D.A. Moritz (Eds.), *Classification of nursing diagnoses: Proceedings of the Third and Fourth National Conferences* (pp. 196–202). New York: McGraw-Hill.

Kennison, B. (1983). *Nurses and patients: The clinical reality of sickness.* Unpublished doctoral dissertation, University of Michigan, Ann Arbor.

Kim, M.J., & Moritz, D.A. (Eds.). (1982). *Classification of nursing diagnoses: Proceedings of the Third and Fourth National Conferences.* New York: McGraw-Hill.

LaMonica, E.L. (1979). *The nursing process: A humanistic approach.* Menlo Park, CA: Addison Wesley.

Little, D.E., & Carnevali, D.L. (1976). *Nursing care planning.* Philadelphia: J.B. Lippincott.

Maas, M.L., Johnson, M., & Moorhead, S. (1996). Classifying nursing-sensitive patient outcomes. *Image: Journal of Nursing Scholarship, 28*(4), 295–301.

Marriner, A. (1983). *The nursing process: A scientific approach to nursing care* (3rd ed.). St. Louis, MO: C.V. Mosby.

Marriner, A. (1979). *The nursing process: A scientific approach to nursing care* (2nd ed.). St. Louis, MO: C.V. Mosby.

Maslow, A.H. (1970). *Motivation and personality* (2nd ed.). New York: Harper & Row.

McCain, R.F. (1965). Nursing by assessment—not intuition. *American Journal of Nursing, 65,* 82–84

McCloskey, J.C. & Bulechek, G.M., (Eds.). (1996). *Nursing Interventions Classification (NIC), Iowa Intervention Project* (2nd ed.). St. Louis, MO: CV Mosby.

Mundinger, M.O., & Jauron, G. (1975). Developing a nursing diagnosis. *Nursing Outlook, 23*, 94–98.

Piaget, J. (1973). *The psychology of intelligence.* Totowa, NJ: Littlefield, Adams.

Popkess-Vawter, S.A. (1984). Strength-oriented nursing diagnoses. In M.J. Kim, Moritz, D.A., McFarland, G.K., & McLane, A. M. *Classification of nursing diagnoses: Proceedings of the Fifth National Conference.* St. Louis, MO: C.V. Mosby.

Rantz, J.R. & LeMone, P. (1995). *Classification of nursing diagnoses: proceedings of the eleventh conference.* North American Nursing Diagnosis Association. Glendale, CA: CINAHL Information Systems.

Shamansky, S.L., & Yanni, C.R. (1983). In opposition to nursing diagnosis: A minority opinion. *Image, 15*, 47–50.

Swain, M.A. (1973). *Curriculum development.* Ann Arbor: University of Michigan, School of Nursing.

Thomas, M.D., & Coombs, R.P. (1966). Nursing diagnosis: Process and decision. *Nursing Forum, 5*, 57–64.

9

Interpersonal Communication in Nursing and Health Care

Accurate observation	**Communication**	**Empathy**
Active listening	**Conflict resolution**	**Information superhighway**
Assertiveness	**Cyberspace**	**Interview**

═══ **Objectives** ═══

After completing this chapter, students will be able to:

Contrast helping relationships with social relationships.

Describe the four roles of the nurse in a helping relationship.

Describe the components of empathy.

Explain the importance of effective communication to quality nursing care and effective collaboration among health team members.

Identify effective and ineffective communication techniques.

Recognize conflict situations and resources for conflict resolution.

Across the room or across the information superhighway of **cyberspace,** communication is the process of messages sent and received and information transferred. Communication demonstrates caring, learning, sharing, and much more. Although cyberspace has revolutionized information processing in a new age of information, communication is one of the oldest and most fundamental processes and activities of daily living. A hallmark of communication in the new information age is its global, indeed galactic, potential. Yet basic concepts and principles underlie all communication and are invaluable to its understanding and application.

You will use communication along with critical thinking to give direct care, teach your clients, resolve conflicts, and demonstrate nursing's contribution to health care.

This chapter introduces the nature and application of interpersonal communication in nursing and health care. The material is appropriate to nurses regardless of practice setting, specialty area, or job title. As Kidd (1990) stated, "Caring can only be demonstrated and practiced effectively interpersonally" (p. 95). A consistent theme in her study of emergency room nurses was communication as a primary instrument for most caring actions. To Benner and Wrubel (1989), "Caring is primary because it sets up the possibility of giving help and receiving help" (p. 4).

Helping relationships within the nursing profession take several forms, with the nurse playing many different roles either separately or in combination. Important and challenging roles related to interpersonal communication are in keeping with nursing's professional emphasis on health. These roles include direct administration of physical care, advocacy on behalf of clients, psychosocial support, and health education and counseling. These roles require the nurse to combine problem-solving and communication skills and to act as a therapeutic listener and resource liaison.

Locked in each person is a wealth of unique experiences, strengths, feelings, and values. Effective **communication** is the master key that unlocks such human resources, enabling a nurse to understand, to care, and to help another person. The client in turn, learns that the nurse does understand, does care, and will assist him or her. Such rapport between two persons, in this case between a nurse and a client, underlies a helping relationship and a most rewarding profession. Although client is referred to in the singular, the importance of family and community is assumed. Indeed, in those circumstances where the client is unable to speak for himself or herself, the family plays an even greater role in the client communication process.

Interpersonal communication is both a science and an art. As a science, it requires a disciplined study of concepts and practice of technique to gain certain skills. As an art, it requires the fusion of the nurse's self with creativity, insight, and practice to achieve style. The distillation of art and science into a personal style of interaction is neither automatic nor innate. Study and practice are required to develop one's own skill and interpersonal style.

Human communication is a complex process in which two or more persons exchange messages and derive meanings. Effective communication occurs when persons exchange messages and derive a mutual understanding of the intended meaning. A general classic principle of communication is applicable to nurse–client interactions as well as to all other interactions, both personal and professional: when the behavior (verbal or nonverbal) of a person is perceived by another, communication occurs. Therefore, one communicates whether intentionally or not.

First, consider nurse–client interactions, and recognize that much of the same information can be applied to communication and collaboration with peers, and also to conflict and conflict resolution.

Nurse–Client Interactions as Helping Relationships

Most nurse–client interactions occur within the context of helping relationships in which a nurse "has the intent of promoting the growth, development, maturity, improved functioning, (and) improved coping with life" of the client (Rogers, 1961, pp. 39–40). In a traditional health care relationship, a client might identify a health problem or illness and seek help from a doctor; the doctor might then prescribe nursing services to assist the client. Examples include counseling in pain management, sexuality, ostomy care, nutrition, management of illness at home, and grief and loss resolution. Today, more clients are seeking nursing care directly in times of crises. Nurses, too, are offering services more directly to prevent a problem or illness and to maintain the health or improve the wellness of the client, the family, and the community. Thus, helping relationships may be client-initiated or nurse-initiated.

Characteristics of Helping Relationships

All helping relationships have the same intent and share certain common characteristics. As professional helpers, nurses exemplify the following characteristics:

- ❏ Awareness of self and values
- ❏ Ability to analyze own feelings
- ❏ Altruism – *unselfish concern for the welfare of others*
- ❏ Strong sense of ethics
- ❏ Responsibility

Genuineness and unconditional acceptance of the other person are essential qualities for those who wish to help persons become healthier in mind and body. In exploring what it means to help another human, counselor and behavioral-science researcher Laurence Brammer (1988, p. 9) described most distressed persons as seeking to meet basic needs, rather than as diseased or ill. This fact often surprises nurses who enter the field to work with "sick" persons and subsequently learn the enormous needs of all deprived persons for nursing services. Brammer outlined the characteristics of an effective helper as follows:

Awareness of self and values—The nurse needs to be able to answer "Who am I? What do I believe? What is important to me?" to help another person answer those questions. A certain level of insight precedes the use of a most important tool in nursing, the "use of self" as a care-giver.

Ability to analyze own feelings—Nurses as helpers gradually learn to recognize and cope with their own feelings of joy and grief, power and anger, accomplishment and frustration.

Ability to serve as a model—To show another person the route to health, a nurse necessarily maintains a certain level of health in mind, body, spirit, and life-style.

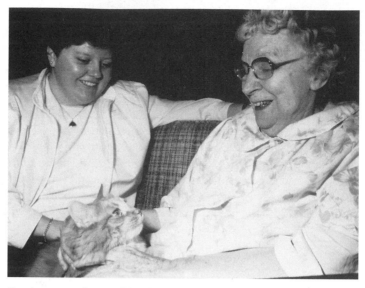

Genuineness and unconditional acceptance of the other person are essential qualities for those who wish to help.

Altruism—Nurses characteristically convey a sense of altruism, that is, they receive self-satisfaction from helping people in a humanistic way.

Strong sense of ethics—Nurses strive to make the best possible judgments based on high principles of human welfare.

Responsibility—Two dimensions of responsibility are inherent in nursing: taking responsibility for your own actions and sharing responsibility with others (p. 16).

Professional Versus Social Relationships

A successful helping relationship between nurse and client represents a different order of interaction than that occurring in a friendship. This difference is not because of any superiority in the nurse but because of the mutual trust and the responsibilities for assisting others that characterize professional relationships. Although many elements of a professional relationship are warm, friendly, and social in nature, there is an underlying purpose in helping relationships that is beyond mutual enjoyment. The nurse's purpose is to enable the person to adapt to changing life circumstances in as healthy a way as possible, and the nurse empowers the person to maximize his or her strengths to achieve personal potential.

A comparison of social and professional helping relationships provides significant contrasts. Perhaps the most important difference between these two types of relationships is also the most basic: professional helping relationships have their origin and reason for being centered on the client's needs or concerns. Nursing process and ethics oblige the professional practitioner both to define problems and to work toward their solution.

The professional accepts the person with unconditional positive regard and is mindful of possible differing values between the professional and the client. The professional is therefore expected to use appropriate communication skills both to understand and to meet the identified needs. Independence of the client is encouraged as appropriate. Similarly, the nurse professional is under professional obligation to use information from the relationship ethically, i.e., to not share it inappropriately or indiscriminately. A professional relationship requires that in return for honest information about personal values and behavior, confidentiality without recrimination is guaranteed.

Recent changes in health care delivery and mass communication have profoundly altered professional helping relationships: clients are becoming more equal partners in the quest for improved wellness or health. Helping relationships in acute care settings occur under time constraints as lengths of stay in acute care settings continue to decrease. Also, and increasingly, such relationships are more apt to occur in community rather than institutional settings. Information about a variety of health conditions is available electronically to health care consumers, although sometimes the quality is questionable and professional interpretation is unavailable.

Additionally, many nurses are convinced that the clients they care for face to face must like them, and that a successful relationship is a friendly one. This attitude, although popular, is neither possible nor advisable in most helping relationships. The effective nurse recognizes this pitfall and avoids developing "favorite" clients toward whom he or she is preferentially affectionate. The nurse also avoids forming negative stereotypes of clients. With either extreme, the nurse would lose the objectivity necessary to give quality care. Watson (1979) identified the helping–trusting relationship as one of her primary carative factors and interpersonal needs as the highest order needs. From this theoretical perspective and also from that of Carl Rogers, the following application is illustrative: when the nurse and client are appropriately engaged in such a relationship, both the nurse and the client are changed by the interaction, i.e., both grow. The nurse assists the client to maintain other relationships that are personal and that provide friendliness and affection. The nurse, however, can openly demonstrate unconditional positive regard for the client and demonstrate friendliness and affection in the context of a professional relationship, i.e., clearly acting as a professional nurse in a professional helping relationship. Despite the constraints and pitfalls, and also the changes affecting helping relationships, nurses of today and tomorrow will experience a variety of helping roles.

Helping Roles

The nurse helps the client by acting in one or a combination of the following roles:

❑ Direct administration of physical care
❑ Advocacy on behalf of clients
❑ Psychosocial support
❑ Health education and counseling

Direct Administration of Physical Care

Direct administration of physical care is the traditional and time-honored role of the nurse. In the 1970s, this helping role evolved from one of performing services for others to one of assisting others to regain or retain the ability to care for themselves.

Nurses provide direct assistance for those clients who are temporarily or permanently unable to care for themselves. Obvious examples of such clients include dependent children, adults whose self-care abilities are altered by surgery or chronic or acute disease, and the frail elderly. The majority of relatively healthy persons retain responsibility for their own health care and use nursing help as they perceive a need. Helping means that control remains with the client even when care is directly administered by the nurse. When the client is unable to exercise control, the family, as advocate, may act in this capacity.

Advocacy on Behalf of Clients

Nurses themselves often act as advocates on behalf of clients. The growing complexity of and rapid changes in the health care delivery system make the client's search for satisfactory answers and solutions more difficult. Nurses perform an invaluable service by searching out the available solutions on behalf of the client as a consumer. In this way, the client can make informed decisions in meeting his or her own needs. Sometimes, the "client" includes not only the individual but also the family. For example, an elderly woman caring for her bedridden husband at home may need to arrange a variety of direct-care personal services, including those of the visiting nurse, and relief for herself as care-giver. Perhaps, this same woman needs the nurse's intervention with family members to examine the seriousness of a health situation to effect solutions to unfinished family business.

Psychosocial Support

The often over-used phrase "psychological support" includes a variety of methods by which the nurse sustains the emotions, morale, culture, and spirituality of a client. Communication skills of empathy and assertiveness are essential to this kind of support. Nurses learn to react to the stress behavior of clients and, generally, when clients show signs of distress, nurses act to comfort and support them. In such situations, skills of problem solving and anticipatory crisis intervention prepare the client by describing what to expect in a stressful situation and by providing sufficient information for the client to make informed decisions and maintain self-esteem and self-control.

Social support is usually found among individuals and groups such as one's friends, coworkers, neighbors, community organizations, and church congregation. Either physical absence or inability to participate may interrupt these networks. Often, the nurse can help reestablish contacts by suggestion or direct intervention.

Health Education and Counseling

The effective nurse motivates a client to learn, grow, and change his or her health behavior as needed. The nurse's role as a health educator and counselor depends on the ability to facilitate—not dictate—another person's growth. For example, the nurse might say, "Use whatever seems helpful. I will support you in your decision." This basic approach to teaching adults can be altered appropriately when dealing with more dependent or unstable clients. Dreher (1987) has provided many concrete suggestions and modifications for interacting with dependent elderly persons that would facilitate communication generally, and specifically assist teaching. The role of the nurse as health educator receives special elaboration in Chapter 10, which is devoted to the learning–teaching interaction.

At any given time, a practicing nurse is likely to be enacting several roles simultaneously. Teaching a new mother about infant care involves constant psychosocial support of her mothering abilities, as well as health education and counseling. Care of a dying person may include advocacy of death with dignity, along with physical care and psychosocial comfort to the dying person and his or her family. The four helping roles of the nurse overlap constantly in caring for, and caring about, people. In all these helping roles the nurse also actively strives to increase sensitivity to the varying meanings of interpersonal communication exchanges within and between diverse cultures. Perfecting this skill requires awareness, sensitivity, and purposeful learning by the nurse. References that may help to increase the nurse's awareness include Barna (1994) and Galanti (1991). The increasing diversity of communities presents challenges for everyday and for professional communications. Given demographic projections, nurses would do well to learn basic language skills for the population they serve as the following example illustrates:

> Volunteer firefighters in a small southern community with a large Hispanic migrant population took it upon themselves to learn basic Spanish. They wanted to understand better the needs of the persons they served, especially in emergency situations. The firemen's initiative was captured by a local photo-journalist and publicized in the town newspaper. Shortly thereafter, the paper also published a letter to the editor by a Hispanic reader expressing appreciation to the firefighters for both their sensitivity and their commitment.

Developing Nurse–Client Relationships

Helping relationships as dynamic interpersonal processes do not automatically exist, but grow much the same way a garden grows. Careful preparation of growth conditions are a necessary first step. The progressive caring, feeding, and supportive direction given in a growth phase help any plant and any relationship to be self-sufficient and productive. Skillful nurses, like skillful gardeners, redirect disabled life back toward health, being ever careful not to neglect, oversupply, or destroy it in the process. Both gardeners and nurses eventually enjoy the satisfaction of a harvest, the closing of one growth cycle and the beginning of another. Throughout, there remains a mystical quality in the growth of a plant, the growth of a person, and in the growth of a helping relationship.

Trust

Growth in the interpersonal process depends on the development of mutual trust. Trust evolves when one person risks his or her own self-esteem, seeks support from another, and finds it. The helper fosters trust, not dependence, by making and keeping commitments, sharing responsibilities with the client, and ensuring confidentiality.

Few qualities of the helping professional are as essential as confidentiality. Imagine the damage to a growing, trusting relationship should a client discover that a nurse has inappropriately spread personal communications. It is unlawful, unethical, and in many cases a breach of contract with the employment agency to break confidence. Sharing information that is vital to the health and safety of the client with other responsible caretakers is essential; however, the client has the right to be informed of a nurse's need to share vital information with others. Note-taking and other types of recording should never be the focus of an interaction, as in, "Hold it, I didn't get all of that down." Secretive note-taking destroys trust, while asking the client's permission to take notes and sharing those notes with the client acknowledges the client's control over the information. It is important to remember that trust flows through any successful helping relationship.

Three Phases of Growth in Nurse–Client Relationships

In a growth process, helping relationships are divided into three phases:

1. Opening (or initial)—Introduction and preparation of the personal growth conditions occur in this phase. In the opening phase of the relationship, the underlying goal of both persons is to adapt to each other and to establish trust.
2. Working (or developmental)—This phase of a relationship fosters growth and change, problem solving, and decision making. Throughout the working phase, both nurse and client strive to maintain trust during stressful decision-making and problem-solving encounters.
3. Closing (or terminating)—The closing of a successful relationship can be considered a harvest of mutual satisfaction between nurse and client. The closing phase requires both persons to redirect trust, often by referral to another care-giver or by agreement that the client is self-sufficient again.

These flexible phases form a chain of interactions, ending at a level higher than they began.

Guidelines for Successful Helping Relationships

Because successful helping relationships do not occur automatically, teaching communication skills is now an important part of any nursing curriculum. As Norris (1986) has reminded us, "The curricular trend which acknowledged communication content as basic to nursing assessment and intervention in all areas of practice was a significant advance in nursing education" (p. 106). Aspiring nurses learn appropriate approaches to developing helping relationships as suggested by the following guidelines for the various phases.

Opening Phase

During the opening phase of a successful professional relationship, both nurse and client prepare to work together by establishing a contract, so to speak. In opening a helping relationship, the use of contracts, as suggested, will help the client (and nurse) adapt to a new relationship and to changes in the relationship.

Contracts may include formal statements such as those used by Steckel (1980) in her interventions with persons with diabetes. Usually, however, they are informal agreements that set the limits for several important aspects of the interaction. Consider the following examples:

1. How often will the nurse and client meet?
   Example: "I will be the nurse caring for you on the day shift all week." Or, "I will be the primary nurse responsible for your care. Even when I'm not on the nursing unit, the care we planned together will be performed by another nurse."
2. What will be the purpose of the meetings?
   Example: "I will be the nurse helping you to plan for the care of your child at home. I will stop by each afternoon for a few minutes so we can work together."
3. How will the confidential information be handled?
   Example: "For me to be most helpful to you, I will need to have you tell me how you honestly feel about caring for your husband at home. Also, what information about your feelings, if any, do you want me to share with your daughter?"
4. What will be the terms for closure of the relationship?
   Example: "We will work together to determine when you can manage on your own."

One characteristic of the opening phase of many relationships is testing behavior, a common prelude to trust. Each person establishes a sense of security in the relationship by testing the limits set by the other. This usually is an adaptive behavior to see if the other person means what he or she says. For example, the hospitalized client may express insecurity by calling the nurse repeatedly; this behavior may reflect the client's difficulty in believing that the nurse is concerned with his or her needs and care even when the nurse is not directly visible to the client. Clients whose life experiences or ethnic backgrounds differ from the nurse's will test the nurse's willingness to understand them, sometimes with queries such as, "How can you know what it's like?" The nurse who replies, "I know just how you feel," may be believed only if an honest example follows: "I've had a similar thing happen to me."

Testing behavior can be a direct indication of the amount of security and trust in a relationship; as interpersonal trust grows, testing behavior subsides. A clear indication of movement into the working phase of a relationship is the cessation of testing behavior. However, the issue of trust is a larger issue than trust in the nurse–client relationship. The nurse recognizes that persons who have not resolved developmental tasks of trust versus mistrust may be genuinely unable to trust the nurse. Reasons for mistrust may be deep-rooted and have little to do with the nurse's interpersonal skills.

Working Phase

At the point of completing a contract with the client, the nurse moves the interaction into the working phase by beginning the helping process. The working phase is the part of the relationship in which helping and growth occur, whether the nurse gives direct care, counseling and teaching, or psychosocial support. The care given centers on the client's needs and problems. Therefore, one of the most useful tools of the working phase is problem solving, the systematic process of identifying, clarifying, and resolving troublesome situations.

Problem solving is widely adaptable to all nursing situations. At times, identifying the exact nature of the problem can be difficult and time consuming, requiring that the problem solver turn the problem around to view it differently or emphasize another part of a complex problem. In working with a difficult family situation, for example, a nurse may begin to question whether the sick member of the family is really the source of the problem, or whether other members of the family, the community, or the environment are really the cause.

It is imperative, however, that the nurse not become involved in problem hunting to the extent of interrogating or otherwise forcing clients to "Tell me your problem!" Many troubled persons, if they do recognize their own concerns or problems, may be unable to verbalize them.

As nurses adopt the concepts of self-care, that is, helping others to help themselves, they recognize that helping the client to solve his or her own problems, whenever possible, is preferable to problem solving for the client. A gentle patient-centered exploration of the client's perception of his problem may be a safe way to begin helping the client to solve problems. What has the client already tried, or what does the client think might help? What are alternative strategies, and what would be likely outcomes? What barriers and blocks must be considered, and what does this suggest about prioritizing approaches? Ask how you could be helpful.

Like the steps of the nursing process, these phases should be viewed as flexible. The beginning practitioner does well to remember that sensitivity to interactions increases with practice and becomes second nature. This client-centered process of assisting clients to solve their own problems builds client self-esteem and independence. This approach can be adapted to many nursing situations, even when the client is ill or debilitated, helping him or her to control decisions about his or her own health. At times, progress may be slow, especially in long-term relationships. Testing behavior may recur as a signal of frustration, unmet needs, or wavering trust.

Closing Phase

Closing gestures are likely to determine the client's perception of the entire interaction and, thus, his or her willingness to enter future helping relationships. Successful closing is planned in advance to provide time for adapting to the loss.

It attaches value to the preceding interaction. The challenge is to focus on the client's achievement as a point of departure for possible future achievements.

Interactions of long duration may end in small celebrations or gift giving. Sometimes patients or their families leave gifts of fruit or candy for a group of health care workers as a token of their appreciation. Occasionally, a patient or family may single out a particular individual for special remembrance. Although some nurses may be more comfortable than others in receiving gifts, it is important to examine the meaning of the gift when deciding to accept it. Gifts may represent gratitude, guilt, or some other more personal and less obvious intent. One such small token of gratitude made a lasting impression: one patient, who was dying of cancer, joined in wedding shower festivities with a small gift of a juice container.

Testing behavior during closing may be an attempt to hang on to the nurse. Testing behavior is a common manifestation of separation anxiety, an insecure feeling of loss occurring at the end of meaningful relationships. In an attempt to protect themselves and adapt, clients may withdraw as if to say, "I'll end this relationship before you leave me." Working through loss can be a growing experience and thus a positive behavioral sign. A realization of waning interaction time often prompts clients (and helpers) to intensify the relationship near the end, and signs of grieving and loss reaction may appear. Just as the opening and each working step is planned, the closing is anticipated, planned, and enjoyed as the fruit of a successful relationship.

Interpersonal Communication Process

Elements of a Human Communication Process

The interdisciplinary study of human communication combines the fields of biophysics, physiology, psychology, sociology, anthropology, and ecology. Indeed, these sciences form the basis of a nursing perspective on communication, and the educated nurse may use all of them to communicate effectively with clients as persons.

Communication has been described as a process, a continuous circular flow of energy. Most models of the communication process contain the following elements: source (also known as stimulus); message; transmitter (also known as the channel, i.e., vision, hearing, touch, smell, and taste); and receiver (also known as response). David Berlo (1960), in a classic work, described the human factors of sociocultural influence, environment, communication abilities, attitudes, and knowledge that modify the process. More recent communication scientists have added the element of feedback to complete a circular pathway of communication (Fig. 9-1). Two contrasting kinds of messages can be differentiated:

❐ When a message proceeds in one direction from the source to the receiver, it is termed a *one-way communication.* A person who uses one-way communication neither expects nor encourages a response from the passive receiver.

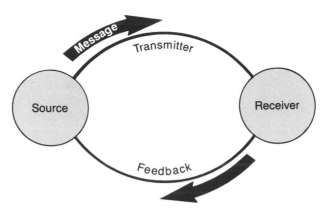

FIGURE 9-1 The communication process.

❏ When the flow of a communication includes a feedback loop, it is termed a *two-way communication*. The receiver is expected and encouraged to participate actively in the exchange.

A traditional lecture, for example, is one way; the question–answer period afterward is an attempt to establish a two-way dialogue. Effective nursing interactions are two-way communications involving both client and nurse as active participants.

Mass, Intrapersonal, and Interpersonal Communication

The field of human communication may be divided into three components:

1. Mass communication—*Mass communication* is the transmission of messages to a large audience of receivers. The modern media communicate information efficiently to the largest possible groups of receivers.
2. Intrapersonal communication—*Intrapersonal communication,* in contrast, occurs largely within the single individual when the mind or the body interprets messages for the person.
3. Interpersonal communication. *Interpersonal communication* is the exchange of messages between two, or a small group of, persons.

Although each is a complex process, the three vary in scope. Effective interpersonal communication requires, in addition, the understanding of the meaning in such messages. The foundation of effective nursing lies in effective interpersonal communication.

Through recent technological advances, even interpersonal communications have entered the cyberspace age as the following examples illustrate. Boehm (1996), in a project called *Hearth,* used a metaphoric hearth (computer keyboard) for patients to communicate:

A patient on chemotherapy wakes up with nausea in the middle of the night. Instead of isolation with this condition, the patient can turn to a metaphoric hearth and communicate with other patients who are on the same medication—or a pharmacist, nurse, physician, neighbor, sister in another state, or whoever is on line (at the hearth) at that moment. The patient can also access additional information from on-line libraries and forums with health care experts or possibly medical support bulletin boards or Internet chat lines.

In another example, Arslanovski, a baccalaureate nursing student, used networked computers and video cameras, i.e., Internet videoconferencing technology. He enabled a young girl, recovering from a bone-marrow transplant for leukemia, to reunite with classmates at her home school from whom she had been isolated for months. The University newspaper headline read, "Nursing student connects patient with friends at home, school" (Finn, 1996). The idea emanated from a homework assignment in a senior nursing course, and as the student explained, "It's all low-cost, consumer-level technology. It's out there, it exists, and it's very easy to integrate into the clinical setting" (p. 8). From simple beginnings, this story made its way to the local television news, CNN, and the International Sigma Theta Tau publication, Reflections.

Interpersonal Process Applied to Nursing: A Theoretical Perspective

Entire theoretical systems for nursing are based on interpersonal process as interaction, and have been detailed by such nurse–theorists as Peplau (1989, 1952) and Orlando (1990, 1961). According to Meleis (1991), the interaction theorists represented a school of thought in nursing theories that was preceded by needs theorists such as Virginia Henderson, and followed by outcome theorists such as Callista Roy. Meleis's analysis helps to clarify the place of the interpersonal process in nursing over time and in concert with the evolution of nursing theory.

The so-called needs approach associated with certain nurse–theorists, however, is not to be confused with the basic needs approach of Maslow detailed in Chapter 4. Rather, the needs of Henderson were more concerned with physical activities of daily living than with growth needs. Therefore, nurses who practiced from this needs approach were primarily physically busy with preplanned activities carried out for the patient, and their communications could be expected to be related primarily to such activities.

The interaction theorists, influenced by humanistic psychology, facilitated the person based on situational circumstances, and were increasingly concerned with psychosocial aspects of nursing care. One might expect the communications of these nurses to be especially sensitive to the client-centered needs of the moment.

The outcome theorists were primarily concerned about how the nurse could regulate the system to foster healthful adaptation. They tended to be more future-oriented, rather than present-oriented, and their communication could be expected to reflect such goals.

From the sciences of linguistics and psychiatry come other theories, such as the theory of Neuro–Linguistic Programming developed by Bandler and Grinder (1975). Neuro–Linguistic Programming postulates that traditional American culture and language exhibit three patterns of language use: (1) kinesthetic, (2) auditory, and (3) visual. Most individuals tend to communicate most comfortably in one of these modes. One challenge for the nurse is to assess which pattern a given client uses most and to apply that knowledge to establishing interpersonal communication. Such awareness of communication patterns or modes is also applicable to principles of learning–teaching as discussed in Chapter 10.

The skillful practitioner will let the nature of the client and the situation determine when it is appropriate to focus most on needs, interaction, outcomes, or other future scientific approaches. All of the theoretical perspectives discussed suggest, however, that there is a range of internal and external variables that modifies the nurse–client interaction and affects communication.

Variables Affecting Communication

Internal Variables: Biophysical, Psychological, and Sociocultural

Within each individual, certain forces facilitate whereas others disrupt the ability to communicate effectively. The level of consciousness affects verbal expression: the unconscious person must communicate his or her needs by body language, and depends on a care-giver to interpret the needs correctly. Other biophysical variables hindering communication are sensory losses, such as hearing and visual impairment; motor impairments; and any biochemical imbalance that causes confusion, especially drug intoxication. In contrast, a biophysical variable that aids communication is muscular coordination, which develops with the growing child into increasingly effective speech and motor expression. Humans of all ages, however, can learn to overcome physical barriers to communication.

Anxiety also affects the ability to communicate. What some observers might view as a client's selective inattention or choice not to hear a message may be something quite different; for example, sometimes the client may be unable to make such a choice or to give evidence of absorbing the message at a particular time. Later, when he or she is able to act, the previously unattended-to message may come into conscious awareness and be used.

The entire realm of perception—the interpretation of stimuli—influences communication. Each human mind learns to perceive stimuli in certain patterns, influenced by personal values and attitudes. A typical example relates to age perception: the adolescent calls anyone older than age 30 "middle-aged," and anyone older than age 50 "old." The 60-year-old perceives himself or herself as "middle-aged," referring kindly to the "old" person of 80 years down the street. Thus, our perceptions are molded by our psychosocial experiences in life.

Sociocultural variables in communication present both obvious and hidden forces. Spoken communication obviously succeeds better if both persons speak in the same language; differing dialects and word connotations of other cultures may prove to be hidden disrupters of understanding. Nonverbal communication also varies across languages and cultures. For example, direct eye contact is viewed as sincere in the American culture, but may be viewed quite differently in other cultures (e.g., Native American or Asian).

Also hidden are individual values, which can block one's ability to understand the other's message. If a nurse values a stoic response to pain, for example, she may not even be able to listen to the whimpering complaints of a client after surgery or be aware of the reason for the client's negative feelings.

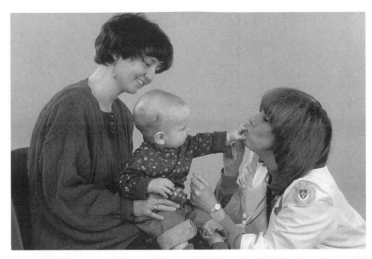

Nonverbal communication techniques include using facial expressions and touch. (Photo © 1997 by B. Proud)

External Variables: Environment

All interpersonal communication occurs within the context of the surrounding environment, as discussed in Chapter 5. Anyone who has tried to concentrate on a lecture while sitting in an uncomfortable chair amid construction noise knows how the environment can hinder communication. This is another opportunity to provide an environment conducive to psychosocial support, as described earlier in Chapter 5. Rather than memorizing rules of environmental structure, such as furniture arrangement, the nurse develops a finer sense of assessment by using empathy in evaluating the physical environment: "If I were frightened or embarrassed in coming to this agency, how would I respond if interviewed in the waiting room? Behind a curtain? In a private room?"

Application of Maslow's hierarchy of needs to interpersonal relations would suggest that the individual might not be ready to communicate highest-level concerns without some provision of environmental comfort and security. Before beginning interactions with a client (especially lengthy ones), the nurse assesses his or her comfort level and feeling of security. This can be done through questioning and observation. Physical comfort is augmented by such measures as body positioning, supplying drink or food, supplying pain medication, rearranging furniture, and controlling room temperature and ventilation.

Security, in this case a feeling of psychological comfort, results from specific relaxation techniques, respect for territoriality, and provision of privacy. The crucial element of confidentiality in interpersonal relations depends directly on the provision of as much privacy as possible. In addition, a private atmosphere lessens distractions to both nurse and client and diminishes interruptions that may connote disinterest. Minimizing distractions can maximize the chances of effective interactions.

Types of Communication Language

Humans communicate meaning to each other through the use of language—patterns of behavior designed to influence others. These patterns of behavior are learned responses and are culturally determined. Communication scientists have distinguished two types of communication behavior:

❏ *Verbal language* conveys meanings through words.
❏ *Nonverbal language* conveys meanings with methods other than words.

For the purpose of this text, we will first consider each of these languages separately. Then, to view humans as holistic beings, we will examine how persons combine verbal and nonverbal languages.

The nurse must first comprehend the verbal and nonverbal components of a client's message to analyze the combined meaning of both. Likewise, the client will seek to understand the nurse's meaning by examining verbal and nonverbal language.

Verbal Language

Consider the dollar bill: a rectangular piece of crinkled paper, it has little significance until someone assigns meaning to it. In this case, the U.S. Treasury has assigned a value of 100 cents to it; other countries value the dollar differently compared with their own currency standards. A dollar bill is a symbol of some worth, a symbol exchanged to meet the needs of individuals.

In a similar way, a word possesses little significance until assigned a meaning within a cultural or subcultural group. A word is a symbol of meaning that a person exchanges to meet his or her needs. Use of verbal language, then, is a symbolization process in which words are chosen as representative of an intended meaning. Commonly, the terms *verbal* and *oral* are used interchangeably and inaccurately: verbal language is the larger concept encompassing all use of words, both oral (spoken) and written.

Oral communication is the most common vehicle of deliberate interchange among persons. As such, the spoken word is subject to many misunderstandings. Nurses should remember this in their oral communications with clients. For nurses, the importance of both speaking and listening is sometimes underestimated. In a study "to discover the specific oral communication skills necessary for success in nursing, and those skills most in need of improvement, according to Directors of Nursing . . . communication skills associated with listening were most important and in greatest need of improvement." (Wilmington, 1986, p. 291).

Written communications are of a higher order, being more formal and permanent than oral communications. Although nurses orally transmit much information about client care, professional and legal responsibility for providing excellent care requires documentation in written form. The need for nurses to develop effective writing skills is crucial. Written care plans not only transmit important information to other health care team members, they are also legal documents.

Nursing publications convey creative and innovative nursing ideas to ever wider circles of practitioners and students. Nursing publications and communication via the internet and world wide web now make global communication an everyday reality. New chat forums are being created daily. The opportunities for and the ease of exchanging ideas among professionals and professional students is unprecedented. That this channel of communication has reached mainstream nursing was evident from such articles as Dubois and Rizzolo's (1994) "Cruising the Information Superhighway," which appeared in the *American Journal of Nursing*.

This electronic medium, however, requires succinct and clear messages, as does all communication that is effective. Additionally, those who access the information must be discriminating consumers, because not all information is of equal quality or merit. Both the credibility and the currency of some sources may be questionable, and communicators exchanging information need to be cautious as well as adventuresome when using this new medium.

Word differences among subcultures may be subtle but significant. A person who believes he or she understands the language of another may discover that words, although identical in sound, differ in their meaning from one subculture to another. For example, the word "bust" is pronounced the same, but quite likely interpreted differently, by a sculptor, a fashion designer, and a drug addict. Words, then, are deciphered in context. Indeed, humans search for the meaning of words in the context of sentences or conversations; taking words or phrases out of context typically leads to misunderstanding. Gray (1992) focused on word meaning and other communication differences between men and women in, *Men are From Mars, Women are From Venus: A Practical Guide for Improving Communication and Getting What you Want in Your Relationships*.

The health professions, as a subculture, have created a language that changes the context of many common words. The use of such professional jargon increases the chance of misinterpretation between clients and professionals. Consider this example: "You're NPO after midnight and you should void 2 hours post-op." The nurse has knowledge of technical terms that may be unfamiliar to the client. The challenge is to establish a common language level by deciphering the technical words for the client and educating him or her about their meaning.

The meanings of words have two dimensions: denotation and connotation. *Denotation*, a standardized meaning, is derived from a cultural consensus on the usage of the term. In contrast, subcultural usage of a word determines its *connotation*, or implies a judgment of its attributes. The noun *nurse*, for example, denotes a person giving care to another in need; various connotations of the word include "handmaiden," "professional," and "manager."

Nonverbal Language

Symbols and actions other than words make up *nonverbal language*. Numerous studies have shown that nonverbal behavior expresses intended meaning, especially feelings, more accurately than does verbal behavior. Yet, nurses sometimes ignore clients' nonverbal expressions. Nonverbal language is culturally determined. To interpret the meaning of a body movement or gesture without consideration of cultural context is equivalent to stereotyping. A client may wish to call the nurse by pet names such as "honey" or "dear," for example, which represent long-standing cultural behavior. Labeling this behavior as rude and condescending is inaccurate.

In clinical practice, the nurse encounters many clients who are unable to use verbal language: the infant and growing child not yet developed in speech, the comatose accident victim unable to speak, and the depressed person not yet ready to speak. The practitioner must use astute observation skills to understand the needs of these clients. For example, many have highlighted the importance of touch as a nonverbal communication technique with elderly clients whose access to other nonverbal communication may be diminished with age. Likewise pediatric nurses, for example, may use unconventional techniques such as a range of smiling and frowning faces to convert children's feelings and nonverbal responses to pain to verbal language.

Sight

Behaviors in nonverbal language that are observed by sight include facial expressions, gestures, and body postures, as well as physical appearance. The finely coordinated muscles of the face often give the most subtle indication of meanings.

The nurse's first observations include the client's eye contact and eye movements. In American culture, eye contact conveys an open, sincere approach to another person. Averted eyes may signal disinterest, diversion, or humility, and often may raise tension in the interaction. In the extreme, however, a fixed and glaring gaze also serves to increase the anxiety of another, as if he or she were being scrutinized. Several barriers, such as surgical masks, hospital equipment, and telephone communication, prevent open-eye contact in clinical situations. The nurse removes a barrier when sitting down to speak to children or to a person in a wheelchair or bed; such a simple action establishes eye contact and avoids the authoritative position of towering over the client.

Posture conveys meanings of interest and disinterest, of alertness, and of withdrawal. Sometimes the client who curls into a fetal position may communicate withdrawal: "Leave me alone." The fetal position may also be a protective behavior signaling, "Take care of me."

Other observations made by sight include those of muscle tension and the rapid-breathing patterns that are characteristic of anxiety. However, each individual manifests anxiety with his or her own pattern of nonverbal behavior—such as chain smoking, nail biting, pacing, and rocking. The nurse's ability to observe and validate such characteristic signs of anxiety increases the probability of understanding the client's meaning.

Appearance speaks of many traits. A professional appearance both reflects and suggests a professional manner, i.e., neatness and cleanliness. Traditionally, white hospital uniforms connoted cleanliness. Today we recognize that color has a language all its own. The current popularity of colored and patterned uniforms, scrubs, and regular clothes seems to connote nontraditional values for some nurses. Although one finds all types of clothing in health care settings, the guiding principle remains: dress appropriate to the circumstances fosters credibility and trust. Color in the physical environment can enhance surroundings for interpersonal helping relationships. Use of brightly colored graphics provides stimulation in children's playrooms and in hospital rooms that are otherwise stark and sterile.

Nonverbal Sounds

The skilled nurse trains the ear to observe speech sounds, because how something is said is as important as what is said. What is not said may be even more important. The skill of active listening involves listening for nonverbal vocalizations such as sighs, cries, and voice inflections accompanying words. Voice pitch, hesitations, and utterances, usually in combination with facial expressions, impart feelings of excitement, surprise, confusion, sarcasm, and mistrust. Such feelings can be heard by perceptive ears.

Silence as a nonverbal behavior holds a range of possible meanings, from boredom to contemplation, anger, or introspection. Clients who are silent during an interaction may cause anxiety in nurses. Yet, silence can be a useful communication tool, because it gives clients time to organize their thoughts and experience their feelings before expressing them. The nurse's silence can convey recognition of individual worth, the importance of being in interaction through silent presence, and the willingness to be present without the need to control a situation verbally. A quiet presence, and perhaps a simple nonverbal clasp of hands, can convey caring beyond words and in a way that the person can quietly accept.

Touch

Nursing is a touching profession: the intimate nature of many nursing tasks requires that caring be transmitted by touch. And yet, nurses have been cited as avoiding touch with seriously ill and aged clients. Touch is as essential for the elderly as for the newborn. The ability to reach out and touch a client may be more common in some cultures than in others. Although a nurse may prefer to know the person better before touching him or her, the nature of many short-term nursing interactions precludes lengthy introductions. For more than 2 decades, Krieger's name has been synonymous with therapeutic touch in nursing. Krieger (1975) believed that therapeutic touch, or the laying on of hands, transfers and mobilizes energy resources, and that by therapeutic touch, the nurse transfers energy to the client and mobilizes client energy.

Space

Touch may intrude as well as soothe, and the observant nurse decides how and when to touch based on each client's response. Threatening touch represents intrusion into the personal space of another. Personal space can be envisioned as a bubble surrounding each individual that forms a part of his or her personal, portable territory. Although we often joke about personal space among friends, this concept can have real professional significance.

Territoriality, or the human's instinctive drive to protect his or her space from intrusion, provokes defensive behavior by the person suffering intrusion. A client may become angry should the hospital nurse touch articles on "his" or "her" bed. In turn, nurses can become defensive when clients or other professionals enter "their" work space. Personal territory provides identity, security, and sensory excitement, as any mother of teenagers knows. Nurses who are aware of clients' territorial needs can use the concept of territoriality to enhance communication. Carl, an 11-year-old child with Down syndrome, underwent open-heart surgery and was required to spend many days in the intensive care unit. When he awoke and found a large poster of his hero, Hulk Hogan, taped to the ceiling above his head, he knew he was in a safe place.

Anthropologist Edward Hall (1966) created the term *proxemics* to mean the use of space in interpersonal relationships. *Space,* or distance between communicators, is an extension of the concept of touch. Hall described four distances for interactions:

1. Intimate distance (up to 18 inches) for privileged touching
2. Personal distance (18 inches to 4 feet) for interaction with familiar persons
3. Social distance (4 feet to 12 feet) for impersonal business
4. Public distance (more than 12 feet) for formal speaking (pp. 109–120)

Nurses are granted intimate distance with a majority of clients, and should maximize this privilege by deliberately maintaining this closeness. The nurse who pulls his or her chair out from behind the desk to talk with the patient and spouse increases the likelihood of an intimate and meaningful exchange. Some nurses fear touch will arouse sensuous feelings in clients. But the mature and secure nurse learns to overcome this concern, learns how to increase the client's own self-esteem through touch, and promotes the use of therapeutic touch—such as massage—for relaxation, pain relief, and sound sleep.

Time

Closely related to special communication is the concept of *temporal communication,* the use of time and timing behavior to transmit meaning. American middle-class time orientation values the accomplishment and performance of tangible tasks. In nursing, sitting quietly with a client is sometimes considered not doing anything. Other cultures, notably the Navaho Indians and Japanese, highly value the vigil of sitting with a distressed person. Much of American culture stresses a here-and-now, present orientation, or an upward-bound, future orientation to time. This explains a sometimes unwelcome tendency to insist that ill or disabled persons look ahead optimistically. We can help the dying person to find satisfaction in his or her past by moving away from a future orientation ourselves.

Other considerations of time involve the length and timing of messages, and the effective communicator will know and not exceed the attention span of listeners. Nurses working with children modify treatments and activities to shorter, more frequent sessions to avoid restlessness. Avoiding interruptions, another element of timing, assists in sending a complete message and prevents frustration and misinterpretation. Cultural variations in time perception need validation—for example, although some cultural groups value punctuality, others do not; this could lead to misinterpretation when tardiness occurs.

Congruence: Matching Verbal and Nonverbal Behavior

To comprehend the holistic person, the nurse observes both verbal and nonverbal behavior and combines these behaviors to analyze their meaning. This analysis searches for congruence between verbal and nonverbal behavior:

> Congruent: "I appreciate your help" (direct eye contact, soft smile).
> Incongruent: "I appreciate your help" (eyes averted, muscles tense).

Especially with distressed clients, the verbal behavior will often be incongruent with nonverbal behavior. Whereas congruence can be interpreted as an indication of open, trusting communication, incongruous messages signal the need for exploration of needs and feelings not expressed. The nurse mobilizes skills of empathy and validation to understand the client's conflicting messages and, in this way, maintains an open, trustful interaction.

Technological advances have blurred the lines between formal and informal, and verbal and nonverbal communication. In cyberspace, persons can both distance themselves through veiled anonymity and bring the world and its peoples to their doorstep or computer work station. Visual images can be shared or withheld to suit the circumstances. Words issued spontaneously, whether through computer charting at the patient's bedside or an informal chat conversation on the internet, hold the promise and threat of permanency. While communication in the cyberspace age is both easier and more complex, the underlying ethical principles of confidentiality and professionalism still apply.

Achieving Effective Communication

Use of Self

Even experienced nurses strive to improve their abilities to become more effective communicators. They try to increase knowledge of communication dynamics as well as self awareness and sensitive perception of others.

The phrase *use of self* represents the nurse's ability to integrate all three abilities to produce successful interactions. Understanding the dynamics of the underlying communication process, its characteristics, and its variables helps prevent communication problems. Nurses also learn how best to assist others when they become more aware of their own values and behaviors. Candidates for nursing often have a basic sensitivity to others; developing and expressing that sensitivity is a challenge throughout nursing practice. Nurses bring themselves, their past experiences, perceptions, and prejudices to their helping relationships. The nurse who also develops a solid knowledge base, self-awareness, and sensitivity brings valu-able resources to the helping relationship. Whereas knowledge is gained by disci-plined study, sensitivity develops by mastering empathy.

*A*chieving Empathy

Empathy is the ability to imagine the life of another person to accurately sense his or her thoughts and feelings. In explaining nursing's unique characteristics that center on caring, Brown (1992) noted specifically "placing oneself in the patient's place, seeing the human side of the person being cared for" (p. 57). Pike (1990) and Layton (1994) also wrote about empathy in present day clinical nurs-ing practice. The nurse attempts to understand clients' lives, their problems, val-ues, feelings, and meanings "to sense the client's private world as if it were your own, but without ever losing the 'as if' quality" (Rogers, 1957, p. 99). Nurses who can separate the client's problems from their own avoid emotional burnout; these nurses offer empathy instead of sympathy. Nurse who try to offer sympathy inappropriately may make such comments as: "I'm so sorry for you. I know just how awful it must be. . . . It's too bad."

Few clients need this awkward compassion. Empathic understanding, which consists of active listening, accurate observation, empathic response, and valida-tion, is much more helpful: "This must be hard for you." "I would be very frustrated if this were happening to me." "I had the same kind of surgery and I remember how much it hurt to cough." "I can suggest some of the things that have helped our other patients with a similar problem." "Other patients with this problem often tell us. . . ."

Active Listening

Active listening is the cultivated skill of deriving meaning from the words or nonverbal expressions of another. Whereas hearing refers to the passive reception of sound waves by the ear, listening encompasses active concentration and percep-tion of another's message using all the senses. Because humans communicate their needs through verbal and nonverbal behavior, the nurse uses sight, hearing, touch, and smell to listen actively.

Listening actively, the nurse may become aware of common themes that give clues to a client's needs. Common themes include the following:

- Self-effacement (attempts to reduce one's significance)
- Poverty of resources needed to cope with a present stressor
- Self-centeredness ("help me"), indicating insecurity
- Wellness or strength to deal with stress (often overlooked in our search for problems)
- Loneliness, creating despair
- Loss manifested in grieving behavior
- Humor, a coping mechanism of tension release

For a helpful discussion, see *Humor and the Health Profession: The Therapeutic Use of Humor in Health Care* (Robinson, 1991) and *Making Sense of Humor*. Green (1994).

Accurate Observation

Accurate observation, the companion skill to active listening, involves not only looking at the client, but also identifying crucial facts about his or her nonverbal behavior. Knowing what to observe and recognizing how you observe are both essential.

How easy it is to jump to conclusions about what we observe, and to offer solutions prematurely! Instead, nurses learn to differentiate an observation from an inference or conclusion to prevent a misunderstanding. For an observed behavior, any one of several conclusions may be valid.

Empathic Response

After careful listening and accurate observation, a nurse responds to the client's message with a verbal, nonverbal, or combination response. Touch is a powerful and effective response to another person; it is often part of an empathic response. Nurses are privileged to hear intimate, painful, and moving accounts of the stresses in others' lives. Successful empathic responses, or feedback, tell the client that the nurse is attempting to understand not only the client's situation but also his or her feelings and values. Empathic responses tend to be responses to situations, feelings, and values in that order of importance and effectiveness.

Validation

It is necessary to gain some feedback from the client to know whether the empathic response is an accurate perception.

> Nurse: "And is it important to you to be at home with your family?"
> Client [nodding]: "We really can't afford a baby-sitter for the entire 5 days I'll be gone. . . ."

The client affirmed her value of being with her children and raised the true concern of expense.

At times, our empathic responses are inaccurate, and the client corrects our understanding.

> Client: "Frightened? No, I've been through this before. I'm just angry that I got an infection the last time I was in this hospital!"

Validation completes a feedback loop, making empathy a two-way communication.

Other Communication Techniques

Nurses learn that there are many effective and ineffective communication techniques. With formal instruction and practice, they learn both to differentiate between these and to develop an effective personal style. Additional techniques useful in maintaining a client-centered interaction include:

❏ Thoughtful use of silence
❏ Stating observations ("You look sad today.")
❏ Reflecting and paraphrasing the client's stated or implied feelings and val-

ues (Client: "I don't know what to do next." Nurse: "You're frightened and confused.")

❏ Summarizing ("So, from what you've told me, you feel confident about managing this new diet plan.")

❏ Seeking clarification ("Tell me what you meant when you said you couldn't go on like this.")

❏ Explaining procedures, expectations, and so forth

Nurses also learn the pitfalls of:

❏ Reassuring falsely ("Everything will be okay.")

❏ Moralizing, preaching, and advice giving ("You really shouldn't. . . .")

❏ Stating their personal value judgments ("I think smoking is a bad personal habit.")

❏ Criticizing and ridiculing ("Your plan is ridiculous.")

❏ Denying client-perceived problems ("Your situation isn't that bad. . . .")

❏ Responding defensively ("I was only trying to help.")

Some techniques, like questioning, can be effective if appropriately used. Exploratory (i.e., what?) questions that invite a response beyond "yes" or "no" are effective for most adults. For instance, "Tell me about your family," rather than, "Are you married?" Children or confused elderly persons, however, may be better able to respond with a simple "yes" or "no." Similarly, harsh, insensitive, or multiple questions by a nurse may confuse, frustrate, or anger patients. Client questions may be direct requests for information or indirect requests for the nurse's empathic response.

Some effective communication techniques, such as humor and daring to be yourself, receive minimal attention in formal nursing literature. Ufema (1987) shared a view about how being yourself can be effective in communicating with dying patients:

> Our ability to make choices is part of what makes us human. Helping the dying patient have a voice in deciding the quality of the remainder of his life can give you some sense of success in working with him. How to talk to your dying patient? Be yourself, be honest and open, and remember that death isn't the enemy. Not recognizing our common humanity is (p. 46).

Interviewing: Putting It All Together

Communication theory and skills have one purpose: producing an effective interview between nurse and client. An interview is an interaction that blends theory and skills with a purpose.

Information-gathering interviews are those in which the nurse seeks information from a client to plan or deliver nursing care.

Helping interviews (also called *therapeutic interviews*) are those in which the nurse tries to help another to problem solve, plan for the future, cope with stress, and so forth. Chapter 8, The Nursing Process, discusses how nurses identify health needs and plan, administer, and evaluate nursing care. Interviewing is essential to that process.

Unfortunately, the connotation of interview has evolved to mean cleverly forcing the other person to confess. Such tactics cannot promote trust in a helping interview, nor is the monotonous, bureaucratic approach of "I just have a few [dozen] questions" acceptable. Successful interviewing uses a healthy balance of verbal and nonverbal behavior, empathy, assertive responses, and client-centered techniques, each chosen specifically to promote trust.

Assertive Communication

Learning to communicate effectively with other persons requires that several interpersonal skills be mastered. **Assertiveness,** a proactive problem-solving and coping behavior, is a verbal communication skill that states one's own rights positively without infringing on others' rights. Effective use of assertiveness prevents interpersonal misunderstanding and solves the inevitable conflicts that do arise.

Interpersonal communication styles can be described as either passive, assertive, or aggressive. The passive communicator abdicates his or her own rights, whereas the aggressive communicator infringes on the rights of others. The challenge for the assertive nurse is to develop a style of interaction that neither passively accepts nor aggressively attacks other persons.

Assertion clarifies your needs, feelings, and thoughts while acknowledging those of another. Assertion also clarifies points of disagreement.

The use of assertive behavior reflects a mature level of self-confidence. A competent and confident nurse chooses to use assertive behavior rather than passive or aggressive behaviors in interpersonal conflicts. Both interactions with clients and the demands of a rapidly changing health care delivery system can challenge the nurse who is attempting to use assertive rather than passive or aggressive communication. The following example contrasts passive, aggressive, and assertive responses:

Client: "Nurse, this soup tastes terrible and it's cold; I won't eat it."
Nurse A [passive]: "Okay. Give it back to me." (Silently thinking, "Why does everyone complain to me?")
Nurse B [aggressive]: "Well, it's not my fault. You'll have to speak to the dietitian. I can't help you."
Nurse C [assertive]: "That's disappointing. You can either have it warmed up or substitute something else. Which do you prefer?" (workable compromise)

Assertive responses require significant practice, because many persons must unlearn habitual passive or aggressive behavior before learning more effective assertive behavior. To help a client become more assertive, the nurse first helps the client acknowledge his or her rights as a consumer of health care services. As an advocate for the client, the assertive nurse protects the client's rights to privacy, confidentiality, and full understanding of the care received. Steps to becoming more assertive include the following:

❐ Use "no" as necessary.
❐ Communicate your intent clearly.

❏ Develop your listening skills.
❏ Attend to body language.
❏ Enhance your confidence and self-image.
❏ Accept critique graciously.
❏ Learn persistence (modified from Anonymous, 1991)

As nurses develop increasingly assertive styles, they learn to respect and protect the rights of others, including clients and colleagues. Communication theory and skills including assertive communication can be applied similarly but for a different purpose in interactions with other health care providers and the public. Nurses use assertive behavior to speak responsibly about what nursing can contribute to health care for today and the future. Florence Nightingale, one of nursing's most forceful and acclaimed communicators, set a shining example: she vividly and persuasively described appalling conditions, asserted health care principles that were profound in their simplicity, and perhaps most important, influenced policy makers. Maraldo, Preziosi, and Binder (1991), in their book *Talking Points*, discussed managing the media of today. Furthermore, they provided examples of helpful facts and recent developments in nursing to use when communicating with legislators.

In many ways, and given scientific and economic advances, health care conditions today are no less appalling than they were in Nightingale's day. Simple preventive measures continue to be inaccessible to many (e.g., prenatal care, vaccines, and condoms), and costs of care are skyrocketing for all. Now, although occasionally nurses broadcast health shows and are seated in Congress, too few practicing nurses use their well-developed communication skills as publicly as Nightingale did. Today, there are more media accessible to nurses than ever before. In addition to professional and public writing (e.g., journal articles, newspaper columns, letters and editorials, articles for lay magazines), nurses can speak before community groups, generate interviews, and call radio and television stations regarding health care issues (Hobdell, Slusser, Patterson, & Burgess, 1991). The challenge for nurses to speak publicly has never been greater. The strategy of transferring familiar communication skills to new situations can give nurses confidence and empowerment to communicate their knowledge and experience more widely.

*E*valuating Communication

Just as evaluating is an ongoing activity within the nursing process, it is also an ongoing activity within the communication process. Both the nurse and client benefit from informal evaluation, which may be simply an indirect question such as, "Let me see if I understand what you are saying." Beginning students may want to note examples of problematic communication in their journals or during nursing care conferences with instructors so they can receive constructive critique.

Barriers to Effective Communication

A number of common barriers are associated with the biophysical, psychological, sociocultural, and environmental variables that affect communication (see Display 9-1). When evaluating communication, the nurse evaluates the extent to which

DISPLAY 9-1 **Barriers to Effective Communication**

Biophysical

Unmet basic needs: oxygen and gas exchange, food, fluids, elimination, rest, comfort, sexual fulfillment
Level of consciousness
Sensory losses, for example, hearing or visual impairment
Motor impairment, for example, speech or writing
Biochemical imbalances, for example, drugs, alcohol

Psychological

Unmet basic needs: safety, security—anxiety and fear, love and belonging, esteem
Ineffective listening and selective inattention
Perception

Sociocultural

Values
Illiteracy
Past experience
Unfamiliar language, including differing dialects and word connotations

Environment

Noise
Uncomfortable temperature, ventilation, lighting
Positioning of communicators
Interruptions

such barriers may be present. Many of these barriers are under the nurse's control. Some personal barriers (e.g., sociocultural values) pertain as much to the nurse as to the client. Person-centered care will be attentive to such barriers and will provide relief to the fullest extent possible. The nurse who breaks confidences both creates a barrier to effective communication and threatens the helping relationship. Inaccurate assessment of the client's developmental state or personal situation may also create barriers. If the purpose of an interview or interaction is unclear to the client, or if a client feels his or her strengths and priorities have been ignored, communication may seem futile. The nurse who is sensitive to any discrepancies between verbal and nonverbal communication may suspect such potential barriers exist. Willingness or invitation to receive feedback from the client about the situation may forestall the development of barriers.

When evaluating communication, the nurse can also reflect on whether the suggested techniques for achieving effective communication are being used consistently. Therapeutic and nontherapeutic techniques are both summarized and compared in Table 9-1.

TABLE 9-1 *Therapeutic and Nontherapeutic Techniques*

Therapeutic	Nontherapeutic
Active listening	Selective or inattentive listening
Accurate observation, stating observation	Stating inference
Empathic response from modeling client's world	Sympathy voiced from perspective of nurse's world
Therapeutic touch	Impersonal distancing
Maintaining confidences	Betraying trusts
Creative use of self	Impersonal interaction
Thoughtful silence	Resistive or fearful silence
Reflection	False reassurance
Restatement	Advice
Summarization	Moralizing
	Approval or disapproval messages
	Criticism and ridicule
	Threats or defensive responses
Well-chosen questions	Questions overused: rapid fire, demanding yes or no answers, direct and harsh queries
Open-ended, except "why?"	
Indirect	

Conflict, Conflict Resolution, and Collaboration

Equally challenging are opportunities for frank and assertive communications among health care workers themselves. Nurses and physicians need to listen to what each can offer to increase care accessibility and control escalating costs. Both professions need to listen to what the public is saying about how they want health care dollars spent. In discussing conflict and communication in health care settings, Northouse and Northouse (1992) stated, "The important question for us to address is not How can we avoid conflict?, but rather, How can we manage conflict effectively and produce positive change?" (p. 215). No one would suggest that improved communication between health care providers and recipients, and among health care providers themselves, is the answer to health care woes. Perhaps it is not unreasonable, however, to suggest that more effective communication could begin to move the players toward solutions.

Barriers to effective communication and the contrast between therapeutic and nontherapeutic techniques are not limited solely to nurse–client communication. These barriers and contrasts also apply to communications between nurses and other professionals, particularly physicians. As McClure (1991), who is executive director of nursing at a large metropolitan medical center, stated, "Obviously, the question of reducing nurse–physician conflict becomes one of improving communications, the age-old solution to most problems" (p. 329). However, she suggested that competence demonstrated through experience minimizes conflicts between individuals. Also important are efforts at communication and understanding between students of both professions, collaborative patient rounds that focus on information sharing and care planning, and mutual problem solving within their shared practice arena.

The cover story in the *Hospitals* April 20, 1991 issue suggested, "Quality improvement is key to changing nurse–MD relations." (Eubanks, 1991). As quality problems are viewed as system problems, nurses, physicians and hospital chief executive officers are challenged to promote collaboration. According to Kowalski et. al. (1991), "The Joint Commission [the accrediting body] is headed toward the whole total quality management focus. I can't imagine how an institution would get there without exquisite collaboration between nurses and physicians. . . " (p. 27).

Of course conflict and conflict resolution apply to many situations beyond M.D./R.N. relationships. Consider some basic ideas about conflict and conflict resolution that may be helpful in a wide variety of personal and professional situations where verbal communication and collaboration are involved.

Defining Conflict

First of all, conflict is neither inherently good nor bad. Neither can it be totally avoided in a complex and diverse society. If we value diversity as contributing to excellence in all facets of society, conflict is inevitable. Not everyone will agree all the time. Although conflict is basically a communications problem, it benefits from the application of critical thinking and problem solving strategies. For example:

❐ Apply critical thinking behaviors actively: listen to alternative viewpoints, entertain alternative solutions, try to understand others' points of view, acknowledge differences. Critical thinking allows opportunities for alternative solutions to "perk" and mature.

❐ Consider what the problem or conflict would look like if it were solved. Remember a problem is the difference between existing circumstances and a more ideal situation. If an "ideal" solution cannot initially be visualized, what would be a partial solution or progress in the right direction?
  a. How is the current conflict alike or different from previous similar problems?
  b. Your conflict may not be unique; what resources might be available? Take advantage of others' previous problem solving.
  c. New problems may need new solutions. An old adage suggests–if you are not part of the solution, you may be part of the problem.

❐ In defining conflict, recognize that who, what, when, and where are often easier to answer than why? Why is not always necessary to answer.

❐ In defining conflict, frame problems in terms of situations rather than people. Situations are easier to change than people! Also, avoid stereotyping, generalizing, and blaming. Consider bad or complex problems and situations versus "bad" people. Critique behavior and action rather than people.

❐ In defining the specific nature of conflict, both problems and perceptions of problems are important. There is often, if not usually, a difference between subjective perceptions and a more objective reality.

❐ Recognize and differentiate between authority (assumed right to control) and influence (the power of producing effects by less visible means). Avoid power struggles.

❑ Recognize and differentiate between issues and pseudo-issues. Issues are problems not easily resolved, or without an apparent right or wrong answer. Pseudo-issues may mask the real underlying conflict.

❑ Neither always be looking for issues to precipitate conflict nor always fail to recognize them. Rather, anticipate problems and recognize situations likely to cause conflict. Pick your conflicts in harmony with your professional and personal priorities.

Some Strategies to Use During Conflict Resolution

The following strategies may be useful in a wide variety of situations:

❑ Recognize the difference between efficient (fast) and effective (correct), and strive for a solution that is both.

❑ Recognize the cultural trend in the management of business and health care toward putting solutions in the hands of those involved, whether professionals or consumers. For a reference that is both current and classic, see Hammer and Champy (1994).

❑ Know your conflict "style"—are you assertive as earlier defined, passive (i.e., easily intimidated and apt to cave-in), or aggressive (i.e., easily provoked or hostilely confrontational)? Are you especially sensitive to gender and/or cultural issues?

❑ Focus on strengths and areas of agreement.

❑ Deal with time-lines and deadlines realistically to decrease pressure.

❑ Avoid escalation, or magnifying seriousness, and also straying from the defined problem. Recognize when to back off.

❑ Leave extraneous psychological "baggage" at home.

❑ Agree on neutral "battlegrounds" or arbitrators. Agree that it is "ok" to both agree and disagree. Being positive and open about differences leads to better communication.

❑ Respect others, but recognize that it is proper and important to take care of yourself.

❑ Recognize "impasses"; recognize also that timing can be crucial, and learn to defuse situations and defer conflicts to more constructive times or places.

❑ Recognize the need for time-outs, cooling off periods and/or strategies to decrease heat and keep emotions in control.

❑ Refuse to be a passive scapegoat or an aggressive abuser of persons and circumstances. Be assertive about personal and professional rights.

❑ In clinical situations, keep patient outcomes as the focus of the resolution.

❑ If conflict is with an individual, address the individual directly and individually under appropriate circumstances.
   Use constructive rather than blaming techniques
   a. Establish ground rules.
   b. Admit your mistakes and acknowledge your feelings, e.g., "When you say or do X, I feel such and such".
   c. Avoid framing differences as right or wrong.

  d. Give factual information and make sure value statements are identi-
      fied as such.
- ❐ Use both formal and informal strategies, e.g., testing possible solutions
  with influential players behind the scenes.
- ❐ Recognize the importance of rules, roles, and accepted channels of com-
  munication.
- ❐ Suggest solutions that make win-win results easier to achieve.
- ❐ Recognize that sometimes conflict requires a crisis for resolution.
- ❐ Recognize the power of: unconditional positive regard, personal needs,
  and values.
- ❐ Learn formal arbitrator/mediator strategies, recognize resources, find ex-
  perts in common.
- ❐ Work on the easiest solutions first, as well as those from common
  ground.
- ❐ Practice what you preach, i.e., be a good role model.
- ❐ Communicate positive results and value collaborative protocols.

Some Additional Thoughts

Remember that some of the above ideas may sound like common sense or may seem old hat. Not all of these ideas are expected to be new—rather, this section may serve as a reminder about new applications of old ideas. Gains from conflict resolution include learning new skills, increasing collaboration, and progressing toward common goals.

In 1990, *The New England Journal of Medicine* carried an item titled, "The Doctor-Nurse Game Revisited" by the same lead author who wrote the classic article 20 years before. Stein (1990) noted changes from hierarchical communication to more collaborative interaction. Stein suggests nursing students are being socialized to relate to M.D.s very differently, i.e.,"Nurses feel free to confront and even challenge physicians on issues of patient care" (p. 548). He also notes among the changes that M.D.s are increasingly likely to be women.

A major reason for learning conflict resolution skills is that they prepare you well for working collaboratively with both nurse peers and other health care professionals. In all areas of managed care, collaborative relationships are becoming essential for professional survival. Collaborative relationships both require and yield better communication. Better communication in both practice and research is likely to yield more satisfying, efficient, and effective outcomes for health care professionals and their clients. Nurses, especially, may find this is a key to having their ideas more widely accepted among other health team members, especially physicians. Increasingly, health education materials, as discussed in Chapter 10, are produced for patients collaboratively by a team of health care professionals. Rather than each health care professional providing a separate communication or instruction sheet which the patient must reconcile with others, a collaborative communication bears the endorsement of all to the patient's benefit. Covey (1990), in the classic *Seven Habits of Highly Effective Persons,* refers to communication as one of the master skills in life, the key to building win-win relationships, and also the essence of professional relationships. Nurses are challenged to improve communication and collaboration in health care, thereby taking a significant leadership role in health care reform.

KEY CONCEPTS

✓ **P**rofessional helping relationships have their origin and reason for being centered on client needs and concerns.

✓ **C**ommunication language includes both verbal and nonverbal language; the latter involves sight, nonverbal sounds, touch, space and time.

✓ **A**chieving therapeutic communication involves using empathy and additional effective communication skills, as well as avoiding communication pitfalls.

✓ **B**iophysical, psychological, sociocultural, and environmental variables can create barriers to effective communication.

✓ **C**onflict resolution skills that can be learned will assist nurses to be effective collaborators in health care delivery and reform.

CRITICAL THINKING QUESTIONS

1. Analyze the communication styles of two persons in your living situation. Compare and contrast passive, assertive, and aggressive communication through examples.

2. What are your strengths or unique personal skills that might influence your interpersonal communication?

3. What are untapped communication opportunities for nurses in your institution and local community?

4. In what specific ways can you prepare yourself for better professional communication with nurses and other health care peers?

5. Analyze your personal strengths and weaknesses for establishing therapeutic communication with persons older than you, younger than you, from another culture, and of the opposite gender.

6. What are the resources in your health care facility that enable communication with clients of diverse cultures?

7. Ms. Jones and Mrs. Alvarez share a patient room in a longterm care facility. Both are visually impaired and have moderate hearing losses. What are some of your communication considerations in providing care?

8. Analyze your personal strengths and weaknesses for resolving conflict situations.

9. A cyberspace pen pal whose native language is not English asks for your specific suggestions about how to best prepare for a visit to your nursing school. What would you suggest?

10. How can cyberspace be used by nurses to further the aims of the profession?

REFERENCES

Anonymous. (1991). Steps to becoming more assertive. *Nursing'91, 21*(3),112,114,116

Bandler, R., & Grinder, J. (1975). *The structure of magic.* Palo Alto, CA: Science and Behavior Books.

Barna, L.M. (1994). Stumbling blocks in intercultural communication. In S.A. Samovar & R.E. Porter (Eds.). *Intercultural communication: A reader* (7th ed., 337–346). Belmont, CA: Wadsworth Publishing.

Benner, P.E., & Wrubel, J. (1989). *The primacy of caring.* Menlo Park, CA: Addison-Wesley.

Berlo, D.K. (1960). *The process of communication: An introduction to theory and practice.* New York: Holt, Rinehart & Winston.

Boehm, S. (1996) Personal communication, August, 1996.

Brammer, L.M. (1988). *The helping relationship: Process and skills* (4th ed.). Englewood Cliffs, NJ: Prentice-Hall.

Brown, M. (1992). *Nurses: The human touch.* New York: Ballantine Books, Random House.

Covey, S.R. (1990). The seven habits of highly effective people: Restoring the character ethic. NY: Simon and Schuster.

Dreher, B.B. (1987). *Communication skills for working with elders.* New York: Springer Publishing.

Dubois, K. & Rizzolo, M.A. (1994). Cruising the 'information superhighway'. *American Journal of Nursing, 94*:58–60.

Eubanks, P. (1991). Quality improvement key to changing nurse–MD relations. *Hospitals, 65*(8), 26–30.

Finn, K.L. (1996, July 9). Nursing student connects patient with friends at home, school. *The University Record*, p. 8.

Hall, E. T. (1966). *The hidden dimension.* New York: Doubleday.

Galanti, G. (1991). Caring for patients from different cultures: Case studies from American hospitals. Philadelphia: University of Pennsylvania Press.

Gray, J. (1992). *Men are from mars, women are from venus: A practical guide for improving communication and getting what you want in your relationships.* New York: Harper Collins.

Green, L. (1994). *Making sense of humor.* Glen Rock, N.J.: Knowledge, Ideas and Trends.

Hammer, M. & Champy, J. (1994). *Reengineering the corporation: A manifesto for business revolution* (paperback ed.). New York: Harper Business.

Hobdell, E.F., Slusser, M., Patterson, J., & Burgess, E. (1991). Showing a profession: Getting nursing on the newsstand. *Clinical Nurse Specialist, 5*(3), 174–177.

Hollinger, L.M. (1986). Communicating with the elderly. *Journal of Gerontological Nursing, 12*(3), 9–13.

Kidd, P.S. (1990). Oral expression and perceptions of care with ethical implications. In M.M. Leininger (Ed.), *Ethical and moral dimensions of care* (pp. 95–105). Detroit: Wayne State University Press.

Kowalski, P. Llewellyn, F.A. & Fralic, M. The staff nurse as quality monitor. *American Journal of Nursing 91*, 40–42.

Krieger, D. (1975). Therapeutic touch: The imprimatur of nursing. *American Journal of Nursing, 75*, 784–787.

Layton, J.M. (1994). *Empathy: Theory, research and nursing applications* (Pub. No. 19-2544, 91-106). New York: National League for Nursing.

Maraldo, P.J., Preziosi, P., & Binder, L. (1991). *Talking points* (2nd ed., Publication No. 41-2287). New York: National League for Nursing.

McClure, M.L. (1991). The nurse executive: Nurse–physician conflict. *Journal of Professional Nursing, 7*(6), 329.

Meleis, A.I. (1991). *Theoretical nursing: Development and progress* (2nd ed.). Philadelphia: J.B. Lippincott.

Norris, J. (1986). Teaching communication skills: Effects of two methods of instruction and selected learner characteristics. *Journal of Nursing Education, 25*(3), 102–106.

Northouse, P., & Northouse, L.L. (1992). *Health communication: Strategies for health professionals.* Norwalk, CT: Appleton & Lange.

Orlando, I. (1990). *The dynamic nurse–patient relationship* (Publication No. 15-2341). New York: National League for Nursing.

Orlando, I. (1961). *The dynamic nurse–patient relationship.* New York: Putnam.

Peplau, H. (1989). *Interpersonal theory in nursing practice: selected works of Hildegarde Peplau.* New York: Springer.

Peplau, H. (1952). *Interpersonal relations in nursing.* New York: Putnam.

Pike, A.W. (1990). On the nature and place of empathy in clinical nursing practice. *Journal of Professional Nursing 6*(4), 235–240.

Robinson, V.M. (1991). *Humor and the health profession: The therapeutic use of humor in health care* (2nd ed.). Thorofare, NJ: Slack.

Rogers, C.R. (1961). *On becoming a person.* Boston: Houghton Mifflin.

Rogers, C.R. (1957). The necessary and sufficient conditions of therapeutic personality change. *Journal of Consulting and Clinical Psychology, 21,* 95–103.

Steckel, S.B. (1980). Contracting with patient-selected reinforcers. *American Journal of Nursing, 80*(9), 1596–1599.

Stein, L.I., Watts, D.T. & Howell, T. (1990). *New England Journal of Medicine 322,* 546–549.

Sullivan, J.L., & Deane, D.M. (1988). Humor and health. *Journal of Gerontological Nursing, 14*(1), 20–24.

Ufema, J.K. (1987). How to talk to dying patients. *Nursing '87, 17*(8), 43–46.

Watson, J. (1979). Nursing: The philosophy and science of caring. Boston: Little, Brown.

Wilmington, S.C. (1986). Oral communication—Instruction for a career in nursing. *Journal of Nursing Education, 25*(7), 291–294.

10

Learning and Teaching

Affective
learning,
affective
behavior
Behavioral
objectives
Behaviorism

Cognitive
learning,
cognitive
behavior
Cognitive
learning
theories

Health
education
Humanistic
approaches
to learning
Learning

Psychomotor
learning or
behavior
Teaching

Objectives

After completing this chapter, students will be able to:

Describe the learning–teaching interaction as a problem-solving communication process.

Recognize behavioristic, cognitive, and humanistic approaches to learning.

Recognize health education as a collaborative activity among the health care team members and with the client.

Describe the various steps of the learning–teaching interaction in the context of the nursing process.

Differentiate behavioral objectives in the cognitive, affective, and psychomotor domains.

Describe learner-centered methods of meeting learning needs for self and clients.

Describe a strategy for life-long learning in a professional career.

Learning–teaching is an essential subconcept of professional nursing. **Learning** involves a change in behavior and implies adaptation to an environmental situation. If nurses believe that persons grow, adapt, and develop to fulfill human potential, as Maslow has suggested, then learning is really the ongoing process of becoming. Nurses need basic knowledge about how their clients learn, which they use both to understand their clients as persons and to understand how learning is sometimes focused to meet immediate health needs. Nurses also need to focus this basic knowledge on the life-long learning that will be required in their own professional careers. Nurses will find that technologic advances are rapidly expanding and facilitating the availability of learning resources for both themselves and their clients. As Carl Sagan (1995) wrote, "In a world in transition, students and teachers both need to teach themselves an essential skill–learning how to learn" (p. 321).

In this chapter, we choose to focus on learning because learning needs precede and determine how nurses teach clients and how nurses plan for their own life-long learning. According to Simms, "Actually one cannot turn off learning, and every encounter is a learning opportunity. Doing or practicing related activities at any age is important in imbedding new learning in one's brain." (L. Simms, Personal Communication, September 7, 1997).

Just as client needs (problems) determine the care nurses give, it is client learning needs that determine what teaching nurses do. Theories about learning come from psychology and are applied in education through the practice of **teaching.** Much of the knowledge about how to teach clients comes from the interdisciplinary study of human communication. We emphasize learning because placing learning first emphasizes what the client is "doing,"i.e., learning. Using this logic and emphasis, the nurse is facilitating client learning, a form of health adaptation. When teaching, nurses incorporate interpersonal communication skills as a nursing action within the nursing process. Thus, teaching occurs primarily during the implementation (i.e., intervention) phase of the nursing process. Many other nursing activities, however, precede teaching—including assessment of learning needs and styles, identifying appropriate nursing diagnoses, and determining expected outcomes.

Facilitating learning is a nursing activity that assumes greater importance as persons take more responsibility for their own health. It is through facilitating client learning that the nurse can function as an influential health educator. Clients need information to make informed choices, control their health situations, and mobilize their strengths. Clients also may need to learn new behaviors, new activities, and different feeling responses to internal and external stressors. Nurses individualize teaching just as they individualize other interventions. A learning need corresponds to other nursing diagnoses; it can be a problem to be solved or a strength to be augmented. To facilitate learning, nurses will use all of their nursing-process and interpersonal communication skills. Therefore, what clients learn is in part an evaluation of nurses' teaching abilities and also of their sensitivity to basic and higher-level needs.

For both yourself and your clients, START WHERE THE LEARNER IS! This chapter starts with yourself as an adult learner and explores your current knowledge of learning/teaching concepts. Since adults learn by "doing", the expectation is that you will "do" as necessary those learning experiences provided. As necessary means according to your current knowledge, past experience, and individual need. Learning experiences are intended to enable and empower you to apply learning/teaching principles to your professional practice and personal development.

Some Assumptions and Definitions Related to Learning

First, some assumptions about you the learner. You are expected to have had:

❏ Unique previous learning experiences.
❏ Minimal experience as a teacher of individuals or groups.
❏ Some knowledge of pertinent terminology and concepts.
❏ Individual strengths, career aspirations, and interests.

Now, some general assumptions about learning:

❏ The learner is the focal point of the learning/teaching process.
❏ Persons learn in common and unique ways.
❏ Facilitating client and personal learning is an important nursing function.
❏ Understanding principles of adult learning can facilitate your own learning, as well as improve your teaching.
❏ You have valuable information about yourself as both a learner and a teacher.

With these assumptions in mind, use the definitions that follow as an easily accessible summary of basic vocabulary related to learning and teaching. These definitions can also help you assess your current knowledge, attitudes, and individual needs.

❏ *Affective learning or affective outcome behavior:* Expresses feelings, attitudes, and values.
❏ *Behavioral objectives or expected outcomes:* Stated learning goals; behavioral objectives or expected outcomes indicate how persons will demonstrate learning (e.g., what they will say or do). Behavioral objectives must be realistic and measurable; often a time frame is explicitly stated.
❏ *Cognitive learning or cognitive outcome behavior:* Demonstrates the result of cognition (i.e., thinking). Examples would be stating effects of a medication or applying learned information to a new situation, e.g., evaluating a plan of care.
❏ *Cognitive learning theories:* Those approaches to learning that emphasize the cognitive processes of thinking, language, and problem solving. Cognitive learning theorists include Piaget, and more recent approaches include information processing and artificial intelligence.
❏ *Distance learning:* Education in which the teacher and learner are separate during most of the instruction. Examples include correspondence courses, interactive television, and virtual reality (electronic simulation through interactive computer technology).
❏ *Health education:* Facilitation of learning for the intent of promoting health and wellness and/or preventing disease.
❏ *Humanistic approaches to learning:* Approaches to learning reflecting "existential" or "third force" psychology, and emphasizing the importance of

a person's affective or feeling responses to learning. Advocates include Maslow and Carl Rogers.

❑ *Knowledge deficit:* "The state in which the individual experiences a deficiency in cognitive knowledge or psychomotor skills that alters or may alter health." (Carpenito, 1984, p. 42).

❑ *Learning:* A change in behavior, adaptation, or coping in response to changing life circumstances.

❑ *Lifelong learning:* Behavioral changes over time that contribute to personal empowerment and career advancement for professionals.

❑ *Mentor:* One who assumes professional sponsorship for a less experienced colleague.

❑ *Motivation:* That which stimulates or moves someone to learn; whereas children are primarily motivated to learn by extrinsic rewards, adults are more likely to be motivated by intrinsic rewards.

❑ *Principle:* An essential element or motivating force that serves as a basis for action.

❑ *Psychomotor learning or outcome behavior:* Learning involving the motor effects of mental processes.

❑ *Social Learning Theory:* Suggests the influence of significant others as a primary motivating factor. A major proponent is Bandura.

❑ *Teaching:* A direct or indirect interaction, the intent of which is to facilitate learning.

❑ *Teachable moment:* A circumstance in which a learner is uniquely motivated or susceptible to motivation.

Theories About Learning

Many theories about learning attempt to explain the phenomenon. We still have much to discover about why learning occurs as it does. Psychologists who support various learning theories offer different explanations of how learning occurs. Instead of considering various theories as being in conflict with one another, it is often more useful to regard them as focusing on different aspects of learning or behaving. As Reilly (1990) suggested, numerous theories are rooted in various assumptions about humankind, the nature of knowledge, and the processes by which persons learn (p. 28). Also, as Reilly and Oermann (1992) suggested, "Cultural determinants are significant in any concept of learning, for they denote the structure of knowledge, its meaning and relationships, and the process by which members of a culture learn" (p. 39). As the cultural demographics change in America, and as nurses also become citizens of the global village, awareness of cultural influences on learning assumes greater significance. References such as Geissler (1994) may prove helpful.

An eclectic approach to learning, which the authors advocate, presumes that no one learning theory is more correct than another. An eclectic approach leads one to select from various theories, using whatever fits best from each source, and being alert to the inconsistencies of different theories. For our purposes, we divide learning theories according to whether they emphasize behavior, cognition or thought processes, or a humanistic–holistic view of the person. A brief discussion of the various types of learning theories will enable us to compare and contrast them.

Behavioristic Learning Theories: Conditioning and Behavior Modification

Behaviorism represents learning as a process of making connections through association. Its origin is the conditioned response. This technique, developed by Ivan Pavlov (1849–1936) with his salivating dogs, was more concerned with neurology than psychology. The contemporary proponent of conditioning and behaviorism was B. F. Skinner (1904–1990), the originator of behavioral technology. Skinner concentrated on the role of reinforcement in establishing conditioned or desired responses. Although Skinner's principles of reinforcement were developed in the animal laboratory with pigeons, they can be applied to the control of health-related behavior by means of behavior modification programs.

Behavior modification, once the domain of psychology, currently is applied to practice arenas as diverse as education, business, and health care. Behavior modification has been widely used to control smoking, and also to achieve socially acceptable behavior in a variety of institutions. Behavior modification involves a carefully planned schedule of positive reinforcement when desired behavior occurs. This reinforcement may involve tokens, approval, or praise from a significant person. The reinforcement must be perceived as positive by the learner as well as the teacher.

Nursing Implications

Behavior analysis, behavior therapy, and behavioral intervention as used by other health scientists holds great promise for nurses, according to Susan Boehm (1992), a noted nurse–scientist. She said,

> Primary areas where behavior therapy can be most critically and successfully applied are in cases requiring behavior change to reduce cholesterol, increase exercise, minimize urinary incontinence, or combat chronic illness. Those are areas where nursing intervention is critical. As nurses, we are constantly looking for ways to help people with these health problems (p. 3).

As Boehm indicated, the nurse possesses much information that the client could use to manage his or her own health behavior. Contrary to the way many people understand behavior modification, the learner's response, not the teacher's stimulus, is the key to behavior change. Additionally, for reinforcement to operate in any setting, the learner must believe that what is to be learned will help meet a particular need. The important formula to remember is as follows: Response → Reinforcement → Future behavior

The initial step for the nurse is to shape learning by reinforcing—it is hoped in a positive manner—the adaptive behavior observed in the client or patient. This reinforcement can be done without knowing either what goes on inside the person or exactly why. It is also possible and appropriate to use the natural setting and the client's response, rather than worrying about contriving artificial stimuli. Because behavioral conditioning focuses on the individual learner's response, the nurse recognizes that instruction, teaching, and facilitation, like other nursing interventions, must be individualized to be most effective.

As persons with health problems become aware of how behavior modification works, they may choose to provide their own meaningful reinforcement. For instance they may use **biofeedback** techniques to reduce stress and promote relaxation. Biofeedback is that altered physiological or psychological state or response (and awareness of it) that can be measured objectively and/or subjectively.

The consumer movement in health care has had the important effect of bringing health information and reinforcement under client or internal control. For example, expectant mothers choose natural childbirth and husbands become helpers in reinforcing healthy birthing behaviors. Programmed learning, which guides learners to desirable responses that are then reinforced, is now available both in hard copy and electronic form via computers. A new educational video series and home reference book, edited by the former Surgeon General C. Everett Koop (The Health Publishing Group, 1996), provides educational materials designed to help health consumers become more knowledgeable about problems so that they will practice healthy behaviors in promoting wellness and preventing disease.

Cognitive Learning Theories

Cognitive learning theorists include the Gestalt psychologists, and developmental psychologists such as Piaget. The Gestaltists were concerned with insight, namely the "Aha!" experience. This insight involves a perceptual reorganization that allows ideas to combine in such a way that $1 + 1 = 3$ rather than the usual 2. In other words, insight makes clear the relationships of puzzle pieces to each other, so that the puzzle makes sense. Nurses often do see persons gain sudden insights into complex and puzzling health situations, as the Gestaltists theorize.

Developmental psychologists' important contribution to learning has been a better understanding of age-linked stages of cognitive development. This understanding has led to teaching children at their appropriate stage of development, rather than as small adults. For example, a pediatric nurse may apply Piaget's theory and use a three-dimensional model to teach a school-aged child about his or her heart function. The nurse knows that the concept of the heart as a pump is insufficiently developed in the elementary school student to be understood through a verbal explanation. The cognitive development of a child at this age is at the stage of concrete operations rather than formal thought. Developmental readiness is a key factor in many cognitive approaches, as is individual readiness expressed as motivation.

Humanistic Approaches to Learning

Humanistic approaches to learning are a rather recent development growing out of humanistic or "third force" psychology. Humanistic approaches to learning emphasize the affective or feeling responses toward learning. This focus remains

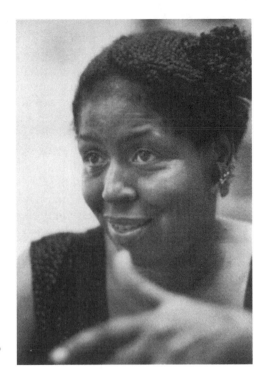

The humanistic teacher listens and responds to her students.

a prime consideration, even if what is to be learned is new knowledge or a motor skill.

A humanistic approach is sometimes also called existential or phenomenologic. *Existential* is a term rooted in philosophy and is concerned with a person's subjective awareness of his or her existence. The existential perspective is a self-deterministic view. *Phenomenologic* refers to a concern for what is happening in the present. From an existential perspective, behavior is dealt with in the present. There is neither the Freudian concern for the past nor the behavioristic emphasis on shaping future behavior.

The humanistic viewpoint emphasizes the importance of the person's view of self, the human's unique potential as a learner, and learning as a product of the person's perception. A hallmark of the humanistic approach is the belief that the human has a basic drive toward health or wellness and self-actualization.

Humanism and Holism

The humanistic view of learning is particularly pertinent to a holistic philosophy of health care, that is, one that focuses on the whole person. The rationale for such an approach is rooted in the belief that understanding one's health problems is essential to adapting to those health problems and moving toward health and self-actualization. This view also assumes that when no health problems exist, a person still learns to manage his or her health care to promote continued and heightened well-being. Although each person is unique, the common basic needs shared with other humans provide the basis for learning needs common to all persons if they are to achieve self-actualization.

Abraham Maslow (1970) and Carl Rogers (1969) represent theorists who advocated humanistic approaches to learning. Their concepts and principles have a special relevance for nursing. Maslow's humanistic approach and hierarchy of needs suggest a way to prioritize nursing interventions so that physiologic needs are met first, followed by safety and security needs, love and belonging needs, esteem and self-esteem needs, and ultimately growth needs. In Chapter 8, we made other applications of this hierarchy to the prioritizing of various nursing interventions. Much of traditional nursing care has involved meeting the physiologic needs that an ill person is unable to meet for himself or herself. Increasingly, nurses are also focusing their care functions on promoting and maintaining health and assisting clients to meet growth needs that foster self-actualization. Nurses are also assisting clients to use their own strengths or self-care abilities. Remember, however, that the *client* must perceive his or her needs (physiological, safety and security, etc.) to have been met at a satisfactory level before growth issues and self actualization are attempted. The nurse takes cues from the client before proceeding with teaching and encouraging learning.

Carl Rogers, humanistic psychologist and teacher, was especially concerned about personalized approaches to the learner. He emphasized the importance of a safe and facilitative learning environment to maximize the learner's self evaluation and hence independence.

Common Selected Learning/Teaching Principles

The nurse using an eclectic or broadly encompassing approach to learning should understand common learning/teaching principles. The following selected common adult learning principles are applicable to your own and others' learning:

- ❑ Learning involves a change in some kind of behavior, e.g., thinking, feeling, or psychomotor.
- ❑ People learn in both common and unique ways.
- ❑ All persons have actual or potential learning needs.
- ❑ Learning is based on need as identified by the learner.
- ❑ Individual learner variables affect learning.
- ❑ Learning is multisensory.
- ❑ Readiness and motivation affect learning.
- ❑ A behavior tends to become frequent when it is followed by some reinforcement or consequence that the learner considers positive.
- ❑ Individual teacher variables affect teaching. For example, these variables may include previous education, basic needs, culture, and values.
- ❑ The environment and learner/teacher interaction variables affect learning.
- ❑ The methods for facilitating learning vary with the learning need.

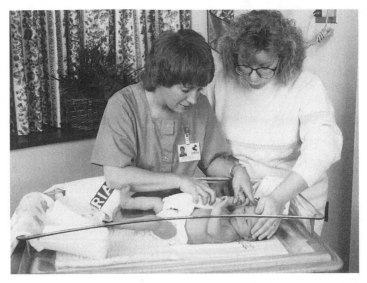

Effective teaching methods are chosen to match the client's learning needs and behavioral objectives.

❏ The learner needs feedback and so does the teacher.
❏ Evaluating learning is an essential part of teaching.

Learning–Teaching Interaction as a Problem-Solving Process

The learning–teaching interaction is not only a communication process but also a problem-solving process. As indicated so many times in previous chapters, the nursing process is the problem-solving process of professional nursing. It is logical, therefore, to approach the learning–teaching interaction within the context and organization of the nursing process. This means the steps of the learning–teaching interaction parallel those of the nursing process:

❏ Collecting data (assessing)
❏ Determining what the assessment means for this client at this point in time (analyzing)
❏ Using the data to identify strengths and to state learning needs (identifying problems)
❏ Clarifying behavioral outcomes (formulating goals/objectives)
❏ Planning (identifying appropriate interventions)
❏ Using teaching methods or strategies (implementing interventions)
❏ Evaluating both learning and teaching
❏ Evolving a learning–teaching philosophy and synthesizing learning theory (aggregating)

Collecting Data To Assess Learning Needs

Assessing the person's strengths and biophysical needs, including growth and development needs, enables the nurse as teacher to identify problems and learning needs that are truly personalized. Assessing learner needs should include the following steps of assessment:

- ❏ Using empathy to anticipate learning needs
- ❏ Assessing level of knowledge, skill, and attitude
- ❏ Assessing level of comprehension
- ❏ Assessing readiness to learn (motivation)

Beyond the basic learning needs, individual learning needs are difficult to predict. An effective nurse–client relationship is crucial to detecting those individual needs. Without open, sensitive, two-way communication, a nurse never learns what the client wants and needs to learn.

The assessment of a client's current understanding, skill, or attitude communicates this message: "You are a competent person. You are capable of learning and adapting. I will help you build on what you already know and do." Consider what message is conveyed to a client when the nurse does not "start where he or she is" but teaches what he or she already knows. Consider also the total breakdown of the helping relationship when the nurse begins teaching far beyond the client's understanding, or prior to meeting basic needs.

Beginning with the hypothesis that all clients are capable of learning and comprehending, the effective nurse–educator sees the challenge as that of discovering how best to facilitate client comprehension. Typically, data on stage of growth and development or on level of vocabulary give a rough indication of potential comprehension. However, the possibility exists for the nurse to stereotype levels of comprehension based on social class, occupation, age, or years of formal education. Inbred perceptions of poor people, unskilled workers, older people, or unschooled clients label them "unable to comprehend" before they have a chance to prove otherwise. Nurses avoid such stereotyped labels. Instead, they recognize the value in full, lifelong learning experiences acquired informally and independently through many crises and changes.

In assessing a learner's readiness to learn, educators speak of a "teachable moment," that is, a period in which a learner is receptive and ready to listen, adapt, and learn. Ideally, then, teaching should be timed to take advantage of a learner's teachable moments so that learning occurs more readily and naturally. At such times, learning is likely to have more personal meaning, and the learner is therefore more aware of how learning may benefit him or her.

These moments can often be anticipated. Indeed, the entire concept of anticipatory crisis intervention is derived from the fact that before a predictable crisis, for example, childbirth, a client is open and receptive to learning and growing. Prehospitalization teaching also attempts to promote learning before a crisis.

In contrast, many other receptive or teachable moments occur spontaneously, informally, and suddenly. Nurses and students sometimes tend to view teaching much too formally, missing many of the constant and unlimited opportunities for informal learning–teaching. A crucial assessment skill is the ability to recognize the client behaviors that indicate learning receptivity. Such client behaviors include direct and indirect questions and other information-seeking behavior. Examples might be regular exercise, which indicates an awareness of the contribution of exercise to health and a possible interest in expanding this activity; breast self-examination, indicating willingness to learn other protective measures such as increasing dietary fiber; or reading lay books about health-related matters. Look also for those behaviors that are already in the direction of where you think the learner needs to go, but recognize, as Reilly and Oermann (1992) suggested, the significance of cultural determinants. Recognize also that although learning needs may be identified at any level of Maslow's hierarchy of needs, clients will strive to have their most basic needs met first. Remember that all behavior has meaning. Remember also that among the many learner variables that affect learning are the following few:

- ❏ Biological/physiological conditions including pain and fatigue
- ❏ Altered sensory perception
- ❏ Growth and development
- ❏ Literacy and language
- ❏ Present knowledge
- ❏ Attitude and skill
- ❏ Poverty
- ❏ Stress
- ❏ Cognitive ability

Once persons have reached maturity, it is not appropriate to treat them as children, even under conditions of diminished cognition or frailty. It is appropriate to recognize that such circumstances may require consultation with experts to derive individualized strategies that are appropriate.

Analyzing the Learning–Teaching Situation

Analyzing the learning–teaching situation involves determining what the assessment means for this client at this point in time. The teacher tries to assess the learner's motivation–the drives, present or future–that would facilitate learning. When a nurse–educator perceives no motivation for learning, it is possible to induce motivation by sustained psychological support. It is important to remember, however, that dealing with other perceived needs may indeed be more important. Often it is possible to provide information after the nurse learns from the client just what needs he or she perceives as most critical at the moment. Needs may loom large to a person and obstruct his or her ability to cope with new information. However, sometimes a very few minutes or a brief discussion will put the need into perspective, and the nurse can move onto other issues. Beginning a teaching session with a questions such as, "Is there something I can help you with before we start?" will increase the effectiveness of your teaching interventions. Remember also that actual information alone is necessary, but an insufficient motivator to change. Therefore, simply telling a person the changes he or she must make in his or her diet will rarely prompt the person to do so, unless that person is able to express what this change in lifestyle means to him or her as a person.

This is the time to analyze motivation. What is the prime motivation for continuing the learning–teaching process? The needs of the client to learn, or the needs of the nurse to teach? Now is also the time to analyze expectations. What are realistic expectations of the learning–teaching interaction? Consider the press of other needs, and also the time and other resources available. Because clients are sicker and hospital stays shorter, this analysis becomes most important. Nurses must make the most of their time to facilitate client learning, if indeed that is a priority. Based on the data collected about the person and other pressing needs, the nurse will analyze whether a suggestion such as group instruction will be effective and efficient for this particular situation.

*S*tating *Learning Needs*

Once the nurse has identified data indicating a client's learning needs, the question arises: "How do I work these data into the nursing process?" The answer is found in the following test: if the assessment demonstrates a learning need, then begin a learning–teaching process within the nursing process. In other words, proceed to state a learning problem or need, set mutually acceptable learning goals, enact teaching interventions, and evaluate progress.

Typically, a learning need can be stated as a problem in a variety of ways, for example:

❏ Limited knowledge of prescribed medications
❏ Anxiety caused by limited ability to perform one's own personal care

Or, using NANDA language

❏ Knowledge deficit related to. . .
❏ Decisional conflict related to uncertainty about. . .
❏ Ineffective coping related to lack of knowledge about. . .

Such problems, as with any problem statement, can be validated with the client or family, e.g., "I wonder if you'd like more information now, or if you have something else on your mind to talk about first?" If the client seems reluctant to talk, you might suggest a subject such as the procedure she will be having the next day.

Clarifying Expected Outcomes

At this point in the learning–teaching process, and within the nursing process, outcomes are formulated to direct the interventions that follow. These goals will clarify the expected behavior changes following teaching or facilitation of learning. Specifically, learning outcomes or goals are called **behavioral objectives.** *Behavioral learning objectives* are statements of what the client will do or say as evidence of learning. You need to be able to identify clearly what is to be learned and also how to evaluate whether it has been. This need applies equally to yourself and to your clients as learners. Behavioral objectives state measurable behavior changes, such as the ones listed at the beginning of each chapter in this text. Standard format reads, "The learner will. . . ."

Because learning occurs in three domains, behavioral learning objectives are stated within each domain:

1. Cognitive
2. Affective
3. Psychomotor

Cognitive learning objectives use verbs demonstrating results of thinking processes: "The client will state how salt affects his (or her) blood pressure." Thinking or cognitive objectives include knowing and comprehending information, and also applying, analyzing, synthesizing, and evaluating. For example, Mr. Jones will verbalize alterations in respiration and appropriate interventions for these. **Affective learning** objectives reflect the client's feelings, attitudes, and values: "The client will express her reactions to her mastectomy scar" or "Mrs. Gonzales will verbalize her feelings about the loss of her pregnancy." However, as you work with affective objectives, take care to begin where your client is at the moment. For example, a client may not wish to express his or her reactions, or feelings of loss right then. Providing an opportunity for the client to do so, or letting him or her know that you will be available to offer support later when the right moment arrives, may be the most effective intervention. If you will not always be available, provide your client with resources to use at a later date. **Psychomotor learning** objectives state actions and skills: "The client will demonstrate clean technique in changing his (or her) dressing" or "Mr. Johnson will take and record his daily blood pressure accurately." The nurse who communicates effectively with the client will have the necessary information to assist in writing realistic and meaningful objectives and deciding which learning priorities are most important for the client. As the health care provider who spends the most time with clients, the nurse is in ideal circumstances to contribute uniquely to the teaching plans of collaborating health care educators. Patient education, like other aspects of nursing care, is rapidly moving to extramural settings, such as outreach education centers in malls and home care. In hospitals, JCAHO standards pay increasing attention to health education outcomes. Patient education is being integrated into critical paths and case management protocols. More learning and teaching will be highly selective, directed, and paced. With more learning resources available through technology and increasing collaboration among providers, instruction will be more closely tailored to client's individual situations.

Identifying and Implementing Teaching Interventions

This step becomes easier when you acknowledge that learners need the opportunity to practice new skills, i.e., what it is you want them to learn. They need to think content, express feelings, or use psychomotor skills. An incredible number of teaching interventions exist, some traditional, some innovative. How do you choose teaching methods and materials? Various interventions or teaching methods can be effective if chosen to match the client's learning needs and behavioral learning objectives. The most creative lecture will not teach psychomotor skills; clients can learn affective expression if there is an opportunity to vent feelings. Clients may also require teaching to learn how to vent and to recognize that they can communicate their feelings and needs to others.

The point of implementing teaching interventions is to communicate information that will enable clients to become more aware and to develop their knowledge or psychomotor actions and skills, feelings, attitudes, and values. Teaching is a special kind of communication intended to empower the learner to learn. Teaching uses basic communication skills such as active listening, empathy, helping responses, and assertiveness. The client who needs to learn how to change a colostomy drainage bag wants the nurse to understand what it means to him or her to do such a procedure. Similarly, the nurse may be called on to teach other than technical aspects of care. The client who wants to learn how to express his or her needs more openly seeks a signal from the nurse that the nurse also recognizes this client priority as an important component of care. Other skills of supporting and crisis intervention are interwoven.

Further consideration of the learner's ability, developmental stage, cultural values, and past experiences aids in the choice of teaching methods. Assessment of the home environment and the potential family members or friends who can help will also assist the nurse to plan more effective teaching interventions. Each client's reading ability, visual and hearing ability, and interest level differs. The nurse chooses reading materials appropriate to the reading level of the client and compensates for sensory losses when teaching. Common problems of ineffective teaching result from methods below or beyond the client's developmental stage. Sadly, sometimes both verbal and written communication miss the mark and cannot be comprehended by the very learners for whom they were intended. In addition, it is wise to have teaching materials available in both regular and large, bold print for clients who may have vision problems.

Children's education progresses with their levels of concentration, abstraction, and coordination. Knowledge of growth and development is applied when teaching children about health. In contrast, children's materials are inappropriate for teaching adults, however dependent those adults may be. When teaching, nurses rely on general guidelines for matching teaching methods to client needs. Many such guidelines have been written, most of them concentrating on the nurse. The learner-centered guide to teaching methods presented in Table 10-1 provides a contrast. This guide proposes that the nurse can facilitate learning by focusing on what the learner or client perceives that he or she needs to learn, rather than on what the teacher or nurse wants to teach. Additionally, the methods in the guide require some form of communication or interpersonal interaction—either ''live,'' or using previously prepared communication materials. Table 10-2 suggests a learner-centered teaching plan for a specific client.

More creative teaching methods evolve constantly. The use of artistic expression in composition, movement, music, and drama has developed, particularly in

TABLE 10-1 *Learner-Centered Guide to Teaching Method*

Learning Need	Method
If a person needs to learn:	**The nurse can facilitate learning by using:**
Awareness of self, own attitudes, and values	Active exercises, questionnaires, values-clarification activities
Awareness of others' situation, attitudes, and values	Role playing, interacting with others with similar conditions or strengths or problems
Awareness of own behavior	Reverse role playing, audio or video playback, analysis of interactions
Basic factual information	Lectures and discussion, reading, self-directed media programs
Concepts and relationships of ideas	Reading, discussion, models and graphics
Application of concepts to practice	Opportunity for guided practice
Manual skill	Skill practice, demonstration—return demonstration, programmed learning
Relating to others	Group discussion, play groups, role playing, counseling
Self-expression, self-confidence	Group discussion; creative arts (music, art, movement); positive reinforcement; role modeling
Decision making, priority setting	Make decisions and receive feedback
Adaptation to life-style change	Counseling, self-help and mutual help groups, contracting

mental health settings. Relaxation methods of controlled breathing, hypnosis, meditation, biofeedback, expressive exercise, and introspection prevail in learning stress reduction, self-control, and pain relief. The ever-increasing use of audiotapes and videotapes for self-instruction in health care settings, home, school, and the workplace has expanded health teaching immeasurably. These and other methods are available for nurses to use in teaching. There are also many traditional library resources to assist nurses' teaching and facilitation of clients' learning. A variety of methods can contribute to multimedia sensory input, self-paced learning activities, and the positive reinforcement that are associated with an enabling learning environment. In addition to audio and video tapes, prominent electronic media include CD-Rom programs, interactive video discs (especially those for nurses that provide clinical simulation and CAI—computer assisted instruction). There is computer software designed to generate individual patient education handouts on demand. Akin to what pharmacists dispense with prescriptions, these handouts commonly cover adult, women's, and children's health and medication information. As a learner in the new information age, you may soon find yourself a participant in what is referred to on the World Wide Web as the cyberspatial educational arena of virtual coursework, a fancy term for distance learning in the new information age.

TABLE 10-2 *Specifics of a Teaching Plan for Ms. Robinson*

Learning Need	Behavioral Objective	Intervention
Cognitive—Limited knowledge of altered respiratory status	Ms. R. will verbalize alterations in respiration and appropriate interventions for these	Explain briefly how respiratory function is compromised by surgery, anesthesia, and pain; explain what intervention is necessary; demonstrate procedure for coughing and deep breathing
Affective—Feelings of helplessness after surgery	Ms. R. will verbalize decreased feelings of helplessness and therefore be receptive to learning	Spend time with her even when she does not talk; help her vent feelings of helplessness; listen carefully to facilitate development of trusting relationship; acknowledge and reinforce all positive, growth-oriented behaviors; assist her to view herself as a total person rather than focusing on limitations; assist both person and family to express their feelings to each other
Psychomotor—Decreased muscle function as a result of surgery, anesthesia, and pain medication	Ms. R. will maintain clear lungs and will gradually increase mobility from a few steps to regular hall ambulation	Assist with coughing and deep breathing every 1–2 hr while awake and every 3–4 hr during sleep hours; assist with ambulation four times a day until able to proceed without assistance; help her walk a bit farther each time

Do you know which of your own characteristics facilitate your learning or affect your teaching? You probably know intuitively your own personal learning style and characteristics as a learner. For example, are you a visual, auditory, or kinetic/physical learner? You can also assess your personal characteristics and apply these to situations where you are the teacher or facilitator of learning. For example, some people are naturally humorous and casual while others tend to be more reserved and formal. Being a good "listener" for verbal and nonverbal clues dropped by learners will carry you far toward beginning where the learner is, valuing the individuality of the learner, and providing a low-stress and psychologically safe learning environment.

Evaluating Learning

If, indeed, the nurse has developed a learning–teaching process within the nursing process, the evaluation component flows logically from the goals and interventions.

Refer again to the example in Table 10-2, which illustrates evaluating learning. Note that the learning needs and corresponding behavioral objectives span all three domains of learning: cognitive, affective, and psychomotor. All three objectives require different ways of evaluating to determine what was learned. For the cognitive or knowledge objective, the nurse will want to evaluate what the client "knows" as a result of the learning–teaching interaction. There are many nonthreatening ways to create situations in which the client can demonstrate his or her knowledge. Based on this information, the nurse will determine whether this objective has been met. The evaluation of affective objectives requires creating the climate and opportunity for voicing feelings. This evaluation, in turn, suggests both that feelings will be expressed and that this expression will be in the direction intended, such as decreased helplessness. In this example, the positive or satisfactory evaluation of psychomotor objectives requires that the client demonstrate both the coughing and ambulating (walking) behaviors.

Imagine that an evaluation of a teaching plan for Ms. Robinson reveals the following: the first two objectives listed were met; however, we conclude that the third objective—the psychomotor objective—was only partially achieved. From oral and written reports, it is evident that Ms. Robinson ambulates when assisted or reminded, but does not take the initiative to ambulate unaided, although she is physically able to do so. As a result of this evaluation, our nursing plan may be as follows:

❏ Continue to provide gentle reminders of the need to increase ambulation.
❏ Acknowledge and reinforce efforts to increase ambulation.
❏ Plan part of the time spent with Ms. Robinson to include ambulation.
❏ Allow additional quiet time together when she can express other feelings or concerns.

Teaching skills develop over time and with practice. Although observation of other teachers helps the novice learn methods and techniques, each teacher must use creativity to develop an individual style. With each teaching experience, a way to learn is to ask these questions:

How would I improve this session the next time I taught it?
Did the client meet his or her goals, that is, the behavioral learning objectives?
If so, what are the factors leading to his or her success?
If not, what happened to prevent this accomplishment?

Although it is possible to measure the client's learning when using behavioral objectives, it is nearly impossible to predict what long-term influence the nurse may have had on the client, or how a single individual may have motivated his or her future learning—for only the learner determines what will be learned. Durbach, Goodall, and Wilkinson (1987) made this same point: "We must also consider whether our quest for measurable learning outcomes really encourages the kind of evaluation of learning and teaching that is most helpful to clinicians and patients. . . . Behavioral objectives tend to favor the concrete and measurable over the abstract and subtle" (p. 88).

Facilitating client learning is what the nursing intervention of teaching is all about. Teaching usually involves a learning facilitation that has many dimensions. Often the more formal didactic presentation or lecture–demonstration is our initial thought about how to teach. With more attention to the matter, many of the learner-centered methods in Table 10-1 may occur to us.

The Nurse as a Health Educator

Health Education

In 1976, President Gerald R. Ford signed into law the National Consumer Health Information and Health Promotion Act, defining six activities of consumer health education:

1. Inform people about health, illness, disability, and ways in which they can improve and protect their own health, including the more efficient use of the delivery system.
2. Motivate people to want to change to more healthful practices.
3. Help people to learn the necessary skills to adopt and maintain healthful practices.
4. Foster teaching and communication skills in all those engaged in educating consumers about health.
5. Advocate changes in the environment that will facilitate healthful conditions and healthful behavior.
6. Add to knowledge through research and evaluation concerning the most effective ways of achieving these objectives (Somers, 1978).

Concepts of clients' rights, advocacy, consumerism, health behavior, adaptation, communication, and research pervade this law.

All health professionals share responsibility for health education, that is, facilitating another person's learning to live and adapt in the healthiest possible style. Nurses are important health educators. Health is, after all, nursing's primary domain. Nurses outnumber the members of any other health profession. In hospitals, where nurses are with clients 24 hours a day, a great potential for teaching occurs; however, shorter hospital stays of greater acuity suggest that much teaching also needs to occur pre- and post-hospitalization, as nurses encounter clients in other settings. The ability of persons to learn health promotion and preventive practices, to learn to manage illness, and to learn to care for themselves and dependents underlies the health of the nation.

Health Education Activities

Health education activities span the entire range of health care: prevention, maintenance, recovery, and rehabilitation. The nurse–educator who teaches schoolchildren basic health habits helps them to learn health promotion and illness prevention. Assisting an older person to regulate and monitor several medications exemplifies health maintenance teaching. Nurses teach pre- and post-operative care to hasten recovery from surgery and, equally important, to shorten hospital stays. Nurses working in hospice programs teach dying persons and their families how to work through their issues and concerns, finish their business, and therefore adapt to the impending death. Because increasing the cost-effectiveness of health care is a national priority, it is important for nurses to document their health education activities that contribute to these efforts.

Health education, then, is a life-span activity that includes many types of professionals, many levels of health care, and many locations. As interest in sports and physical fitness, healthy nutrition, and aging increases, relatively unexplored areas for health teaching become obvious.

*H*ealth *Education Categories*

The scope of health education activities spans the following six categories, each succeeding group representing a slightly narrower focus:

1. Community health education
2. Occupational health education
3. School health education
4. Group health education
5. Family health education
6. Client–patient education

In their broadest form, immunization campaigns and stop-smoking media campaigns, for example, attempt to teach large communities of persons. Health teaching done in businesses, industries, and schools attempts to promote healthy workers and students. Such teaching may be concerned with helping persons to make their health needs known or helping them to learn strategies for maintaining wellness and resolving lifelong developmental tasks. Persons who are ill receive care and teaching in both formal and informal education sessions. Such teaching may instruct about how to increase functional abilities given personal limitations.

Although nurses have focused traditionally on client and family teaching, the opportunities increase yearly for teaching throughout the broad scope of the six categories and across the entire life span. The efficient use of teaching opportunities will also need to increase. With increasing severity of illness and decreasing length of stay in traditional hospital settings, past methods of delivering health teaching could be caught in the squeeze. Facilitating client learning in the optimal way will be a challenge to all nurses' effective communication, nursing-process skills, creative teaching methods, and use of modern instructional technology. All nursing diagnoses have associated client/family teaching as a component of the interventions. The diagnosis may present as lack of knowledge or decisional anxiety. The following example presents an illustration of how a particular group of nurses sought to address lack of knowledge and related decisional anxiety:

> Registered nurses taking a course to complete their BSN degrees planned a series of health promotion programs for TV. One such program, centered around issues of parenting, gave parents guidelines for when to take a sick child to a doctor or emergency room. They suggested having available a telephone list including the local poison control center and doctor and hospital numbers, a thermometer, and infant ty-

(*text continues on page 348*)

DISPLAY 10-1   **Patient/Family Education Record**

Questions to _____ patient or/and _____ family member (name(s) _____)

1. Unable to assess patient at this time (date/time _____) due to _____
2. Are you ready to learn about . . . (health problem)? _____ YES _____ NO/explain _____
3. How do you best learn? _____ Watch TV/video _____ Listen to Radio _____ Read Newspaper/Books _____ Follow Pictures/Diagrams _____ Learn by doing
4. Is there any religious or cultural practice that you observe which could affect what we teach or how we teach? _____ NO
   _____ YES/explain _____

Barriers identified from Admission Assessment: _____ NONE _____ Language (_____) _____ Vision _____ Hearing _____ Motor Skills
_____ Short term memory loss _____ Emotional _____ Age/Developmental Level _____ Unstable Condition (unable to assess) COMMENTS:
_____

INITIAL ASSESSMENT (name/title/date) _____

LEARNING NEEDS:

1. Special procedures/Rehab techniques
2. Special equipment
3. Recognizing complications
4. Activity level/limitations
5. Meal planning/diet modifications
6. Medication regimen
7. Access to health profession/community resources

8. Follow-up care and prevention measures
9. Diagnostic tests
10. Disease process
11. Other:

EXPECTED OUTCOMES - Patient/family (as appropriate) will be able to:
1. Perform procedure(s) or rehab technique(s)
2. Explain how to obtain, operate, and care for equipment needed
3. Identify signs/symptoms of possible complications
4. Discuss activity level and restrictions
5. Describe diet (preparation and/or restrictions)
6. Name meds, dosage, reason for taking, schedule, side effect(s)
7. State when/how to contact health professional and/or how to access community resources
8. Identify time and place for follow-up care; acknowledge prevention
9. Cite patient's role in preparing for/participating in test
10. Acknowledge patient's need to participate in health regimen
11.

(Courtesy of Margaret R. Pardee Memorial Hospital, Hendersonville, North Carolina.)

(continued)

344

KEY: Place letter(s) or number(s) in box which corresponds to appropriate heading

Learner		Method		Evaluation		Follow-up (f/u)	
P	= Patient	E	= Explanation	S	= States or identifies key points or facts	NA	= Not applicable
S	= Spouse	D	= Demonstration	V	= Verbalizes understanding	1	= None needed
M	= Mother	V	= Videotape/CCTV	D	= Demonstrates skill independently	2	= Re-teach
F	= Father	R	= Role play	DC	= Performs skill with verbal/physical coaching	3	= Reinforce content
D1	= Daughter	P	= Physical model	I	= Inadequate or incorrect skills/knowledge	4	= Repeat demonstration of skill(s)
S1	= Son	W	= Written material	N	= No indication of learning (see Comments)	5	= Assist w/ practice of skills
X1	= Other	A	= Audiocassette	N/A	= Learning not evaluated (see Comments)	6	= Other (see Comments)
		O	= Other (explain)				

Reassess:

Date/Time	Need/Outcome	DEPT	Learner	Method	PATIENT EDUCATION	EVAL	f/u	Comments	Initials
	NA	Nsg		V,W,E	*ADVANCE DIRECTIVES* (ask pt/family if any questions)				

DISPLAY 10-2 Patient/Family Education Record (Side Two)

KEY: Place letter(s) or number(s) in box which corresponds to appropriate heading

Learner

P	=	Patient
S	=	Spouse
M	=	Mother
F	=	Father
D1	=	Daughter
S1	=	Son
X1	=	Other

Method

E	=	Explanation
D	=	Demonstration
V	=	Videotape/CCTV
R	=	Role play
P	=	Physical model
W	=	Written material
A	=	Audiocassette
O	=	Other (explain)

Evaluation

S	=	States or identifies key points or facts
V	=	Verbalizes understanding
D	=	Demonstrates skill independently
DC	=	Performs skill with verbal/physical coaching
I	=	Inadequate or incorrect skills/knowledge
N	=	No indication of learning (see Comments)
N/A	=	Learning not evaluated (see Comments)

Follow-up (f/u)

NA	=	Not applicable
1	=	None needed
2	=	Re-teach
3	=	Reinforce content
4	=	Repeat demonstration of skill(s)
5	=	Assist w/ practice of skills
6	=	Other (see Comments)

Reassess: Date/Time	Need/ Outcome	DEPT	Learner	Method	PATIENT EDUCATION	EVAL	f/u	Comments	Initials

(continued)

(Courtesy of Margaret R. Pardee Memorial Hospital, Hendersonville, North Carolina.)

| Comments: | | | | | | | | | | Initials | Signature & Title | | | | Initials | Signature & Title | | | | Initials | Signature & Title | | | |

lenol. They explained how to watch a child with a fever, abdominal pain, nausea, or diarrhea, all common childhood problems for which young parents often use emergency room facilities inappropriately. The nurses also suggested interventions for the parents to try for these problems and included time lines for when to call the doctor or seek emergency treatment appropriately.

Nurses, as "health" professionals, must assume considerable responsibility for educating their own clients and also for health education in the U.S. Nurses, as the most intimate and consistent caregivers, have a unique opportunity to be leaders in health education. Health education teams commonly include nurses, physicians, therapists of various types, social workers, dietitians, and pharmacists. Displays 10-1 and 10-2 illustrate a patient/family education record used by multiple disciplines in one community hospital. The nurse can shape such collaborative facilitation of client learning to assure that person-centered caring and a health/wellness focus prevail. In addition to collaborative members of the health care team, other stakeholders in the learning process include institutions and organizations, accrediting bodies, managers and leaders, and the learners. Evaluating outcomes of learning is necessary to justify educational activities as an integral part of health care delivery.

Clinical Example Synthesizing Communication and the Learning–Teaching Process

Nurses often have the opportunity to combine their skills in communicating and teaching in ways that create remarkable results. The following clinical example provides such an illustration. It demonstrates the learning–teaching interaction as a special application of interpersonal communication and problem solving, and teaching as the facilitation of client learning.

Example Mr. Smith was a 76 year old man referred to the Patient Educator for self-catheterization instruction due to continued history of urinary retention, with resulting UTIs. Mr. Smith owned and operated an apple farm in rural western NC with is sons. He was very negative about receiving instruction for something he felt was "no big problem" but which had cost him several days of work and reduced revenue. He was also initially resistant to the nurse's attempts at instruction. She was young, female, and he stated, "You ain't from around here" which immediately set barriers between the teacher and learner.

To overcome these barriers, the nurse questioned him about his life on the farm and allowed him to "teach" her about apples. The nurse asked Mr. Smith how the orchards received water in dry weather.

"Got me an irrigation pond", he replied. "And how do you get the water out of the pond?", she said. "With pipes of course-an inflow and outflow circuit." The nurse continued the questioning with, "And what would happen to the pond if the pipes got clogged or couldn't move the water?" "Well", he mused, "the pond would get stagnant." "Exactly!" she said, This analogy was then discussed in terms of Mr. Smith's condition and how his bladder gets "stagnant" from "poor outflow".

(continued)

By utilizing principles of adult learning, the nurse was able to overcome learning barriers and provide Mr. Smith with a meaningful teaching session. He was more receptive to self-catheterization because he was able to understand why this procedure was important to his well being.
Nina Lovern, BSN, RN, C, CDE
Patient Education Coordinator

In this example, the nurse communicated with and taught the client. The communication was effective and the learning was confirmed, as the illustration validates.

KEY CONCEPTS

☑ Learning/teaching is an important subconcept of professional nursing.

☑ Major theories about learning originate in psychology, and include behavioristic, cognitive, and humanistic approaches.

☑ Understanding common learning and teaching principles can assist nurses with their own learning as well as that of their clients.

☑ The steps of learning/teaching interaction parallel those of the nursing process.

☑ Behavioral objectives state goals or expected outcomes and the actions necessary to demonstrate learning.

☑ Nurses are well prepared and positioned to assume leadership in health education.

CRITICAL THINKING QUESTIONS

1. Write an original behavioral objective for each of the learning domains:
   a. Cognitive—thinking
   b. Affective—feeling
   c. Psychomotor—action or skills

2. Review patient education materials available in a local health care setting. What are their strengths and weaknesses in relation to the patient population served?

3. Pick a behavioral objective for a course you are taking. Generate several alternative ways of demonstrating your competence in achieving that objective.

4. Provide a rationale for each of the following knowledge and attitude statements which are generally accepted as true and can be applied to students, nurses, and clients.
   a. In behavior modification, it is the learner's response and not the teacher's stimulus that is the key to behavior change.
   b. Good teaching can be learned.
   c. The process of learning is as important as the product.

5. Write a brief statement on the topic "How I Learn Best" that you could share with a teacher who is facilitating your learning.

6. Assess what you need to learn professionally as a lifelong learner. Consider your short and long term goals, your strengths, and also areas where formal or informal learning is needed.

7. Identify the benefits to be gained by taking a more active role in your own learning.

    a. Identify specific actions (assessing, intervening, evaluating) that you could take now and in the future.

    b. Seek a mentor who can provide continuous mentoring help or facilitation over time.

REFERENCES

Boehm, S. (1992). Behavioral intervention, a strategy for nursing practice, says U–M Scientist. *The University of Michigan News & Notes.* p. 3.

Carpenito, L.J. (1984). *Handbook of nursing diagnosis.* Philadelphia: J.B. Lippincott.

Durbach, E., Goodall, R., & Wilkinson, K. (1987). Instructional objectives in patient education. *Nursing Outlook, 35*(2), 82–83,88

Geissler, E.M. (1994). *Pocket guide to cultural assessment.* St. Louis, Mosby.

Maslow, A.H. (1970). Motivation and personality (2nd ed.). New York: Harper & Row.

Reilly, D.E. (1990). *Behavioral objectives: Evaluation in nursing* (3rd ed.). New York: National League for Nursing.

Reilly, D.E., & Oermann, M.H. (1992). *Clinical teaching in nursing education.* New York: National League for Nursing.

Rogers, C. (1969). *Freedom to learn.* Columbus, OH: C.E. Merrill.

Sagan, C. (1995). *The demon-haunted world: science as a candle in the dark.* New York: Random House.

Somers, A. (1978). Promoting health, consumer education and national policy. *Nursing Digest 6,* 1–11.

The Health Publishing Group (Eds.). (1996). Dr. Koop's Self-Care Advisor. New York: Time-Life Medical

Nursing Ethics and Legal Aspects

Objectives

After completing this chapter, students will be able to:

Describe basic human rights.

Describe a person focus for bioethics.

Identify examples of personal bioethical issues that are of particular concern to you.

Identify major ethical issues confronting nursing, other health professionals, and society.

Describe accountability.

This chapter introduces you to some of the many ethical and legal aspects of nursing and health care. Ethical issues and legalities of health care are subjects of comprehensive nursing books. Obviously, this discussion is only fundamental, presenting some of the more common ideas, terms, and concepts that are relevant to nursing practice. For specific legal advice, nurses consult lawyers or primary sources of legal information. Similarly, difficult ethical issues stimulate a need for interdisciplinary consultation, discussion, and consideration of varying ethical viewpoints. The field of bioethics is growing rapidly both in scope and prominence.

Nurses need to be well-informed about its development, and involved in shaping the relationship between bioethics and nursing practice.

As Davis and Aroskar (1978) wrote, "Moral philosophers beginning with Socrates, Plato, and Aristotle have for centuries attempted to answer the two major questions of ethics: What is the meaning of right? of good? and, what ought I to do?" (p. 20).

The lay use of the term *moral* generally means conforming to the rules of right conduct defined by a particular social group. Morality is one type of social regulation of behavior. For some issue areas, morality and law are similar. In other areas, considerably more variation in conduct is culturally influenced. For example, before the revolution in socially acceptable sexual conduct, sexual morality was equated with virtue or chastity, especially for females. In recent years a trend toward returning to more restrained behavior has been noted, although laws have changed little. Many cultural influences other than concerns about AIDS have contributed to this trend.

Ethics is a discipline involved with good and bad, moral duty, obligation, and values. Ethics is also concerned with social and political philosophy and the philosophy of law. Only recently has biomedical ethics been a well-recognized discipline. Because biomedical ethical issues have implications for other life and health sciences, we prefer the term **bioethics** to designate those health issues of an ethical nature that concern nurses.

The professional use of the term **ethics** implies a high standard of moral quality of professional practice. Accepted practice standards of one's peers are professed in occupational codes of ethics for nursing, medicine, law, and so forth. (See Chapter 2 for the Code for Nurses.) Ketefian (1987) identified a dimension of moral behavior for nurses called "professionally ideal moral behavior," which was defined as, "professionally valued and ideal nursing behaviors that are congruent with the principles expressed in the Code for Nurses" (p. 13). Bioethical issues are of increasing social and economic significance. As cost-cutting practices dominate health care, physicians and nurses may feel pressured to compromise ethical standards in return for bonuses or gain-sharing for cost cutting. The person, however, is the primary and major focus for our initial consideration of ethical issues and their implications for nurses. This approach is consistent with nursing's professional code and person as a major concept in the paradigm of professional nursing.

The concept of client autonomy is a recurring theme in ethical issues. *Autonomous* means independent and self-governing. Autonomous describes an essential quality of "person" as well as a type of behavior. The autonomous person can be described as being rational and unrestrained. This indicates that the person is self-governing and independent regarding his or her decisions and activity.

Persons who are unaware or irrational may be unable to demonstrate autonomous behavior. However, autonomy remains an essential quality of their person, that is, a part of human character, integrity, and holism. Preserving that autonomy becomes a concern for nurses as professional care-givers of such persons. When clients are not independent regarding either decisions or

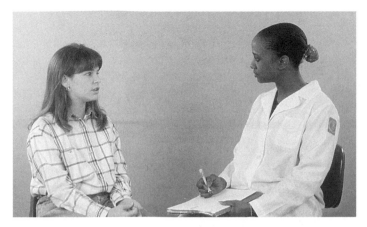

The nurse ponders the concerns of her client before applying the principles of ethical decision making. (Photo © 1997 by B. Proud)

activity, nurses intervene. Nurses help persons do those things that they would do unaided if they had the necessary strength, will, or knowledge. Nurses do this in a manner that enables the client to be as independent or autonomous as possible.

To ensure that they do not impose their personal goals on clients, nurses develop self-awareness about their own continuous growth and development. Self-awareness also helps to guard against exercising any personal need to control or have inordinate authority over others. Whenever students or graduate nurses find themselves labeling clients—calling them "stubborn," "uncooperative," or "noncompliant"—it is instructive for them to take stock of their own expectations and behaviors. These situations are common warning signals that a power struggle may be developing; they are particularly inappropriate and suggest that nursing is not being practiced from a perspective that values clients' abilities for self-care and autonomy. The nurturance or nursing of these self-care powers is the ultimate goal of nursing judgments and action. Some would actually call this the nurturance of autonomy, a state of knowing and freely exercising persons' actual reality-based choices.

Many persons who seek the services of health professionals may believe that their autonomy is threatened because of their dependency on others for care services. The current economics of health care, including constraints imposed on accessing some services and providers, may contribute to this belief. Further, ill and hospitalized persons are especially likely to believe themselves constrained even when they are aware and rational.

Two particular constraints that may be of concern are lack of ability and coercion. An example of lack of ability is the elderly person who lacks the strength to resist heroic lifesaving measures. Constraints on a person's autonomy are sometimes, as an exception, appropriate to protect either the client or the public. More generally, however, fatherly interference with a person's autonomy is a form of control called **paternalism.** Although we usually think of paternalistic interfer-

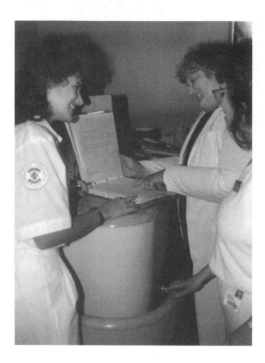

Nurses learn to review charts as part of ethical decision-making.

ence as compromising or constraining the rights of clients, it may not be intentionally limiting, and often goes unrecognized.

Values

The concept of values is a basic notion underlying both the scholarly discipline of ethics and the practical application of ethics in a profession. In Chapter 4, the idea of values was introduced as a characteristic of persons that both makes them unique and defines the beliefs they share with other persons. A *value* is a belief or custom that frequently arises from cultural or ethnic backgrounds, family tradition, peer group ideas and practices, political philosophies in one's country, and educational and religious philosophies with which one identifies. Values, therefore, help explain similarities and differences between individuals and groups.

Values are often based on intangibles rather than on fact, and may be so strongly held as to be worth dying for—examples include honor, freedom, and family. Values are powerful motivators of behavior. To determine persons' values, we can observe how they use their personal and material resources. The following questions are examples of those we might ask: How does each client care for his or her physical body? How does he or she use time and money? How does he or she relate to other people?

We commonly use the term *value* in such a way that it is attached to the person rather than the thing valued. Things or ideas generally valued by many people, such as health and friendship, come to be labeled as valuable in and of themselves, hence the use of adjectives to describe cultural, scientific, and humanitarian values.

Development of Values

Values are both simple and complex and vary in the degree to which they are believed to be important by the person. Because values are learned, they parallel other learned behavior, taking shape in early life and being influenced first by early caregivers and family. Later, peer experiences, formal learning, and societal institutions shape values. As people become more autonomous in behavior, they act on not only those values personally held, but also on those they understand to be acceptable to the larger social system of which they are a part. The more important values become a part of personal moral conduct. At this point in our discussion of developing values, it is appropriate to consider two currently prominent and differing approaches to ethical issues, as exemplified by Kohlberg (1987) and Gilligan (1993, 1989).

Moral Developmental Approach to Ethical Issues

Moral development begins with the transition from instinctive thought to a higher form of thinking based on logic. Kohlberg (1987) presents one such hierarchical organization for understanding moral development (Fig. 11-1).

This representation is somewhat similar to both Maslow's hierarchy of needs and Piaget's stages of cognitive development (see Chapter 4). Kohlberg's three-level model helps one to relate individual moral growth to an accepted pattern of moral development for persons in contemporary American society. This model further divides moral development into six stages—two in each level—as detailed in the following discussion. Not every person achieves the highest level of moral functioning, just as not all persons achieve self-actualization as described by Maslow.

Level 1 moral development (preconventional) occurs in early childhood, with the beginning of value development. At this age, the self depends completely on adults for nearly all aspects of existence—from physical needs of food and shelter to other needs such as safety and love. In the first stage of level 1, moral behavior becomes equated with performance to avoid punishment. Deference to the power of certain individuals in an unquestioning way characterizes the second stage of this level. At this age, the child accepts the labeling of behavior by significant others, whether they are parents or caregivers. We can use this model to understand the children's behavior in the much-publicized child molestation accusations against a California child-care center several years ago. Given these stages of moral development, it is not surprising that the preschoolers involved were not vocal about alleged incidents. The children believed their behavior to be good or bad as labeled by the adults in authority. This is more obvious after the fact, and when viewed from Kohlberg's theoretical perspective.

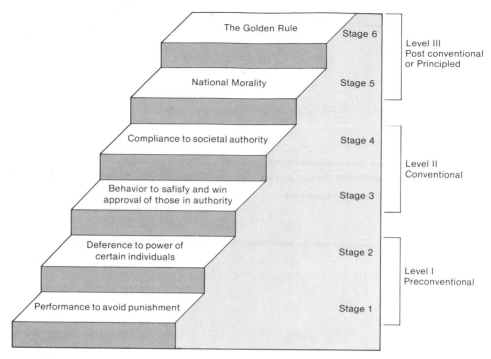

FIGURE 11-1   Hierarchy of moral development (according to Kohlberg).

Level 2 development (conventional), according to Kohlberg, occurs at a time when children are moving from concrete operations to the formal operations of adult thought. This shift enables persons to envision various hypothetical alternatives relating to issues. The transition to formal thought occurs at different ages for different individuals, and for some persons, the cognitive shift precedes the growth of moral development by several years.

In stage 3 of level 2, the norm for interpersonal rules is still the behavior that satisfies individuals in authority and wins their approval. One can imagine that a child in the health care system who is at stage 3 may be reluctant not to do as asked, even if frightened, angry, or hesitant for other reasons. In stage 4 of level 2, in which compliance to societal authority becomes a more accepted mode of behavior, reluctance to ask questions may have a different etiology.

Level 3 development (postconventional or principled), the challenging of conventional morality, is an adolescent characteristic. Stage 5 of this level is sometimes called the stage of national morality, and has been identified as the governmental morality that affects national health care policy. The legalistic orientation that characterizes this stage is directed toward rights and obligations expressed in contracts between professionals and parties being served. This last level of moral development is also labeled the autonomous or principled level. Principles apply not just for their law and order values, but because they express society's consensus about what is right. Stage 6 of level 3, moral development, goes beyond a circumscribed national view and pertains to humankind in general. This stage also has been characterized as applying the golden rule.

For most nurses, the initial socialization to professional values occurs during late adolescence or early adulthood. At this point, many persons may still be in earlier stages of moral development. Thus, adding professional responsibilities complicates coping with ethical issues. It is usually comforting to students to realize that professional faculty understand this developmental process and, furthermore, that they are eager to assist students in making this transition. According to Kohlberg's theory of moral education, growth beyond the stages of conventional morality makes one sensitive to universal ethical and moral principles, as well as to the value of unique persons and their differing views.

Gilligan (1982) presented a somewhat different theoretical perspective of moral development that was heralded by feminists and also nurses. In contrast to what she saw as a male-referenced moral viewpoint (i.e., Kohlberg), Gilligan proposed an ethic conceived in care and practiced in relationships. It emphasized understanding the concerns of others and evaluating situational factors over applying rules and universal principles. If a universality is applied from Gilligan's moral development, it is that care and ethical behavior modeled after maternal or early care enables individuals to experience others positively and also to grow as autonomous persons.

Such an alternative feminine or humanistic morality harmonizes with the Primacy of Caring Theory of Benner and Wrubel (1989) and theories of Watson (1988) and Leininger (1990). Leininger (1990) wrote, ''Nurses who are responsible for human care must discover and establish ethical and moral principles, standards, and guidelines to help them make appropriate judgments and decisions, within the perspective of nursing'' (p. 9). Leininger furthermore reminded us that ''nurses are expected to know, understand, and function effectively with people from many different cultures, demonstrating sensitivity to and knowledge of diverse ethical values and practices'' (p. 9). Such a reminder cautions us about imposing our ethnocentric ethical values, and suggests a focus for lifelong learning.

Values Clarification

Moral judgments in both personal and professional life are made in relation to values, not facts. Because any person holds individual and shared values, both clients and nurses hold wide ranges of values. Given this reality, it is apparent that often nurses and their clients will hold dissimilar values. Dissimilar values can contribute to misunderstanding or serious conflicts. If nurses are going to give person-centered care, they will need to find ways to accommodate these differences. This accommodation must be achieved both for the sake of their clients' health care and also for the sake of nurses' own personal and professional well-being. Understanding one's own values can be a first step that helps a nurse to identify, understand, and learn strategies that accommodate these differences.

Values clarification is clarification of what values are important to a person. It is a self-awareness process that not only identifies what values represent ''me,'' but also asks the individual to prioritize or rate different values to determine the most important values. This detailed self-assessment gives a more complete picture of one's total individual value system.

Values clarification exercises can be oriented toward both personal and professional values. Questions in personal values clarification exercises might include the following examples:

Name five things that are most important to your life today.
List five goals you would most like to achieve in your lifetime.
How did you spend your time last week? Divide the time into 5% blocks
   for major activities. Compare how this time allotment relates to the
   things you think are most important and the goals you hope to achieve.

Questions nurses might ask regarding professional goals include:

How much do I value nursing as a commitment to a lifelong career of
   learning and competence?
Do I like to care for some kinds of clients and not others? Do I prefer
   healthy to ill? Young to old? Physical to psychological disabilities?
Can I maintain the ethics of my profession with the threat of economic
   pressures?

A first step in accomplishing such exercises is to reflect on the questions privately. A second and more enlightening step is to participate in values clarification activities with nurse peers, other health professionals, and lay persons outside the health professions.

Many specific reasons exist for nurses to examine their value systems:

❏ Some inconsistencies in personal values are not apparent until consciously examined.
❏ Some inconsistencies may cause problems if conflicting values are caught
   in the decision-making process.
❏ Personal values may conflict with certain professional practice responsibilities.
❏ Examining values can guide ethical choices in professional practice.
❏ Values clarification contributes toward functioning at a higher level of
   moral reasoning.

Values clarification for professional nurses is increasingly important in an era of many conflicting professional pressures as well as various efforts to curtail or diminish professional nurses' nuturing and caring functions.

A Person Focus for Bioethics

A person focus for the bioethics of concern to nurses makes logical sense, because persons are indeed the recipients of nursing care. Although nurses care for persons both as individuals and in groups, they do so in ways that are always mindful of individual dignity, values, and rights. Because of this immense concern for

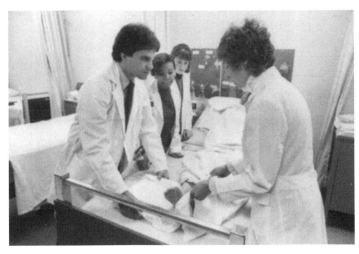

Nurses learn appropriate precautions to ensure client safety.

individuals, not only by nurses but by other professionals and clients themselves, the concept of autonomy is a recurring theme of ethical issues.

Rights of Person/Group

The term *rights* has an ethical connotation as well as a legal definition. As Davis and Aroskar (1991) wrote, "Rights as entitlements, are claimed *to* privacy, to life, to die, to a healthy environment, and to health care. Special rights *of* various groups, such as children, the poor, and the elderly, are also claimed" (p. 70).

The idea of personal rights is clearly related to concern and respect for the individual member of society. Who gives, monitors, and protects which rights and for whom is not so clearly defined. Claims about rights might be viewed as assertions or demands intended to influence and change social and legal boundaries of health care policy. For example, some claim the right to health itself, whereas others argue that access to health care is the issue.

The concept of individual rights becomes an issue or problem when the values of individuals or rights of individuals conflict. Individual (clients, client and care-giver) may have conflicts. Or situations may arise in which an individual is in conflict with the rights of society, for example, a psychotic person capable of injuring others. Conflicting rights are illustrated by persons' rights to confidentiality in conflict with the public good and society's rights in reporting gunshot wounds, venereal disease, and child abuse. Similar but less obvious conflicts might include persons' rights to engage in behavior that interferes with gaining or maintaining health. For example, substance abusers, the overweight, drunk drivers, and persons refusing to wear seat belts or motorcycle helmets inflict a potential economic burden on society for their care when illness or injury occurs. Recently, some women have alleged discrimination against their health rights;

specifically, they find the male domination of the medical profession and control of health care policy to be offensive.

The issue of individual rights is also buried in larger health care issues discussed later in this chapter. For example, the burgeoning cost of the Medicare system has created a crisis. The diagnostic tests, drug treatments, and high technology that have revolutionized health care have accounted for one third of the rise in the cost of the Medicare program in recent years. In this example, the rights of certain individuals seeking high technology for extraordinary care (e.g., dialysis and transplant) threatens the right of society to fund a system of ordinary basic care for the elderly and the poor. Also compromised by these escalating costs is general health promotion and illness care for the entire population.

Perhaps the best-known declaration of rights is that published by the American Hospital Association (1990). This Patient's Bill of Rights serves to raise the consciousness of both clients and health care providers (see Chapter 7). Some see this declaration as a well-meaning document without a mechanism for enforcement. Others have charged that the statement does no more than pay lip service to an ideal, and is thus a mockery. Certainly the stated rights offer a moral challenge to health care providers to act in the spirit of the intent. Documents that declare the rights of other specific groups also serve to raise consciousness. These documents include the following:

❏ Declaration on Rights of Mentally Retarded Persons (United Nations, 1971)
❏ Declaration on Rights of Disabled Persons (United Nations, 1975) and the Americans with Disabilities Act of 1990
❏ Declaration on the Rights of the Child (United Nations, 1979)
❏ Patient Self-Determination Act of 1990

These documents are only some of many such documents. Others speak to a range of special interest groups including pregnant women and senior citizens.

Personal Bioethical Issues

A person focus for bioethics emphasizes that there are a number of bioethical issues concerned with the essence of persons along a conception-to-death continuum. Many of the life-and-death bioethical issues center on the underlying question, "When is a person not a person?" Names like Louise Brown (the first test-tube baby), Karen Quinlan (a long-term comatose young adult), and Dr. Jack Kevorkian ("Dr. Death") remind us of this underlying question about the nature of person. An ad hoc committee of the Harvard Medical School (1968) proposed that irreversible coma, rather than the cessation of vital functions, be the criterion for death. Their decision became timely when improved resuscitation and life-support measures maintained the lives of many who otherwise would have died. This action acknowledged the loss of personhood and, incidentally, made lifesaving transplant organs more readily available. Of interest also is that a California referendum, Proposition 161 (1992) to allow assisted suicide, was soundly defeated by the citizens despite the fact that the issue has surfaced in many other states and nationally.

Exploring the nature of ethical dilemmas may help you to understand moral values different from your own. To some professional nurses, the ideas of test-tube babies, termination of life-support systems, assisted suicide, abortion on demand, and partial birth abortion are particularly distressing. The following discussion is an introductory sample of issues along the conception-to-death continuum. Issues cluster at the beginning and end of life, with remaining concern focused on the quality of the intervening life. These issues involve conception, pregnancy, the rapidly developing area of high-technology neonatal care, bioengineering in its many facets, the psychological competence of persons, and the termination of life. Although these topics are presented in the context of person as client–patient, some implications for nurses as caregivers are also raised. For additional consideration of ethical issues along the conception-to-death continuum, refer to Benner, Tanner, and Chesla (1996), Bishop and Scudder (1996), and Bandman and Bandman (1995),

Pregnancy

The issues of pregnancy are related to its facilitation, prevention, and normalcy. For most of the history of civilization and in most parts of the world today, the dominant issue has been how to prevent pregnancy, childbirth, and overpopulation, rather than how to facilitate new life. Even today, the facilitation issues are mostly the concern of persons seeking the benefits of modern science in curing their childless states. The delay in marriage and childbearing of independent-minded, career-oriented couples will undoubtedly cause this issue to become more prominent in this group. Some women are postponing attempts at pregnancy until an age when fertility has naturally decreased. Many of these women do not fully realize the possible implications of their decisions. The need to be in control of their lives has led to their independence; the same need has also likely made them believe that infertility happens only to other people.

Although science has made great strides in facilitating pregnancy, the ability to induce fertility without the likelihood of multiple births is less well controlled. For health care providers and society at large, the issues concerning multiple births are related to the demanding and extremely expensive care that multiple premature births require. Hospital bills of several hundred thousand dollars are commonplace for each pregnancy episode that may or may not yield a desired outcome for the client. In 1996, an English woman gained international notoriety when octuplets aborted late in pregnancy. Newly perfected in vitro techniques are diminishing the chance of unwanted multiple births. However, a technique that aborts some among several fertilized eggs also raises additional ethical issues, and so does the ability of a mother without ovarian function to conceive from donor eggs.

Prevention issues center around how to avoid conception or intervene afterward to prevent live births. The control of reproduction is both a personal issue and a societal issue. The encompassing ethical questions concern both overpopulation and the allocation of scarce resources. The control of reproduction ranges from permanent sterilization, to temporary contraceptive measures, to abortion. All of these methods create ethical issues for at least some clients and some health care providers. Many cause considerable societal and political discord. Sterilization raises such issues as personal autonomy, societal control, and tampering with the human genetic pool. Contraceptive issues include access to pregnancy control related to age, religion, and economics. Traditionally, women have been held responsible for birth control, which probably accounts for lack of research on male birth control and only recent acceptance of vasectomy. Now, male sterilization—widely available through such a simple procedure as vasectomy—raises questions of contraceptive responsibility (his or hers). Male sterilization also gives men opportunities for more visible and permanent participation in pregnancy control.

The sexual revolution among young people, especially teenagers, forces the issues of teenage contraception into the open for both the public and health professionals. The introduction of more permanent contraceptive devices, such as intrauterine devices, has blurred the issues between contraception and abortion, because the mechanism of interference with pregnancy is one that occurs after conception. Long-term medical contraception with the pill raises ethical issues of solving one health care dilemma (unwanted pregnancy) and creating others, ranging from weight gain to serious cardiovascular complications including stroke. Morning-after abortion pills, such as RU-486, the French abortion pill, have been easily available abroad for years and raise yet other issues, including the monitoring of their use.

In all types of pregnancy prevention, the issues of autonomy, right, and coercion are prominent. These issues share the common foundation, "What is the essence of persons?" In allowing abortion, the Supreme Court favored the view of a fetus as biologic life, and not a "person," before the age of viability. The Court also reaffirmed the rights of a woman to autonomy and control of her own body. Interestingly, although men have recently assumed greater responsibility in controlling pregnancy, the Supreme Court view basically disregards any paternal rights.

Perspectives about abortion range from conservative to liberal, from the extremes of prolife to complete freedom of choice. Additional intermediate perspectives relate to saving maternal life and providing relief in cases of rape and potentially defective children. Because nurses are called on to be both caregivers and counselors, a clear understanding of one's own personal values and religious beliefs is necessary to make decisions about professional involvement in abortion issues. In their edited anthology *Professional Ethics in Nursing,* Thompson and Thompson (1990) present many informative essays that can help begin that understanding.

Recent issues surrounding conception and pregnancy have been revealed in the press as unprecedented in a variety of ways, including the following:

What is a woman's right to use a sperm bank's holding of her dead husband's donation?

What should be the fate of preserved embryos conceived by parents now deceased?

What should be the role of surrogate pregnancy in rescuing products of unwanted conception?

What should be the care of an anencephalic (without viable brain tissue) infant whose organs would benefit others?

What should be the use of fetal tissue in treating disease (e.g., Parkinson's)?

What should be the justification for amniocentesis and post-amniocentesis abortion?

When parents divorce, who gets custody of any embryos? What happens if the parent with custody wants to implant and develop the embryos? Who is responsible? What if the other parent does not agree? Even if one parent has custody, what are the rights of the other parent, the rights of the embryos?

Neonatology

Many of the issues related to neonatology have their origin in issues of pregnancy and contraception related to potential or known defective offspring. The ethical issues in this area have grown with the burgeoning technology of modern health care, which has the potential to rescue not only premature infants but viable products of abortion and miscarriage. Again, the positions vary about what is appropriate care for both potentially normal and defective neonates. They range from conservative to liberal views and from ordinary to extraordinary means. The contrast between views can be as stark as that between partial birth abortion and an extraordinary life-saving intervention perspective which maintains that if a life can be saved, it should be. At one extreme are the prolife, right-to-life advocates and at the other, the freedom-of-choice advocates.

Although a person-centered perspective might tip the scale toward a quality of life ethic and away from a mere existence, many questions would still remain:

If the answer is not to save lives at all costs, then what factor determines which lives to save? Who decides?

What is the role of the parents? Of health professionals? Of society at large in ethical decision making?

What economic costs are reasonable and who should bear them?

What research is justifiable?

What are other rights of the neonate regarding the quality of his or her life?

How do you give person-centered care in instances in which the medical decision is to rescue a severely compromised infant or in which the withholding of basic needs or other treatment becomes an issue when family members cannot agree?

In 1988, the American Nurses Association (ANA) Committee on Ethics released guidelines on withdrawing or withholding food and fluid. Especially in instances such as infant care, the committee concluded that it is the moral and professional responsibility of nurses and others to determine whether providing food and fluid is in the person's best interest. The committee furthermore concluded that in almost all cases such a decision should be made if doing so provides comfort.

At first glance, it may appear that modern medicine and its technology have been the sole reason for increased neonatal survival. However, the role of highly skilled nurses with advanced education should not be overlooked, nor should the increased ethical burdens borne by around-the-clock caregivers, such as nurses, go unnoticed. Increasingly, nurses are assuming more proactive and collaborative involvement in ethical decision-making processes for their client–patients. Nurses are also asserting themselves among peers to receive the collegial support that sustains caregivers in such demanding situations. Recent ANA publications include the following: (1993) *Ethical Dilemmas in Contemporary Nursing Practice;* (1994) *Guidelines on Reporting Incompetent, Unethical, or Illegal Practices;* and (1995) *Annotated Bibliography for Ethical Guidelines.*

Bioengineering

The issues of bioengineering begin with genetic screening and counseling. They range from manipulation of genes and embryos to organ transplants and artificial replacement of body parts. Over the years, genetic counseling has evolved from intervention after infant death or defect to preconception screening. Genetic screening involves testing population groups for genetic problems. The ethical issues of screening include privacy, confidentiality, and individual versus societal rights. Truth telling, human experimentation, informed **consent,** the potential for political evil, and the conflict between medical and religious viewpoints are also issues. **Eugenics** is the science of improving human genes. Gene therapy, i.e., genetic repair or engineering, is thought to have the potential for good or evil. For good, it might replace a defective gene with one that is healthy, forestalling cancer or chronic illness. For evil, it might create animal–slave mutations. There is also some fear that deoxyribonucleic acid (DNA) experimentation will create killer bacteria or human clones. The global interest in gene therapy is especially reflected in the Human Genome Project, an international project to identify and map human genes. Clearly the moral, ethical, and social aspects of such a project assume global proportions also.

Artificial insemination (AI) with donor semen might be considered an early form of bioengineering, even though conception occurs in vivo (in life). The clear intent was to conceive a normal child by carefully selecting the donor. Within recent years, the element of engineering has increased: fertilization now occurs within the laboratory in vitro (in glass). The growing blastocyst is then transplanted to the mother. The engineering element is also in evidence when one considers the laboratory failures that preceded the success.

Using techniques from biotechnology and genetic engineering, powerful monoclonal antibodies can now be created. The experimental drug NEBACUMAB was a first-generation example of drugs that can save lives using molecular biology and, for example, can produce miracle cures for lethal blood poisoning. Although NEBACUMAB may be a miracle cure, likened to penicillin, its initial cost of $3700 per dose raised ethical questions such as, What is the cost per life or life-years-saved? How should the drug be rationed? Who should pay? One might also ask what makes a drug like this so expensive and who benefits from such an amount of money? Another question might be, How is something that could benefit so many being monitored for such exorbitancy? In a discussion about how ethical conflicts will intensify in critical care nursing, Dente-Cassidy (1992) wrote, "Rationing of health care will become one of the most urgent issues of the nineties"(p. 45).

Organ and body part replacements are both natural and mechanical. Generating natural organs for transplants can impinge on the rights of donors. The enormous cost of transplants, both natural and mechanical, adds additional issues related both to resource allocation and responsibility for payment. Transplants of organs such as kidneys, and the replacement of joints such as knees and hips, are becoming commonplace. Their success rates and less serious ethical issues have made them quite acceptable. Heart transplants, however, continue to be fraught with both technical and ethical problems. To donate one of two kidneys to a close relative is a sacrifice of sorts. It is, however, quite another circumstance for one human life to be lost so that another can be saved. Furthermore, the idea of keeping donors alive until their organs are harvested may be unpleasant to many persons despite the potential lifesaving benefits. To both caregivers and family members, such practices are seriously disturbing. Cases of anencephalic babies who were kept alive to donate other healthy organs illustrate the point. This practice gained considerable publicity partly because of the prominent medical center involved. Clearly, whatever the future holds, the ethical issues related to bioengineering successes and failures will only increase. One factor affecting the increase will be the changing age demographics. Consider the following example related by an older gentleman contemplating liver transplant:

> When he was younger, Mr. Carter would never have thought he would welcome or even consider a liver transplant as a senior citizen. At age 74, however, and faced with fatal liver failure, he felt differently. As his wife noted, he indeed was a "young 74". Although currently in rapidly declining health, Mr. Carter was willing to travel across the continent just for evaluation when encouraged by his specialist and family physician that he might not be too old to have the surgery. Even if he was deemed to be a satisfactory candidate after the evaluation, Mr. Carter was faced with the return home and then a wait of unknown duration until a donor was found. At that time he would then be expected to travel across country again and remain in a strange city for six weeks for surgery and initial recovery. Given an 85% chance of a successful transplant, he could expect perhaps to live another eight years, whereas the specialist who diagnosed his worsening organ failure thought his remaining life expectancy without the transplant might only be two years. (name changed for anonymity)

Psychological Competence

In a person-centered approach to nursing care, a person in his or her physical, mental, and spiritual totality is the recipient of nursing care. The psychological status of a person includes cognitive functioning or thinking, affective functioning or emotional feeling, and also behavioral or psychomotor functioning. **Psychological competence** then refers to the ability to function adequately in all these areas. Personal bioethical issues spanning a wide range contain at least some element of psychological competence related to these cognitive, affective, and behavioral domains.

Apart from the broader issue of competence to be considered in relation to "**informed** consent," mental retardation is perhaps the most often cited topic involving ethics and the cognitive domain. From a person-centered perspective of nursing care and health promotion, the label "mental retardation" is unfortunate, given the varying degrees of functional ability that remain for the persons so stigmatized. About 3% of the general population is classified as mentally retarded. The causes of mental retardation can be divided between genetic and acquired. The genetic cause is illustrated by Down syndrome (a chromosomal disorder) and Tay-Sachs disease (a disturbance of lipid metabolism). Acquired mental retardation can occur prenatally with maternal afflictions and in the neonatal period or in childhood from such varied causes as the aftermath of infections, poisoning, or social deprivation (Davis & Aroskar, 1991, p. 192).

Regardless of the cause of retardation, the rights of mentally retarded individuals to humane and adequate physical and psychological care become an ethical concern for nurses. These rights guide nurses' assessment, analysis, planning, intervention, and also their evaluation of nursing care. Providing for mentally retarded persons in the community rather than in institutions both highlights and blurs the assistance needed. Assistance may be needed to secure the rights of both to have families and to live in a family style group home rather than an institution but also to secure appropriate educational and employment opportunities. At times of hospitalization, special concerns arise regarding client education, informed consent, and research participation.

Ethical issues related to diminishing cognitive competence may also arise during serious illness or with the care of elderly clients. Nurses, as around-the-clock caregivers, make around-the-clock observations. They are often aware of confusion and diminished mental skills that other episodic caregivers do not notice. This diminished cognitive competence may affect decision making and informed consent. Often nurses are also the first professionals to note when the label of confusion is inappropriately applied to clients. Such labeling may pose serious ethical dilemmas by interfering with client autonomy. Erroneously assuming that persons are unable to make decisions may violate their basic rights and deprive them of the control that they could assume for their care and behavior. On occasion, a somewhat confused client can participate in decision making when he or she is facilitated by caregivers and supportive family members.

Persons with a wide range of psychiatric and mental health problems may pose other ethical dilemmas for nurses. Many such persons have temporary or permanent disturbances in all areas of psychological functioning: cognitive, emotional, and behavioral. The principles guiding ethical decision making in the care of such clients support persons as individuals, emphasize remaining strengths regardless of functional deficits, and recognize the basic human needs shared in common with all persons.

The question of what degree of participation clients with psychological dysfunction can and should have in determining their care is a common and complex one. Mental health reform has emphasized voluntary treatment and humanization. The questions remain about whether behavior change by psychosurgery, behavior modification treatments, or psychotherapy meet primarily the needs of individuals or the collective needs of health professionals and society. Nurses are assuming more proactive involvement in psychotherapy and increasing their potential for influencing ethical decisions in this realm of health care.

Death and Dying

Most persons in our society die in hospitals, nursing homes, or other institutions where nursing care is given. The related ethical issues concern both the process of dying and the actual event of death itself. Not the least of the associated ethical dilemmas is the lack of a precise definition of death or agreement about what death is. A major turning point regarding the definition of death came from the irreversible coma or brain death definition proposed by the Ad Hoc Committee of the Harvard Medical School in 1968. The four determinations that were to be made only by a physician included the following:

1. Unreceptivity—that is, stimuli produce no response
2. No movements or breathing during observations made for at least 1 hour; if the patient is on a respirator, the machine may be turned off for 3 minutes to determine any effort to breathe spontaneously
3. Absence of reflexes
4. Flat electroencephalogram recorded for a 10-minute minimum and repeated at least 24 hours later without change (in actual practice, this may be optional, but prudent).

The death determination is considered valid in the absence of hypothermia or drug intoxication. Recently, one midwestern state accorded nurses the legal right to make a death determination in the absence of a physician. This legislation was passed in large part because of the efforts and expert testimony of a hospice nurse.

Despite such a definition, it is not surprising that ethical issues continue to surround the cessation of life just as they do the precise beginning of life. Here again, the essence of person remains the underlying question to be answered. A person-centered nursing ethic seeks a consensus decision that involves the person, the family, and health care providers whenever possible. Such an approach does not preclude weighing the best interests of both the person and society. The questions often become, Is it living or dying that is being prolonged? For whom? And why? In arguing the conflict of client self-direction and professionals doing good, Davis (1990) suggested: "When we use principle-based ethical reasoning or when we use ethics of caring, we must first ground our concern and questioning in the concreteness of a given situation" (p. 30). The Patient Self Determination Act of 1990 makes many demands of health professionals and health care organizations including the following:

❏ Policies are on file that address all provisions of state law.
❏ Information is to be provided to patients upon admission.
❏ Patient wishes are to be documented in the medical record.
❏ Hospitals cannot "condition" care.
❏ There must be compliance with all related state laws.
❏ Education is to be provided for staff and the community.

The questions related to death care sometimes seem easier to cope with when persons have already lived a long and full life. The hidden dangers of this view become more apparent as the issues of an aging population, burgeoning technology, and escalating health care costs become more thoroughly entangled. These dangers remind us of a science fiction film in which humans were allotted only a 30-year life span and then targeted for annihilation as part of the social plan.

Two concepts that are associated with death and dying are *benemortasia*, meaning good or kind death, and *euthanasia*, also meaning good or pleasant death. Benemortasia is sometimes used in describing the ethics of caring demonstrated especially in the hospice movement. Euthanasia has been the center of much controversy for years in legal, religious, and ethical discussions.

Euthanasia has been divided into *passive euthanasia*, meaning allowing to die or not interfering with a death process, and *active euthanasia*, which is either killing or actively assisting in the death process. As Thompson and Thompson (1981) stated, "The ethical concern is a question of the direct versus the indirect. Direct killing is generally held to be wrong and even called murder. Indirect killing might be called neglect, or an accident, or simply an act of God, or the Natural Law. 'Letting die' is sometimes related to passive euthanasia" (p. 187). Additionally, the terms *voluntary* and *involuntary* are sometimes used. With voluntary euthanasia, the client is able to give consent about active or passive means. With involuntary euthanasia, the client, because of his or her condition, is unable to be involved in the decision-making process. These designations lead to four types of euthanasia, sometimes described as follows:

1. Active voluntary, for example, suicide or mercy killing
2. Passive voluntary, for example, refusing treatment
3. Active involuntary, for example, mercy killing
4. Passive involuntary, for example, letting die

Some ethicists suggest that such labeling is not helpful or clarifying. In reality, many ethical issues arise unlabeled in everyday health care. For example, nurses weigh the ethical consequences of giving pain relief medication that may contribute to a fatal respiratory depression. More sensational are such issues as the assisted suicides by persons calling themselves "obitiatrists." An early and widely publicized obitiatrist, Dr. Jack Kevorkian, was quickly labeled America's "Dr. Death." Less widely publicized has been the Netherlands' liberalized legal system, which has openly and benignly neglected to prosecute such practitioners since the early 1970s.

The same issue of whether to use ordinary or extraordinary means to support life applies at the end of life as it does at the beginning. Some older persons and their families have proactively responded to this issue by preparing a "living will." Such a document asks health professionals to comply with the person's request for life with quality and death with dignity (see Display 11-1).

Nurses and clients should obtain legal counsel to determine the status of such living wills in their state. Most states have passed living will legislation. The Patient Self-Determination Act of 1990 is a federal statute that intends for patients to have the necessary information so that they are able to exercise their rights and options if they so choose. It requires that institutions receiving Medicare and Medicaid funds provide patients with written information about their right to prepare **advance directives** and the institution's policies regarding their use. Advance directives are "documents such as Durable Powers of Attorney and Living Wills that allow a person to plan for the management of health care and/or financial affairs in the event of incapacity" (Singleton, Dever, & Donner, 1992, p. 42). Although all states do not have living wills, all 50 states and the District of Columbia do have **Durable Power of Attorney** legislation. A durable power of attorney lets patients "appoint representatives and alternates to make health care decisions for them if they become incapacitated and to declare which treatments they'd accept or reject" (Badzek, 1992, p. 59). Although advance directives are not without certain disadvantages (e.g., they do not apply to mentally incompetent persons and minors), information about whether patients have executed

---

DISPLAY 11-1   The Living Will

To My Family, My Physician, My Clergyman, My Lawyer:

If the time comes when I can no longer take part in decisions for my own future, let this statement stand as the testament of my wishes:

If there is no reasonable expectation of my recovery from physical or mental disability, I,

request that I be allowed to die and not be kept alive by artificial means or heroic measures. Death is as much a reality as birth, growth, maturity, and old age: it is the one certainty. I do not fear death as much as I fear the indignity of deterioration, dependence, and hopeless pain. I ask that medication be mercifully administered to me for terminal suffering even if it hastens the moment of death.

This request is made after careful consideration. Although this document is not legally binding, you who care for me will, I hope, feel morally bound to follow its mandate. I recognize that it places a heavy burden of responsibility upon you and it is with the intention of sharing that responsibility and of mitigating any feelings of guilt that this statement is made.

Signed_____   Date_____
Witnessed by:_____
_____

any advance directives is increasingly important assessment data to gather. Weber and Kjervik (1992) suggested that the Patient Self-Determination Act of 1990 ''presents nurses with an opportunity to be proactive in their roles as advocates . . . (and) exercise their political savvy to influence the system to respect the patient's wishes'' (p. 6). Patients anticipating hospitalization can be alerted to bring such documents with them at admission. In one city with a large senior citizen population, the local hospital made detailed information regarding advanced directives available to the community in well-publicized educational programs at their outreach health education center in the local mall.

Clients make other attempts to be proactive in meeting the issues of death and dying, including refusing treatment for certain conditions determined to be fatal and participating in hospice movements. Such constructive approaches to inevitable death became more commonplace after a widely read and discussed classic work by Kubler-Ross (1969). She presented stages of dying positively as developmental achievements. More recently, however, the healthy death approach has created often unfulfillable expectations that do not fit social, physiologic, or hi-tech reality. Realistically, Benner and Wrubel (1989) noted,

> Clearly, the death awareness movement and the notions of ''comfort care'' and ''appropriate death'' all create possibilities for making death less isolating and the subject of death less of a taboo. However, in this context of high expectations, the nurse will be required to coach the modern patient on the realities often associated with death even while trying to maximize comfort and minimize mental confusion and suffering for the patient and family. (p. 289)

Nurses are proactively addressing the issues surrounding death and dying. They are becoming better informed and also confronting feelings and anxieties about death and dying individually and with others. Table 11-1 summarizes the various areas of bioethical issues discussed previously. For each, several related topics are listed.

Ethical Conflicts

Personal and Professional Values

Personal values are related to societal values, which undergo change over time. Individuals are affected by the value programming of family, schools, churches, and significant role models. Traditional and challenging values vary from generation to generation. Socialization to a profession exposes individuals to professional values.

Nurses need to feel comfortable that their personal values are generally compatible with those values associated with the profession. This does not mean that personal and professional values are always congruent. Indeed, ethical conflicts between personal and professional values occasionally occur. Because of the vast practice opportunities available in nursing, however, most nurses can find a comfortable fit between their personal style and values and professional demands.

TABLE 11-1 *Personal Bioethical Issues*

Issue or Event	Topic

Pregnancy
  Prevention
  Interruption
  Facilitation
	Contraception

	Sterilization: male and female
	Abortion
	Selective abortion of multiple fetuses
	AI
	In vitro fertilization
	Surrogate pregnancy
	Rescue of unwanted products of conception
	Preserved embryos
Neonatology	Birth defects
	Withholding nutrition
	Withholding lifesaving interventions
Bioengineering	Genetic screening
	Manipulation of genes and embryos
	Organ transplants
	Artificial organs and joints
	Eugenics
Psychological competence	Informed consent
	Behavior modification
	Psychotropic medication
	Psychosurgery
	Mental retardation
	Paternalism
Death and dying	Truth telling
	Promise keeping
	Euthanasia
	Refusal of treatment

Considerable variation exists in client populations to be served, settings for practice, and acuity of illness. For example, nurses who might be uncomfortable in abortion situations will not choose employment in agencies where such procedures are likely to be performed. If one occurs unexpectedly, the nurse preferably will participate but then make arrangements to avoid future episodes. The effect of exercising such choice is to avoid the circumstances that are known to cause major ethical dilemmas regularly. Although such self-selection may forestall major dilemmas, minor ethical issues will invariably remain. Table 11-2 lists selected bioethical issues and examples of related questions.

There are several reasons for including a chapter on ethics in this book. Readers may learn the nature of the ethical dilemmas and demands in nursing.

TABLE 11-2 *Selected Bioethical Issues*

Issue	Related Questions
Truth telling	Should a patient be told he or she is going to die if the person seems unable to cope? If family members do not want the individual to be told?
Promise keeping	Should a nurse promise not to divulge a patient's awareness of impending death?
Behavioral control or modification	Is patient welfare or staff convenience the intent of control? Are patient priorities considered?
Suicide	Under what circumstances, if ever, is suicide morally defensible? Does the nurse have the right to interfere?
Euthanasia	Is a severely defective newborn better off dead? Should a brain-dead person be considered a dead person? How can a living will preserve the dignity of a person?
Refusal of treatment	What if the nurse disagrees with the person's decision to refuse life-saving treatment?
Irreversible coma	Is it morally right to hasten the death of a person kept alive by machines to transplant vital organs?
Opposing loyalties	Is the nurse obliged to keep hospital beds open if care for individual patients is compromised?

Perhaps they will also discover that such dilemmas raise intriguing and stimulating philosophical and practical problems. Such an introduction may confirm that nurses do not have to struggle alone with ethical issues. They can receive professional peer support in trying to resolve such dilemmas.

Whether they recognize it or not, nurses self-select their profession, a reality that has several implications. Most persons who choose nursing may be described as persons who are broadly interested in people and health, can forgo immediate personal gratification to assist another in a caring way, believe in service to humanity, and do not consider monetary gain as the primary motivating factor in selecting a life work.

Client and Professional Values

Nurses bring their personal values to their professional education. The development and clarification of values section was included to acknowledge the importance of both clients' and nurses' values. Values clarification, sometimes called values conflict resolution, and addressed in professional education, can help nurses understand many kinds of potential values conflicts.

Nurses respect client values and choices even when they do not agree with them. This respect is the essence of a principle called *unconditional positive regard*. As Rogers (1961) stated in his classic work, "It is an atmosphere which simply demonstrates, 'I care'; not 'I care for you if you behave thus and so'" (p. 283). Another important related principle is that behavior has meaning. In other words, what persons are doing at any particular time is serving some useful purpose. That is, it makes sense to them from their model of the world and, furthermore, the behavior reflects values actually held.

Nurses learn to accept that their clients may have religious and cultural values that differ from their own, but they guard against imposing their personal values on their clients. Nurses need to recognize where values come from and recognize and understand their own values as such. Then they can differentiate between their own values and those of their clients.

Values Among Health Professionals

Medicine and nursing have long held varying values for cure and care. This is not to imply that nurses do not value cure, nor that physicians are uncaring. Rather, it is a belief that "cure as an end in itself" as well as "doctor as the agent of cure" have been values that both attract and hold professionals in medicine. Increasingly, medical care has drifted from charitable and altruistic values to industrial values and services characterized now by product-line marketing and bottom-line cost-effectiveness. Again, we can draw on the principle that behavior has meaning. For the most part, American society has tolerated—if not enthusiastically supported—the health care system favoring cure. If the choice between care and cure could be viewed as an either/or decision, this situation would be more understandable. However, the human is not physically immortal, and technology has limits. Therefore, it would seem that a system that supports care and cure more equally would serve more people better over time. Carers and curers can work collaboratively toward that end. This would reduce the care–cure dichotomy between nurses and physicians that has been reflected in their practices. As Fagin (1992) indicated, "The challenge for physicians and nurses to work together to address the very real health care problems of our present and future has never been greater" (p. 302). With health care reform, another issue that has gained prominence is how to resolve nursing care definitions that contradict nursing's Code and values.

Theoretical Approaches to Ethical Issues

Theoretical Models

Most traditional ethical theories belong to one of two opposing and mutually exclusive classifications: teleological or deontological. A **teleological** theory is one in which the ends justify the means. The outstanding example of a teleological approach is **utilitarianism**. The utilitarian approach is sometimes described as advocating the greatest good for the greatest number, or choosing the least evil or least bad outcome. As you might guess, applied medical research supports this theory. The opposite approach in its most extreme form is **deontological** theory. Using this theory, the moral right or wrong of an act is considered completely apart from the goodness or badness of its consequences.

Teleological and deontological approaches can be illustrated with regard to abortion. In a teleological approach, saving the mother's life justifies taking the unborn life. On the other hand, in a deontological approach, any purposeful termination of life is morally bad; thus, the fetus would be spared.

A third traditional approach, sometimes called a moderate deontological approach, is also called Natural Law and derives from the work of St. Thomas Aquinas. It bases the goodness or badness of human actions on their agreement with the general nature of human beings. Aquinas believed that the universe is structured so that each creature has a goal and a purpose. He also believed that humans possess a trait that no other creature does, i.e., reason. The full development of human potential as well as the fulfillment of human purpose requires that we follow the law of reason.

Egoism is a fourth traditional position. The egoistic perspective uses self as the measure for right and wrong. Decisions in ethical dilemmas are made in the interest of the self. This means that in nursing, nurses would act in their own self-interest rather than in the interest of their clients. Putting personal needs or comfort before that of clients is generally inconsistent with and contrary to nursing's professional code of ethics. Also, because the self rather than universal principles is the point of reference, this ethical perspective does not provide for moral development as proposed by either Kohlberg or Gilligan.

Additional contemporary positions offer modifications of the earlier traditional views. Davis and Aroskar (1991) summarized the following approaches as being applicable to nursing:

- ❏ Frankena's theory of obligation—Built on the following two principles:
  Principle of beneficence—A proactive attempt to do good and not evil
  Principle of justice as equal treatment—An attempt to distribute benefits and burdens equally among members of society; fails to specify whether the criterion should be merit, equality, or need
    If and when the two principles conflict between the priorities of individuals and society, ideally inputs of multiple individuals will yield a consensus.
- ❏ Firth's ideal observer theory—Requires an all-knowing, impartial moral judge (person or machine) to make decisions that are equal for all and consistent over time
- ❏ Rawls's justice as fairness theory—Built on the following two basic principles of justice:
  Each individual is to have the same right to the most extensive system of liberty for all.
  Social and economic inequalities are to be to the greatest benefits of the least advantaged and open to everyone under equal conditions of opportunity (pp. 34–38).

One might reasonably ask, What is the reason for identifying so many ethical approaches when none tells specifically what a nurse should do in any given situation? Perhaps the major reason is to highlight some assumptions that we as experienced practitioners and educators make and that we hope may influence your approach to ethical decisions.

The assumptions are:

- ❏ All nursing practice involves ethical decisions.
- ❏ Person-centered care demands a willingness to confront ethical dilemmas.
- ❏ Personal and professional values influence ethical decisions.
- ❏ Persons (caregivers and clients) can be assisted to achieve higher levels of moral reasoning.
- ❏ There is no one "correct" ethical theory.

The questions of applied ethics, that is, what to do in everyday practice, are of most concern to nurses and nursing students. The traditional and contemporary theories of ethics in combination with awareness of personal and professional values and the data of individual situations can assist nurses to develop strategies to cope with ethical dilemmas. Gordon and Fagin (1996) remind us of the importance of "Preserving the moral high ground."

Even religious doctrines, which previously advocated one right ethical answer to life and death issues, are being challenged by scientific technology and the individual assertiveness of clients and health care providers. Perhaps traditional ethical decision making could be characterized as general ethical approaches of broad and rigid rules applied deductively to specific situations. Increasingly, individual situations are influencing relaxation of old rules through inductive reasoning and a care ethic that is situation specific. However, even personal and societal ethics are subject to swings of the pendulum from conservative to liberal and back again. Recent trends showing the resurgence of conservative influence in health care should be noted:

- ❏ A return to *family values* movement
- ❏ The "squeal" rule of the Supreme Court, requiring parents to be informed by health professionals of contraceptive advice to underaged teenagers
- ❏ An increasing involvement of family (however defined) in health care decisions
- ❏ Renewed interest in the quality, not just high-tech maintenance, of human life
- ❏ National and local attempts to constrain abortion

A *Practical Strategy for Considering Ethical Dilemmas*

With the prior discussion in mind, we suggest a practical approach to ethical decision making as presented in Thompson and Thompson (1990) and modified slightly by the authors. This approach is similar to both the scientific method and the nursing process presented earlier. The nursing process phases corresponding to various aspects of this ethical decision-making approach are indicated in parentheses. The suggested approach illustrates that its various aspects may relate to more than one phase of the nursing process. For example, the steps labeled diagnosis (steps 3 through 6) require a considerable analysis before the identification. This approach also illustrates that much of the essential nursing activity is mental thought that precedes and accompanies visible action.

1. Review the situation as presented.
   a. Determine what health problems and individual person strengths exist. (Assessing)
   b. Identify what decision(s) need to be made. (Assessing, analyzing, diagnosing)
   c. Separate the ethical components of the decisions from those issues that can be resolved solely on a scientific knowledge base. (Analyzing)
   d. Identify all the individuals/groups who will be affected by the decision(s). (Analyzing, diagnosing)
2. Decide what further information is needed before a decision on a course of action can be made; gather this information from primary sources, if possible. (Analyzing, assessing)
3. Identify the ethical issues involved in the situation as presented. Consider the historical, philosophical, and religious bases for each of these issues. (Analyzing, diagnosing)
4. Identify your own values/beliefs (moral stand) regarding each of these ethical issues and your professional responsibilities indicated by the Code for Nurses. (Analyzing, diagnosing)
5. Identify values/beliefs/possible rights of other people involved in the situation. (Analyzing, diagnosing)
6. Identify the value and rights conflicts, if any, in the situation. (Analyzing, diagnosing)
7. Discuss who is best able to make the needed decision(s) and identify the nurse's role in the decision-making process: Who owns the problem? (Planning)
8. Identify the range of decisions/actions that are possible and the anticipated implications of same to all people involved in the situation. Identify how closely the suggested actions conform to the Code for Nurses. (Planning)
9. If appropriate, decide on a course of action as the nurse in the situation and follow through. (Planning, implementing)
10. Evaluate the results of the action for achieving the client and societal goals. (Evaluating)
11. In retrospect, evaluate and review the results of the actions or decisions and keep them in mind for future situations of this type. (Aggregation)

Nurses may find organizational as well as social constraints to practicing according to the professional code of ethics. For example, the majority of nurses continue to work in hospitals and are under contract to their employers, whereas the code of ethics supports "clients" being the unit to which nurses are primarily accountable. Similarly, the social relationships, bureaucratic hierarchies, and economic pressures of managed care may make adherence to the code and the preceding strategies difficult. These constraints suggest that nurses under contract may need to negotiate their "right" to perform according to their professional code when they perceive that they are hindered from doing so.

Public Policy for Health Care Issues

A **policy** is a purposefully chosen plan of action (or inaction) aimed toward some end. Such a course of action by government is called *public policy*. Policy making can be aimed at various levels of complexity (i.e., micro, subsystem, macro). For example,

Micropolitics involves few people and has limited impact.

Subsystem politics focuses on broader policies and may have greater impact, but policy makers still have relative independence in developing and implementing policy. Such subsystem activity recognizes that policy makers within the larger (macro) system have varying levels of interest and expertise regarding different issues.

Macropolitics focuses on national issues that are broad and have much public interest (Kalisch & Kalisch, 1982).

Incremental policy making of the past, which tried to remedy issues of access to health care, has brought us to the 1990s with access issues still remaining and health care cost crises dominating the national scene. What the role of the federal government will be in resolving these crises is a key issue. At one extreme would be an unrestrained market system and at the other, a socialized plan for health care. Governmental involvement to set levels of health care costs according to some prepayment or prospective payment plan (rather than paying ever-escalating charges after the fact) is a middle-of-the-road intervention that, although already under way, promises to change shape over time. One such major government intervention was the catastrophic health care insurance recently added to Medicare.

The development of nursing as a full profession is caught amidst the reform of the health care system under managed care and the conflicting vested interests of other health professionals. The commercial aspects of health care have catapulted it to one of the nation's largest industries. Economic realities suggest that the delivery of person-centered care by a primary nurse in a traditional manner to a small caseload is not feasible. What are the alternatives and how will they be determined? As always with finite resources, some difficult choices will need to be made. Some of the priority setting for nursing care should come from nurses who are informed and able to suggest cost-effective nursing care alternatives. Nurses, who understand the foundations, principles, and potential of person-centered care, are the largest group of health care providers. Now they must document nursing care outcomes as economical and develop new economic and political savvy. Acting collectively, they can influence public policy to support health care and nursing care alternatives that are humanistic as well as economically feasible. The partnership between the ANA and the Consumer Coalition of Quality Health Care, a watchdog consumer group, illustrated the kind of action that will be necessary by coalitions seeking consumer protection. If the consumerism movement that brought hospice and renewed interest in person-centered care is to survive bottom-line health care economics, such action will indeed need to be most vigorous.

Major Health Care Issues Needing Ethical Resolution

When one reaches a stage of moral development characterized by awareness of universal ethical principles, a tangle of more abstract and larger ethical issues emerges. Although the same or similar questions may have arisen earlier, they assume greater significance when considered from an ethical perspective. Some of these questions are as follows:

> How should burgeoning technology be used?
> How do all citizens get access to health care?
> What should be the quality of health care?
> Who should control health care decisions?

How Should Burgeoning Technology Be Used?

The burgeoning technology of health care is evident in virtually every hospital, whether a sophisticated university health science center, a local division of a large, commercial health care conglomerate such as Humana, or a community hospital struggling to provide local service. New technology makes last year's high-tech model of the ever-changing equipment obsolete before it is paid for. Cooperative efforts are beginning and must progress rapidly. These are necessary to determine which center should provide which services. Such planning is mandatory for survival in the conglomerate, corporate world of high-tech health care.

Aside from the ethical issues related to economics, technology has amplified ethical issues related to access and the control of public resources. As always, technology challenges us to make ethical decisions about its use. Examples, characteristic of this decade of technology, are as follows:

> A president pleads for a liver transplant for a singular infant who is only one of many in similar circumstances.
> A judge orders castrating drug treatment for a convicted sex offender.
> The Persian Gulf War reactivates discussion of the "ethics" of nuclear war.
> In 1996, President Clinton named a 15 member National Bioethics Advisory Committee. A prominent nurse educator and President of the National League for Nursing was among the members named.

Surely such illustrations are just the tip of the iceberg.

How Do All Citizens Get Access to Health Care?

If access to health care is a right of all, inequality of access denies this right to some. Thus, inequality of access becomes an ethical issue. Two specific problems related to access are as follows:

1. Health care services are geographically clustered. This distribution creates an advantage for the suburban middle class and a disadvantage for many elderly and poor people living in rural or inner-city areas. What is nursing's responsibility and opportunity to serve underprivileged areas?
2. Access to health care, once controlled largely by physicians giving illness care, is increasingly controlled by insurance companies and managed care providers striving to cut costs. If nurses are capable of certain health care management, are they ethically responsible to try to have this management designated as part of the nursing role? Nursing would then assume privileges of both control and accountability and become more equal partners in primary care.

Managed care forces nurses and other health care providers to work together to provide access to both health and illness care, better distribution of services, and affordable health care. Access to affordable health care means that options other than the most expensive care must be appropriately available. In the past, many persons used an emergency room for nonemergency problems, such as a sore throat, because it seemed the only service available. Managed care gatekeepers have halted this practice. However, screening in less expensive neighborhood clinics that could reduce the need for such gatekeeping was slow to develop. Nurses assist clients to use health care facilities appropriately and have worked to make such neighborhood clinics available. Rather than making *less* services available to gain economic advantage under managed care, this approach improves access to and emphasizes a *different* kind of service.

The high cost of health care creates opportunity and a competitive edge for nurses as primary care health professionals. Nurses have many needed primary skills and cost less than physicians. However, this high cost also offers a considerable threat to nursing as a profession. Nurses are the most expensive item in the personnel budget, especially in acute care settings. And in all settings, professional nurses are more expensive than lesser trained assistive personnel. For public opinion to influence this issue, nurses must "Tell the world what you do" as suggested by Buresh and Gordon (1995). Then perhaps the full range of nursing services will be assured in all settings.

What Should Be the Quality of Health Care?

Quality of health care becomes an ethical issue because it is related to quality of life. The issues of access and quality are also, of necessity, related. If one does not have access to the system, the chances of receiving quality care are low. From a technologic or medical perspective, the quality of health care may be high for those with access. The quality of life is compromised, however, by dehumanizing, depersonalized, and unwanted interventions—these may even cause those with access to perceive the quality of health care to be low. To provide quality health care and access to all persons is an ethical goal. It would require major reordering of our national social and economic priorities. If we allot fewer health care resources than needed, how shall we decide who gets quality care?

Who Should Control Health Care Decisions?

The concept of client autonomy is a recurring theme in ethical issues. A person-centered nursing perspective affirms the client–patient as the focus of ethical decision making. High-level wellness is both relative and individual. Therefore, the client can be expected to make personal health care decisions based on what the client, not the professional, defines as his or her concept of health. If the professional accepts this premise, then how the individual client views his or her health care becomes important. The criteria for judging the success of clients' health care decisions will change also. Effective coping and positive health care decisions will be acknowledged by health care professionals. Many trends, including the consumerism movement and home care for birth and death, suggest that persons are interested in controlling their own health care decisions.

Tax dollars ought to support the health care delivery that persons want and need. Despite the billions of dollars poured into tertiary (i.e., specialized) care, most persons will have only a minimal need for such services during their entire lifetime. It is possible that every state has more beds in nursing homes than in hospitals. Yet conditions in many nursing homes are such that one would not wish himself or herself or a loved one cared for there. Nursing is the one health profession in a unique position to help persons use advances in scientific health care and reasonable self-care practices to increase their control over health care decisions. The use of tax dollars to finance tertiary care is just one illustration of the fact that broader ethical issues related to health care are difficult to resolve. Resolution would require a profound social commitment, national priority for equality of human rights, and the valuing of individual persons.

Accountability

As the previous discussion suggests, accountability to the profession to uphold its standards is an ethical issue. Accountability is also a major introductory legal concept. From your life experiences, you have internalized an everyday definition of accountability. Being answerable for professional conduct extends the concept to another dimension.

Standards

Accountability means responsibility or the obligation to account for one's behavior or acts. Persons are generally held accountable in relation to a peer group: a group with similar educational preparation, experience, licensure, specialization, certification, and so forth. Standards are both professionally and legally defined. Novices or learners are held to different standards than licensed experts.

In the introductory clinical nursing course of one baccalaureate nursing program, faculty members identified the following eight general behavioral objectives related to accountability and reliability. The student will:

1. Assume responsibility for own actions.
2. Demonstrate self-discipline in meeting commitments and obligations, for example, keeping appointments and submitting written assignments on time.
3. Prepare in advance for clinical experience.
4. Report unsafe client–patient practices.
5. Demonstrate awareness of client–patient rights.
6. Demonstrate commitment in meeting client–patient needs.
7. Follow standard regulations and rules.
8. Apply safety measures to nursing interventions.

The first objective, to assume responsibility, takes on new meaning for the professional nursing student. Although being a student gives a license to learn, certain prudent behavior is expected nevertheless, as indicated by the other objectives. The principle of reasonable care is considered in determining whether one has exercised such prudent behavior.

Reasonable care means that level of competent performance and knowledge generally used by similarly educated and experienced health practitioners in one's community. This standard of reasonable care can be applied to students as well as to licensed practitioners. Thus, just as a faculty member is expected to exercise appropriate judgment in making clinical assignments and supervising a student, so too is the student expected not to proceed without appropriate supervision if uninformed or unable to perform a certain skill. Clients have a right to expect a student to perform at a safe level, if not as skillfully as a licensed practitioner. Licensed practitioners themselves demonstrate accountability through consultation with informed peers, and in a number of other ways.

Professional nursing standards are a means by which nurses regulate nursing practice. Nursing standards for licensed practitioners are generated and published by a professional organization (ANA). Licensed registered nurses (RNs) are understandably held to high professional standards. The American Nurses Association first published general standards of nursing practice in 1973. Since then, *Standards of Clinical Nursing Practice* (ANA, 1991) and a variety of standards of specialty practice have also been published.

The state provides another form of regulation, that is, legal regulation through practice acts and licensure. The relationship of professional and legal regulation of nursing practice is shown in Figure 11-2.

Accountability is a demanding professional and legal responsibility to assume. However, as the previous discussion suggests, accountability has many dimensions. The expectations about its demonstration change over the course of both professional education and career development. Potential nurses who wonder about whether they can meet these ethical and legal obligations are not alone in

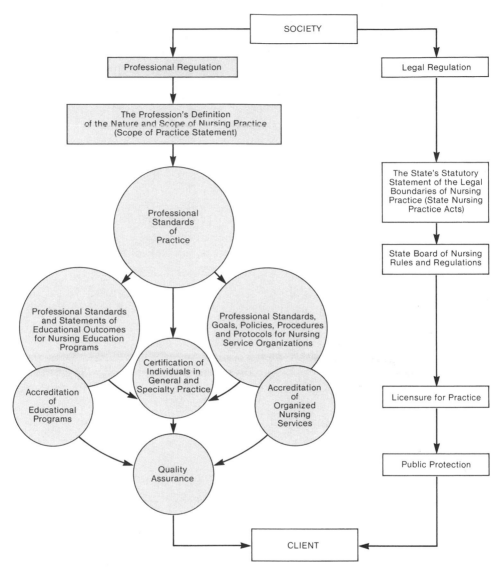

FIGURE 11-2 Professional and legal regulation of nursing practice. (Hirsch, I. L. (1988, April). Statement on nursing's scope describes how two levels of nurses practice. The American Nurse, 13).

their concerns. Probably most nurses, as well as other professionals, have had such questions early in their careers. Most practicing professionals as well as educators can provide reassurance. There are many safeguards built into both educational and professional systems to make ethical and legal practice less troublesome. Legal security for the nurse is enhanced by such diverse strategies as record keeping and documentation, contracts in education and practice, effective interpersonal communication as discussed in Chapter 9, the Good Samaritan laws, and professional liability insurance.

Documentation

Documentation is literally the collecting or supplying of written information for future reference. A diploma signifying educational achievement and a state license to practice as an RN fit this definition. These credentials document an initial competency attested to by experts or their representatives. Nurses document their actual clinical practice in written narratives about patients' conditions and the administration of medications and treatments. They also document accountability with signatures or initials indicating access to controlled substances. Students, practicing under both direct and indirect supervision, could be thought of as practicing under the professional license of the supervising educator. It should come as no surprise then that even introductory clinical courses hold students to course objectives of beginning accountability.

Health care records, which vary greatly among agencies, are legal records and provide documentation about health care given. They are admissible in legal court proceedings to document care given. If care is not documented, we have no basis for assuming that an action was taken. This applies specifically to concrete actions such as dispensing medications, changing dressings, taking vital signs, etc. Responsible health care providers demonstrate their professional accountability with such documentation. Therefore, such documentation needs clear entries that include the nurse's name, the date, time of entry, any significant change in the person's progress, and the nurse's observations and actual interventions. See Mandell's (1994) ''Not documented, not done.''

Documentation in the past has often taken the form of handwritten notes. Increasingly, computerization enables documentation to occur electronically at the client's bedside. In this day and age of continuous commercial surveillance, one can imagine video documentation of provider care as a realistic possibility.

Practice Acts and Licensure

The laws that govern nursing practice are state laws. The first nursing practice act was made state law in North Carolina in 1903. It was a **permissive licensure.** Such laws permitted nurses to practice without a license if they did not claim licensure or use the RN initials. Currently, **mandatory licensure** for nurses requires all persons who nurse for compensation to be licensed. Many state practice laws underwent major revision in the 1970s. In 1972, New York's nursing practice act boldly defined nursing's professional practice as ''diagnosing and treating human responses.'' This or similar wording has been a model for many other state law revisions. This definition was also central to the social policy statement by the ANA (1980).

Nursing practice acts define nursing practice and requirements for licensure in a particular state. They also create a board of examiners and specify their responsibilities. One of the requirements of licensure is passage of the National Council Licensing Examination. All the state boards of nursing contract with an independent agency, the National Council of State Boards of Nursing, for the provision and scoring of the test. The national passage rate for first-time takers is approximately 86%. During the mid 1990s a movement to create a multistate license for nurses gained momentum, due in part to the exploding technology that created telehealth systems.

Having the same examination for all states now facilitates state-to-state movement of RNs. The rationale of having one examination taken by graduates of associate degree, diploma, and baccalaureate programs was debated for many years. Perhaps there was one redeeming argument for a single examination: the purpose of licensure is to protect society by ensuring that professionals demonstrate a minimal level of competence. Remember, according to the state, RN is intended to designate the professional nurse in a legal sense only. RN is not intended to mean professional according to the definition and criteria for a profession. Movement to have different exams for different levels of preparation is in progress, as is additional licensure for advanced specialty practice beyond what is already regulated (e.g., for nurse–midwives). Some states have been more receptive than others.

Many states are considering ways to test competency for RN renewal of licensure. It is, however, proving particularly difficult to find a definition of professional nurse competency about which there is agreement. It is even more difficult and threatening to decide how competency should be measured. Nurses have a moral obligation, if not a legal one, to update their knowledge of nursing science and practice through some form of continuing education or learning.

Negligence and Malpractice

Before beginning this discussion, it is necessary to consider some basic legal terminology. *Laws* are the civilized principles and processes by which people in society seek to resolve disputes and problems. **Criminal law** is concerned with behavior detrimental to society as a whole. **Civil law** deals with legal rights and duties of private persons. A **legal right** is a claim that is recognized and is enforceable by law. Nurses and clients have legal constitutional rights. For example, persons who are hospitalized retain their constitutional rights, including those granted by amendments related to freedom of thought and speech, due process of law, and protection of minorities and the handicapped. The contrast between criminal law and civil law can be illustrated as follows: criminal law is basically the State versus John Doe, whereas if Nurse Naylor were sued by Client Smith, the civil case would be Smith versus Naylor.

Generally, health professionals are concerned with the category of law called **torts.** This concern is added to the legal rights and responsibilities the professionals retain as private citizens. Torts are civil wrongs that may be intentional or unintentional. The underlying concept of torts is the violation of reasonable behavior.

Two commonly confused terms relating to torts and reasonable behavior are negligence and malpractice. **Negligence** is the more general concept. Although we often think of being negligent as being careless, the two are not necessarily synonymous. For example, Student Baker, who injured Client Jones by attempting a new procedure for which he had not received instruction, would be negligent even if he did it carefully. Negligence applies to laypersons as well as to professionals. **Malpractice** involves negligence in carrying out professional services by persons who are licensed to perform such services. Technically, malpractice applies only to the professional already actually licensed to practice.

The term **liability** means responsibility because of position or particular circumstances. Thus, health professionals are liable or legally responsible for their professional behavior. Even though they proceed carefully, they could be found negligent as students or licensed professionals. Their performance must be prudent in comparison with what similarly prepared health professionals would have done in the same circumstances. Again, the standard for judgment is that of the reasonable and prudent person. However, the reasonable and prudent standard for malpractice involves a comparison with other similarly licensed practitioners. Malpractice is the specific type of negligent behavior for which professionals are uniquely liable because of their education and licensure.

Common Problems

Negligence related to nursing commonly includes such acts as failure to take appropriate precautions, failure to recognize dangers, or failure to report hazardous conditions. The nurse is responsible both for error in dependent nursing functions, such as administering medications, and in professional judgment regarding more independent functions, such as assessing client responses. The duty to take affirmative action when presented with a deteriorating situation (e.g., unusual bleeding) refers to taking positive steps to bring such a situation under control. Common problems related to legal issues can be the result of such seemingly simple errors as the failure to properly identify persons who are the recipients of care. These identification errors could result in wrong medications and diagnostic tests, or untherapeutic interventions by a variety of health care workers.

Avoiding Litigation

Although opportunities for negligence abound, a formal charge is likely to be brought and a trial to occur only if harm results. Such a trial in court to settle issues is called **litigation.** Increasingly, clients pursue litigation if they believe they have suffered mental or physical harm. Therefore, even careful students and RNs need the protection of liability insurance. Both the professional organization, ANA, and the student organization, the National Student Nurses' Association, provide such insurance service to their members at a reasonable cost.

Although liability insurance is strongly advised, some of the strategies for avoiding litigation are surprisingly simple and often overlooked. A most basic strategy is not to undertake, without supervision, any procedure or intervention for which you have not received appropriate instruction or assurance that you are able to practice on your own. This advice is equally true for students and licensed practitioners. An extension of this strategy is not to practice or proclaim practice for which you are not licensed. For example, nurses cannot practice as licensed midwives or pediatric nurse practitioners unless they are legally licensed for that expanded practice. Furthermore, nurses cannot practice medicine in ways restricted by law or practice nursing in states in which they are not licensed.

Nurses, as well as other health professionals and ordinary citizens, are afforded protection to act in emergencies by what are called **Good Samaritan laws.** Under these laws, which vary from state to state, persons who give emergency care, such as at the site of an automobile accident, are regarded as a protected class.

Another often neglected strategy for avoiding litigation is effective interpersonal communication. The importance of this strategy cannot be underestimated. Faulty communication can create both ethical and legal problems. For example, informed consent is required for clients' participation in varied therapies and also in research investigations. Informed consent has both ethical and legal dimensions. Even when informed consent has been appropriately obtained, something occasionally goes wrong. Nevertheless, certain clients are less likely to take their disappointment and frustration to a court of law for minor problems. Often, these are the clients who believe they have been treated humanely and thoughtfully and have been communicated with appropriately. Some actions in the care of clients might be considered assault (threat to do bodily harm) or battery (committing bodily harm). These are actions taken when the client's consent has not been obtained or his or her communication to resist the nurse's action has gone unheeded.

Even when they attend to the suggestions above, nurses and students are sometimes involved in lawsuits, as the following example illustrates:

> Through a lawsuit against a large academic medical center, a plaintiff (patient) pursued a claim of professional negligence directed at a senior nursing student. The allegation related to a hip fracture that the patient had suffered. The nurse manager asked the instructor to investigate the alleged incident with the student. The student was amazed, declaring that nothing untoward had occurred during her care of the patient.
>
> In cases of professional negligence, the plaintiff has the burden of proving the existence of each of the elements of negligence: duty, breach, damage, and causation. The patient's clinical record was the primary documentation regarding care. During the subsequent trial, the patient altered her story about the care several times. There was no doubt that the fracture had occurred during hospitalization, but there was no evidence that it related to the student's care and/or negligence. To the contrary, x-rays and documentation confirmed that it occurred after the student's care of the plaintiff.
>
> Noting that emphasis was placed on chart documentation in this litigation, the nurse manager commented, "We were fortunate that our nursing and medical documentation was complete and descriptive. The progress note documentation indicated assessment of the patient's pain, but was without statement of hip pain, until after the fracture was diagnosed. Since it was unlikely that we were all involved in covering up the injury, it seems that the injury had not occurred until just prior to

its diagnosis." As this case illustrates, charting, which documents the meeting of the standard of care, is one of the most critical bases for a convincing legal defense.

Several lessons were learned from this experience by both the professional staff and the nursing student. They included the following:

❏ Basics are important: Objectivity, thoroughness, and precision are documentation imperatives.

❏ Expect the unexpected: The nurse manager and staff believed that they had had good rapport with and had been extremely supportive of an admittedly challenging patient.

❏ The unexpected is generally explainable: Not only was the client "challenging" during hospitalization, she had an extraordinary personal history prior to hospitalization.

❏ The psychology of litigation is manageable: Although challenge to professional practice and integrity was anxiety provoking, there were legal, collegial, and administrative supports sufficient to meet the defendants' needs.

❏ There is no substitute for professional care: The client had been carefully assessed prior to and following her fracture. In addition to the existing documentation, several other professionals substantiated professional care, including conferences to plan consistent care.

❏ Never underestimate the importance of relationships: Although positive relationships were not enough to prevent the lawsuit, the relationships among the nurse manager, instructor, student, and Dean of Students were excellent. These helped to make a difficult situation more bearable.

Legislative Process

Affecting Nurses

Perhaps the preceding discussion has suggested that all details of nursing practice are indeed legislated or come into being by the making of laws. In reality, "custom and usage" may be equally important. Often it is the changing practice according to local custom that serves as the impetus for changing law to regulate that practice (e.g., nurses doing venipuncture to initiate intravenous hydration). With such notable exceptions as midwifery and nurses administering anesthesia, the law generally does not prohibit nurses from functioning in more independent ways consistent with their education.

The Nurse Training acts of 1943 and 1971 authorized the creation of the U.S. Nurse Cadet Corps in the U.S. Public Health Service, which supported and expanded the training of nurses.

In addition to legislation, state and local, which specifically regulates nursing, nurses have recently worked more actively to shape broader legislation directly related to professional interests, e.g, quality of care. For example, the ANA strongly supported HR 3355 (The Patient Safety Act of 1996), which was intended to ensure that health care agencies would disclose information related to staffing levels and patient outcomes.

Shaping Policy

Political participation can benefit both nursing and society. Policy changes that appear to be primarily self-serving for any professional group are understandably suspect. However, the detailed discussion of this chapter has identified a number of bioethical issues that, by their very nature, may be of more concern to nursing than to other health professions. These issues relate primarily to preserving the essence of persons amidst growing technology and ever-increasing economic pressures.

The 1970s and 1980s have been characterized by their attention to personal welfare over social welfare. In the 1990s, many Americans are concerned about social welfare issues. Nursing offers an outlet for social expression. Nursing also offers a community of professionals who value social welfare, especially as it relates to health concerns. Nurses are prepared by education and privileged by social mandate to promote social welfare. To do so fully, nurses will need to become partners in the legislative process. Nurses shape policy when they vote, inform themselves and legislators about health care matters, and offer resources to political candidates evidencing ethical and humanistic support of pressing health care issues. Becoming politically active is identified by McIntyre (1991) as a professional growth activity.

Nursing students can make a difference in the professional and legal systems that apply to nursing. Professionalism is important for the future well-being of the profession, its practitioners, and for society. As students adhere to professional standards, including an ethical code, they renew the professional commitment of nursing to society. As they practice ethically and legally, they encourage society's reaffirmation of the nursing profession's valued place in society. Baccalaureate-prepared nurses and students who practice to the full extent of their educational background make an important professional statement. They demonstrate the value of this level of education, that is, society's investment in them. They also demonstrate that society will be enriched by making this level of educational investment in all nurses who aspire to serve society as professionals.

The following example, reported by the former president of a nursing school student government, shows the impact that students can have on both their communities and health policy leaders:

> Getting involved in leadership as a student opened doors and opportunities that I never could have imagined. While an undergraduate, I had the opportunity to serve as the first nursing co-chairperson of the Medstart Coalition. Medstart is a student organization that serves underrepresented children and educates the community about these children's needs. Medstart was founded in 1990 by students, in hopes of improving their own knowledge base, while simultaneously improving the lives of children in their communities. It began with a single conference, totally generated by student leaders. The conferences have become nationally renowned in child health advocacy circles.
>
> Expanded programming has served teen mothers, pediatric health promotion for underserved communities, and violence prevention. Some of the speakers included the U.S. Surgeon General, the mayor of a major metropolis, and the president and founder of the Children's Defense League. Letters of support have come from the

Secretary of Health and Human Services, a state Governor, and even the President of the United States and other local and national officials concerned with child health. And, a quadriplegic teen, victim of random gunfire, launched a national speaking tour and violence prevention organization with the support of the Medstart organizers. [Jeffrey M. Adams, R.N.]

Baccalaureate nurses (and students) who practice to the full extent of their education also serve society in other ways. They innovate practice in ways that change the legal boundaries of practice. This expansion furthers the profession but, more importantly, benefits society by giving it the full range of nursing's potential service (e.g., nurses in independent practice who collaborate with physicians).

Students can also make a difference in the legal system by influencing and shaping legislative process. Aspiring nurses can work for candidates who are nurses or who support nursing's position in health care issues; equally important, they can inform the voting public about nursing's potential as a profession and its political health care agenda.

KEY CONCEPTS

A person focus for bioethics is consistent with nursing's theoretical metaparadigm and also nursing's professional code of ethics.

Bioethical issues are health care issues that are resolved through moral decision making. They have personal, professional, political, social, and economic implications.

Ethical conflicts arise from differing values among clients, between clients and professionals, and among health professionals.

Practical strategies for analyzing ethical issues require both critical thinking skills and ethical decision making.

Accountability demands personal responsibility to educational, legal, and professional standards.

Legal aspects involve laws governing nursing practice and liability of nurses for their professional behavior with clients.

CRITICAL THINKING QUESTIONS

1. How do you feel about clients making ethical decisions with which you do not agree?

2. What ethical responsibilities does nursing as a profession have for the collective action of its members?

3. What responsibilities does the nursing profession have to influence health care legislation?

4. Choose an ethical issue of interest. Compare its discussion in current medical and nursing literature.

5. Apply the Thompson and Thompson ethical decision-making strategy to a specific ethical issue from your clinical or personal experience.

6. Compare and contrast the Nursing Code of Ethics with that of another profession.

7. For you, what health situation, if any, would make living intolerable?

8. What have been the sources of value programming in your life?

9. Watch one of the current health care TV shows and analyze the ethical and legal issues raised by the episode.

10. Familiarize yourself with periodical literature outside of nursing (e.g., the Harvard Medical School Health Letter or Kennedy Institute of Ethics Journal). Monitor and discuss with faculty and peers ethical issues of concern to professional nurses.

REFERENCES

American Hospital Association. (1990). *A patient's bill of rights*. Chicago: Author.

American Nurses Association. (1995). *Annotated bibliography for ethical guidelines* (Publication No. D-97). Washington, D.C.: Author.

American Nurses Association. (1994). *Guidelines for reporting incompetent, unethical, or illegal practices* (Publication No. NP-91). Washington, D.C.: Author.

American Nurses Association. (1993). *Ethical dilemmas in contemporary nursing practice* (Publication No. NP-81). Washington, D.C.: Author.

American Nurses Association. (1991). *Standards of clinical nursing practice*. Kansas City, MO: Author.

American Nurses Association, Committee on Ethics. (1988). ANA comments on withholding food and fluid. *American Nurse, 20*(3), 26.

American Nurses Association. (1980). *A social policy statement* (Publication No. NP-63 35M). Kansas City, MO: Author.

American Nurses Association. (1973). *General standards of nursing practice*. Kansas City, MO: Author.

Badzek, L.A. (1992). What you need to know about advance directives. *Nursing '92, 22*(6), 58–59.

Bandman, E.L., & Bandman, B. (1995). *Nursing ethics through the life span* (3rd ed.). Norwalk, CT: Appleton & Lange.

Benner, P.E., Tanner, C. & Chesla. C.A. (1996). *Expertise in nursing practice, caring, clinical judgment and ethics*. New York: Springer.

Benner, P.E., & Wrubel, J. (1989). *The primacy of caring: stress and coping in health and illness*. Menlo Park, CA: Addison-Wesley.

Bishop, A.H. & Scudder, J.R. (1996). *Nursing ethics: therapeutic caring presence*. Boston: Jones & Bartlett.

Buresh, B. & Gordon, S. (1995). Tell the world what you do. *American Journal of Nursing 95*, 18–19.

Davis, A.J. (1990). Are there limits to caring? Conflict between autonomy and beneficence. In M.M. Leininger (Ed.), *Ethical and moral dimensions of care* (pp. 25–32). Detroit: Wayne State University Press.

Davis, A.J., & Aroskar, M.A. (1991). *Ethical dilemmas and nursing practice* (3rd ed.). Norwalk, CT: Appleton & Lange.

Davis, A.J., & Aroskar, M.A. (1978). Ethical dilemmas and nursing. NY: Appleton-Century-Crofts.

Dente-Cassidy, A.M. (1992). Predictions for critical care nursing. *Nursing '92, 22,* 43–45.

Fagin, C.M. (1992). Collaboration between nurses and physicians: No longer a choice. *Academic Medicine, 67*(5), 295–303.

Gilligan, C. (1993). *In a different voice: Psychological theory and women's development.* Cambridge, MA: Harvard University Press.

Gilligan, C. (1989). Remapping the moral domain: New images of self in relationship. In T.C. Heller, M. Sosna, & D. Wellbery (Eds.), *Mapping the moral domain* (pp. 3–19). Cambridge, MA: Harvard University Press.

Gilligan, C. (1982). *In a different voice: Psychological theory and women's development.* Cambridge, MA: Harvard University Press.

Gordon, S. & Fagin, C. (1996). Preserving the moral high ground. *American Journal of Nursing, 96,* 31–32, March '96.

Harvard Medical School. (1968). Report of the Ad Hoc Committee of the Harvard Medical School to examine the definition of brain death: A definition of irreversible coma. *Journal of the American Medical Association, 205*(6), 85–88.

Hirsch, I.L. (1988). Statement on nursing's scope describes how two levels of nurses practice. *American Nurse, 20*(4), 13.

Kalisch, B.J. & Kalisch, P.A. (1982). *Politics of nursing.* Philadelphia: J.B. Lippincott

Ketefian, S. (1987). Moral behavior in nursing. *Advances in Nursing Science, 9,* 10–19.

Kohlberg, L. (1987). *Child psychology and childhood education: A cognitive–developmental view.* New York: Longman.

Kubler-Ross, E. (1969). *On death and dying.* New York: Macmillan.

Leininger, M.M. (Ed.). (1990). *Ethical and moral dimensions of care.* Detroit: Wayne State University Press.

Mandell, M. (1994). Not documented, not done. *Nursing 94, 24*(8), 62–63.

McIntyre, E. (1991). Becoming politically active. *Nursing '91, 21*(10), 116–122.

Rogers, C.R. (1961). *On becoming a person.* Boston: Houghton Mifflin.

Singleton, K.A., Dever, R., & Donner, T.A. (1992). Durable power of attorney: Nursing implications. *Dimensions of Critical Care Nursing, 11*(1), 41–46.

Thompson, J.B., & Thompson, H.O. (1981). *Ethics in nursing.* New York: Macmillan.

Thompson, J.E., & Thompson, H.O. (Eds.). (1990). *Professional ethics in nursing.* Malabar, FL: Robert E. Krieger Publishing.

United Nations. (1979). *Declaration on the rights of the child.* New York: Author.

United Nations. (1975). *Declaration on rights of disabled persons.* New York: Author.

United Nations. (1971). *Declaration on rights of mentally retarded persons.* New York: Author.

Watson, J. (1988). *Nursing: Human science and human care: A theory of nursing.* New York: National League for Nursing (Pub. No. 15-2236).

Weber, G., & Kjervik, D.K. (1992). Legal and ethical issues: The Patient Self-Determination Act—The nurse's proactive role. *Journal of Professional Nursing, 8*(1), 6.

Part Four

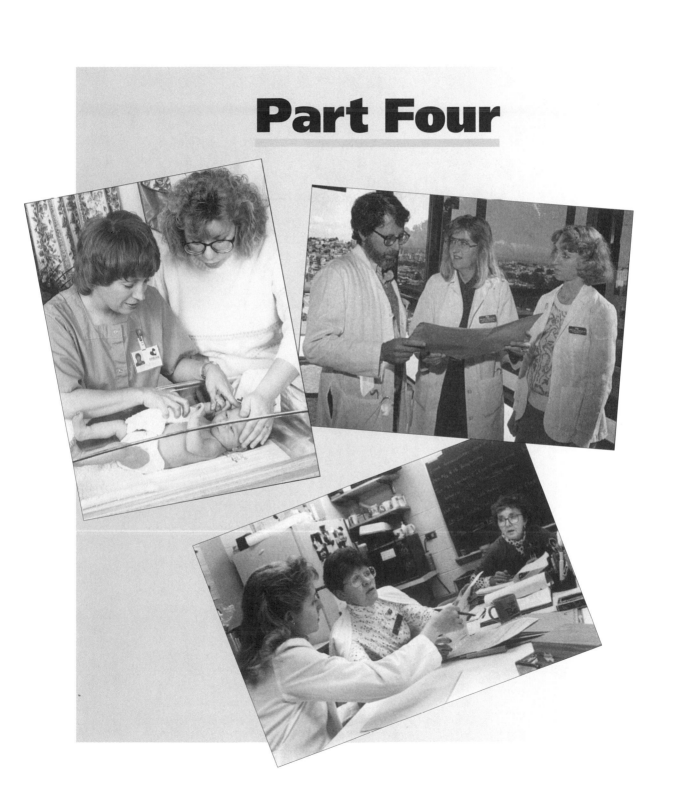

12

Opportunities and Challenges

Career development   **Goal**   **Novice**
Expert   **Mentor**

After completing this chapter, students will be able to:

Identify several career and personal opportunities available to professional nurses.

Identify several challenges facing the nursing profession.

Explain how the challenge to humanize health care also offers an important opportunity for the nursing profession.

Identify personal characteristics and attitudes that are compatible with professional nursing.

Nurses have served a social need during all of recorded history. Nurses have sometimes been men, although more often they have been women. Throughout history, nurses have been educated in a variety of ways: history has recorded nurses who were self-taught as well as nurses who pursued all avenues of formal education. Regardless of gender or education, interpersonal care has been the hallmark of nursing service. What nursing will become in the future is a function of social need and also is influenced, to a great extent, by nurses themselves.

> WANTED: Diverse, quality persons to make a difference in the health care of the future. Creative opportunities and challenges in all health care settings. Applicants must like people and analytical thinking. No experience necessary, but maturity and adaptability helpful.

Nurses fulfill a myriad of career aspirations in general practice and by specializing within nursing. They also may blend nursing with other fields or unique personal abilities for "dual careers." This chapter summarizes the issues, opportunities, and challenges facing nurses and the nursing profession currently and in the future. The challenges presented in this chapter also can be viewed as opportunities of a different nature. Under the challenge to humanize health care, two explicit health problems (acquired immunodeficiency syndrome [AIDS] and care of older persons) receive brief but special emphasis. These health problems create particular windows of opportunity for organized nursing. The care strategies for self-development at the end of the chapter assume that career management begins with the recognition of opportunities, challenges, and individual potential, whether one is a student or an experienced practitioner.

Nursing Professionalization at a Crossroad

The criteria for professions and the brief historical perspective of nursing's development can help us understand modern nursing and its relation to other professions and society at large. We might conclude the following about nursing as a profession:

- ❐ Nursing has a briefer professional history than the traditional professions of law, medicine, and theology.
- ❐ Nursing has been and continues to be primarily a woman's occupation.
- ❐ Nursing's ranking on the criteria commonly used for professions is the subject of considerable debate.

This final point argues for the individual growth and activities of nurses as crucial to the continuing professionalization of nursing. Current and aspiring nurses who are the present and future nurse leaders will need to be the ones who provide, preserve, and develop today's nursing for tomorrow.

Problems Common to Nursing and Other Professions

If nurses are to control the service they provide to society, they will need to address current problems and issues vigorously. In general, the problems faced by nurses and other professionals originate from the characteristics of professional occupations—autonomy and independent decision making, career commitment, collegial relationships, and professional worth or rewards. Issues, in contrast to problems, are larger questions for which no consensus exists about a right answer. Issues, therefore, are questions not easily answered with a simple yes or no. Contemporary nursing issues and health care reform issues create a crossroad of decisions that affect the continued professionalization of nursing.

Contemporary Nursing Issues

The challenges and opportunities that await nursing at the close of this millennium and beyond are posed within the context of the issues that have faced nursing during its quest for professional independence. Briefly summarized, these are as follows:

Control of Nursing Practice

One of the pressing issues facing nursing is that of who shall control nursing practice. Control is a primary issue determining whether nursing will continue its professionalization toward independence and autonomy. Forces both within and outside nursing challenge the obvious answer that nursing should control its own practice. For example, medicine and health services administrations would gain much from controlling nursing, and some nurses are unwilling to assume this responsibility of "control." If nurses do not assume control of nursing, all issues related to future practice will be decided by whatever group does control it.

Control of nursing practice has led to controversy about the so-called extended and expanded roles for nurses. A *role* is a pattern of behavior associated with a distinctive social position. An *extended role* is a role lengthened in a unilateral manner. For example, the role of the physician is extended through the use of another health care worker, commonly known as a Physician's Assistant or PA. In this case, the authority base for extension is from the physician. *Role expansion* is a multidirectional spreading out. For example, an expanded role for the nurse, such as a Nurse Practitioner, may involve some extension into the physician's role, but this is a lesser part of the expansion. The authority base of expansion is primarily nursing knowledge and clinical expertise as demonstrated by the nurse practitioner and clinical nurse specialist. The assistive personnel who have surfaced during health care reform are a manifestation that this issue of control is yet to be resolved.

The boundaries of medicine, nursing, other health professions, and auxiliary occupations will be altered as sciences develop and practices change. Boundaries will also be affected by a surplus of some health care professionals, e.g., specialty physicians and acute care nurses, and undersupplies of others, e.g., primary care physicians and registered nurses who are primary care practitioners. Roles in particular practice areas may be especially affected, for example, obstetricians (physicians) and nurse–midwives (RNs). The issues may be not only ones of managed care and professional control, but also of consumer preference for certain health care choices. It may be to nursing's advantage that its professional care better fits both client pocketbooks and consumer priorities.

RELATIONSHIP OF "CONTROL" TO OTHER ISSUES

Four other important issues will continue to affect nursing as a developing profession:

1. What services should nurses provide?
2. How should nurses be educated?
3. What payment should nurses receive for their services?
4. What should be the influence of organized nursing on American health care policy?

If nursing claims its autonomy and retains control, then nurses, with their clients and society, will decide these issues together. Answers to the four questions, in turn, will influence organized nursing's impact on even larger national and international health policy issues. Many issues are more intertwined than they may appear on first inspection.

What Services Should Nurses Provide?

Those who contend that nursing is moving toward professionalization would argue the following principle: the profession, with help from the society it serves, should decide what services to offer. Clearly managed care and professional competition may also be factors. Many health care problems, especially chronic conditions, require other than medical management. The number of persons who require supportive nursing services to adapt to the lengthening life span will continue to increase greatly.

How Should Nurses Be Educated?

Differences in education currently undermine the unity and development of the profession. Although the baccalaureate degree is advocated as the preferred professional preparation, associate degree programs prepare approximately half the graduating RNs. The AD approach to education is often used by persons with a variety of other life challenges. Thus, in two years such persons will be licensed and continue their education while working and earning the money they need. This may also be an approach for persons who are unsure of their interest in nursing. They have an opportunity to try the profession and to use their AD preparation as a base for additional education. AD nurses are often highly motivated. With the clinical background they obtain after working for a while as an RN, they offer new dimensions to professional nursing from their varied life experiences. Additionally, these nurses may move from the AD preparation directly into Masters' programs when such programs are accessible to them.

Even though many employers do not differentiate among RNs in the workplace, baccalaureate graduates should seek employment that will use their skills fully and compensate them for their additional preparation. Of course, nurses who have undergone a more expensive education should offer something obviously different and important.

The shift in education to the graduate level for other health care disciplines magnifies the fact that only a small percentage of RNs are prepared with either master's degrees or doctorates. There is a need for master's-prepared nurses as clinicians, managers, administrators, and instructors. Doctoral-prepared nurses are needed as leaders in all specialty areas, including education and research. If one assumes that each facility in which nursing care is provided would benefit from having doctoral-prepared nurses to stimulate research and practice, the shortage becomes apparent. It will be increasingly difficult for nurses to be peers with other health professionals who have had more advanced education.

These issues present both challenges and opportunities. Therefore, nurses prepared at all levels need to expect to continue professional learning and career growth through formal education, continuing education programs, and individual self study. To meet both the challenges and opportunities all nurses also need a better understanding of the basics of economics and business, politics, cultural diversity and international affairs, and the humanities.

Former ANA President Lucille Joel correctly observes that most nurses practicing today, "were educated for a profession that, in a way, no longer exists. . . We'll have to nurse through assistants in many situations and do so with confidence. We'll take on functions that were once the province of other disciplines" (1996). [source:http://www.ajn.org/guide96/g6xx008e.1t] Although Joel is not explicit, nurse practitioners in expanded roles, for example, perform activities such as routine assessments and health care that once were the province of physicians.

What Payment Should Nurses Receive for Their Services?

The whole health care payment scheme has changed in recent years. Retrospective reimbursement or governmental payment of actual cost after the fact is now prospective prepayment. Such prepayment for hospitals and physicians is limited to "reasonable" cost based on averages, because health care cost containment has become a critical national economic issue. Many persons believe that the concept of *managed care* should have been named *managed cost* because of its cost containment origins. These authors, however, continue to believe that costs can be managed without sacrificing the quality of care, and therefore see managed care as a goal as yet unmet.

Salaries for entering nurses are competitive with those in other service occupations. Because nursing provides around-the-clock service, shift differential wages usually prevail. Few other health or social services fields offer comparable earning power while pursuing advanced career preparation. Although differences in basic education may not affect initial earning power, advancement to better paying positions favors those persons with advanced degrees. These persons will assume leadership positions of increased responsibility in specialized practice, management and administration, teaching, and research. Although salary increases over time are somewhat compressed in nursing, there are other economic compensations, e.g., expanding job markets in nontraditional settings and advanced positions. A few nurse administrators in large organizations make salaries in the six-figure range. Opportunities for nurses as health care entrepreneurs are increasing daily.

Clearly, some of the rewards for service are not monetary. As one colleague wrote, "Aren't we truly blessed in being able to contribute to others and our profession through our knowledge and experience?"

What Will Be the Influence of Nursing on Health Care Policy?

Despite the many issues facing the profession and the occasional lack of organized nurse power, nursing is beginning to value equally the caring and scientific components of the profession. Nurses are recapturing the autonomy and indepen-

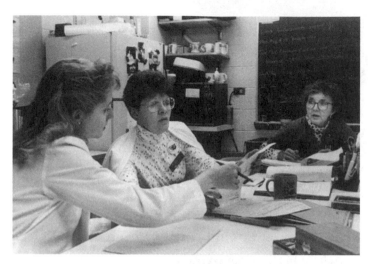

Nurses empower each other to influence health care policy.

dence that many of our nursing ancestors had. We are learning to put forth a nursing model of health care so that we will be viewed as colleagues of other health professionals rather than as extensions of them. We could learn much about influence from some of our nurse predecessors; Florence Nightingale, Margaret Sanger, and Lillian Wald did not sidestep the issues of their day when they intervened to halt the miseries of the battlefield, unwanted pregnancies, and urban poverty. They also did not always agree with nursing or medical colleagues, or find support from them. Wald, for example, also did not always agree with politicians or financial backers. These nurses persevered, however, because they believed they were right about the essence, nature, and value of nursing service to society.

We need to remember that nursing is not the only profession with issues about unique services, educational preparation, and payment for services. Not only is medicine oversupplied in certain specialties—increasingly, physicians are being salaried rather than receiving unrestricted fees for professional services. Dentists, once in great demand, are finding society has greatly diminished needs for traditional dental services. Nurses should also remember that issues and crises can be growth producing. Nursing is growing as a profession and its practitioners can grow as professional persons. From this perspective, many professional issues can be understood better as having maturational and situational aspects, as do other crises. Optimistically, nurses are taking the best of nursing art and melding it with scientific nursing to create a better health care future. See Ellis and Hartley's (1994) *Nursing in Today's World: Challenges, Issues and Trends* and McCloskey's (1994) *Current Issues in Nursing* for other perspectives.

Changing Images

Diversity

Because most nurses are white and female, there is a great need for multicultural diversity as well as more men in nursing. As one young man who is now an R.N. reported,

> Five years ago I made a decision to become a nurse because I believe that the nursing profession provides countless opportunities to help others, especially the sick. The nursing program is demanding, vigorous, and somewhat stressful; however, I did enjoy my nursing education. In fact, the program itself not only provided students with excellent nursing knowledge but also gave us a lot of opportunities for personal growth and interpersonal relationship development. . . When I was a second year nursing student, I started to volunteer and I have been actively involved in my church to help coordinate health promotion programs. . . Nursing can help make a person more sensitive and compassionate to others, and most important of all, in some instances, it offers what medicine does not offer to patients when caring is needed and cure is not possible.
>
> Before entering nursing school, I hardly understood what a sick person might feel or what it is like to be sick, because I had been blessed with good health. . . Compassion is the heart of nursing, or it is not nursing if without compassion. I strongly feel that all our technologies can never replace the human touch. As a nurse I respect individuals' value and dignity. I can sense my patients' pains. I also empathize with what they and their families are going through. I can still clearly remember my emotional reactions when I was doing my pediatric med-surg rotation: as I was caring for the little and young patients with cancer and seeing the painful procedures that they had to go through, I had tears in my eyes and would want to go into the restroom (so no person would see me crying). I am a man and I cry for my patients. Caring for suffering patients makes me really understand the true meaning and importance of compassion. . . Can men be in nursing?—absolutely— yes! [*Andy Chan, BSN, RN*]

Specialty Areas of Practice

The specialty areas of practice for nursing are of two basic kinds: clinical specialty and functional specialty. Clinical specialty parallels the specialization that occurred in medicine and other components of the health care delivery system. There are nurse specialists for the following specialties:

- ❑ Age groups—that is, pediatric, adult, and geriatric
- ❑ Illnesses—for example, coronary disease, diabetes, and cancer
- ❑ Abilities or disabilities—for example, midwifery, sexuality, burns, rehabilitation
- ❑ Locales—for example, ambulatory care units, operating rooms, emergency rooms or trauma centers, home-care, and community health

Some specialists in clinical areas are certified. Certification may be public, with state licensure, or private, that is, voluntary—such as through professional organizations.

Functional specialty refers to the following activities: management or administration, research, and teaching. All clinical specialty areas have opportunities for nurses to combine a clinical specialty with a functional one. In recent years, the trend has been to consolidate functions so that it is unusual to practice solely as a clinical nurse specialist without taking on functional responsibility (e.g., as a coordinator for staff or patient education). Other trends include consolidation of specialties (e.g. women's health, family practice) and consolidation of services across various settings to provide *seamless care.*

Traditional and Nontraditional Career Options

Traditional career options exist in acute-care settings and community health, and parallel the traditional medical specialty areas, including medical and surgical nursing, obstetric and pediatric nursing, psychiatric mental health nursing, and operating room nursing. These options increasingly reflect the consolidation mentioned above.

Several trends related to practice options are as follows:

❏ More practice options are possible than ever before.
❏ There is a trend toward more advanced preparation (i.e., BSN or master of science in nursing).
❏ External barriers (traditions and legalities) to practice options are presently decreasing, but have the potential to go either way.
❏ More attempts are being made at collaborative practice among health professionals.
❏ The growing movement toward primary care and community and home health care provides tremendous potential for nurses.
❏ There is increasing emphasis on wellness programs in schools, residential living communities, and industry.

Some nursing practice options include the following, which require educational preparation beyond the initial R.N. licensure:

Nurse–practitioner: an ambulatory care nurse with advanced skills in assessment of the physical and psychosocial health and illness statuses of persons in a variety of settings.
Clinical nurse specialist: an expert in a particular practice, such as psychiatric mental health or medical–surgical nursing.
Nurse–midwife
Nurse anesthetist

Another role sometimes seen as the domain of nurses is that of *case manager* or *clinical manager.* Some nurses might argue that nursing case management has long been a general function of nurses. New emphasis on cost containment compels even greater care efficiency. Now nurses may hesitate to choose these roles out of concern that management efficiency will erode clinical nursing care. If nurses do not assume case management, however, others will do it in the name of efficiency. Nurses can view this reality as an opportunity to exert control over nursing practice, influence health care policy, and demonstrate both efficiency and effectiveness of nursing care. Master's-prepared nurses with advanced clinical and management skills may be ideally suited to this role. Cody (1994), however, suggests another possibility: "The role of *case manager*, if the term is taken literally, seems to this author to fit only one person per "case"—and that is the *person* whose "case" is at issue" (p. 181). Under managed care, the care being managed is not just nursing care. Therefore, some organizations do not see this role as within the domain of nursing.

A *physician's assistant* (PA), a role sometimes occupied by nurses, is NOT an expanded nursing role! It is actually a dependent medical role, i.e., that of physician extender.

Future of Practice Options

Nurses themselves must take a leadership role in deciding what part of health care is nursing, and then follow through to control that nursing care. Retaining control requires initiative and diligence for a number of reasons: 1) Because nurses are mostly female, it is often assumed that they will take the dependent or assistive role; 2) Most nurses have fewer years of formal education than other health professionals have; and 3) There are large numbers of nurses who do seem to prefer to be directed rather than to take initiative. Given the size of the health care industry, nursing leadership must come not just from nurses prepared in graduate programs, with master's and doctoral degrees, but from baccalaureate graduates and other R.N.s as well.

Although some employers do not differentiate among associate degree, diploma, and baccalaureate graduates, nurses need to find or generate job opportunities that allow them to practice as prepared and to grow to their full potential. Many students begin to explore practice options through part-time employment as a nurse assistant during their formal education. The realities of the workplace look different from the student and the employee perspectives. The opportunity to observe how a variety of nurses practice in different ways can be instructive.

*N*ursing's Independent, Interdependent, and Dependent Functions

Function is the kind of action or activity proper to a person. To describe some-one's function, we would note the person's behavior. Let us look at what characterizes independent, interdependent, and dependent behavior in nursing. Traditionally, nursing has assumed a subordinate position in health care and has performed functions auxiliary to medicine that were detailed in Doctors' Orders, an old term for the medical plan of care. Thus, historically nurses' functions were seen as dependent on medical definition and nurses were seen as demonstrating dependent behavior. Undoubtedly, such labeling was largely a reflection of social custom and the roles that women often assumed.

Dependent nursing behavior is performed under delegated medical authority or supervision, or according to a priori routines. Routine administration of prescription medications without attention to side effects or clients' learning needs might be an example of a dependent nursing behavior. Historically, much of traditional nursing activity has been giving care or doing treatments according to the dictates of the physicians' or doctors' order book. The current image of the professional nurse, as advanced by nurse leaders, is that of a baccalaureate graduate who is a more independent career colleague of the physician.

Independent nursing behavior is initiated as a result of the nurse's own knowledge and skills, rather than as a result of delegated authority from the physician. Although some nurses may practice independently, it is not the norm for practice options. Even if most nurses do not believe that independent practice is currently feasible or something they want to do, they may be interested in independent behavior.

Mundinger (1980) preferred the term **autonomous** nursing practice to *independent* nursing practice. She believed that although nursing may encompass some physician-directed activities, both nursing theory components and unique nursing practice will be involved. Mundinger differentiated autonomous function from dependent function in the following way:

> Knowing why, when, and how to position clients and doing so skillfully makes the function an autonomous therapy. But, if physicians order it, how can it be autonomous? If physicians order an action nurses would not do in the absence of those orders, if they do not know why or when to do so, it is probably a dependent rather than autonomous function. But if the nurse has the knowledge and the skill to initiate and carry out the actions and answer for the results, then it is autonomous (p. 4).

Nursing has independent, interdependent, and dependent functions, as do many professions. It was also a reflection of earlier times in nursing history that physicians' dependence on nurses to fulfill their medical plans was seldom acknowledged.

Remember that health care is medical and nursing care. Remember also that medicine and nursing differ in their major foci of cure and care respectively. Although medicine and nursing are separate, they are not always distinctly so. **Interdependent nursing behavior** designates overlapping functions shared between nursing and medicine and speaks to the desirability of collegial relationships in which each profession contributes according to its knowledge, skills, and focus. Overlapping functions may occur in many areas. Nurses, by law and also by virtue of their education, experience, etc., practice within certain limits, as do all professions. In some settings, the limits are more flexible: in some third world countries, there are few physicians, and even in more rural U.S. settings, on-site medical assistance is limited. In these areas nurses may practice quite independently. In other areas, especially in critical care units and primary care centers, activities such as monitoring complex equipment or ordering diagnostic tests may seem more independent, but strict regulations or prior agreements about steps to be taken in special circumstances may leave little room for autonomous decision making.

If nursing is a profession, most of the practice should consist of independent functions. Nursing as a profession has only recently begun to assert its autonomy.

Professional autonomy requires that nursing find ways to expand practice options to accommodate independent behavior of students currently being prepared. The profession should research more vigorously ways to increase the cost effectiveness of nursing care within managed care, and also to function within the hospital setting without loss of professional identity .

Educational Opportunities and Requirements

Just as aspiring nurses should know about practice options, they should also know about the educational opportunities and requirements in nursing. Nursing is one of the few fields in which such a wide range of formal programs educate practitioners who have the same legal registration, that is, RN. In the past, the opportunity to enter licensed practice in nursing was available to persons with little, if any, formal education beyond high school. Such programs preparing licensed practical or vocational nurses, however, are being phased out, or increased to two-year programs.

Currently, the minimal educational preparation for RN licensure is 2 years of college study, culminating in an associate degree. Such programs are widely available in community or junior colleges. Associate degree programs in nursing also may be available in colleges and universities offering the baccalaureate degree. A widespread move is under way to require the baccalaureate degree for eligibility to receive professional licensure. With this move has come a clear intent to exempt persons who do not have this educational preparation but who were already practicing as RNs before the change. This exemption would mean that when the legislation goes into effect, all those persons previously prepared for this level of licensure with lesser education will be accepted as "professional." A similar exemption provision has been made for persons who practiced a clinical specialty before the introduction of specialty certification requirements. This practice of *grandfathering* or *accepting* results from legalities that control practice rather than from the generosity of women trying to be nice. Likewise, the very term *professional* as a legal adjective has a meaning different from that intended when differentiating among occupations.

Diploma or hospital schools once offered the most common programs to prepare nurses for RN licensure. Today, most nurses are being prepared with associate degrees in institutions of higher education offering regular college credit. For those persons who are academically qualified and economically able, initial enrollment in a college or university program leading to the baccalaureate degree with a nursing major (BSN) is highly recommended. Other so-called generic baccalaureate programs may offer the bachelor of science (BS) or bachelor of arts (BA) degree. There are also undergraduate programs in nursing that enable persons who are already RNs to complete the baccalaureate in nursing through RN Studies or RN Completion programs, for example. Because nursing as a profession values mature practitioners, increasing numbers of universities are offering the first professional degree at the graduate level. These programs enroll persons who are not RNs but who already hold an undergraduate degree in another field. A variety of educational opportunities are available beyond baccalaureate preparation in nursing. They usually require 1 or 2 additional years of full-time study (or the equivalent) for the completion of a master's degree.

Basic educational programs in nursing prepare nurses for generalist, entry-level staff nurse positions. After graduation from state-approved schools, nurses take a state licensing examination before receiving recognition as RNs. All RNs are expected to have certain basic skill competencies. Increasingly, hospitals recognize the gap between the best of educational preparations and the demands of nursing in the real world. It is in the best interest of hospitals to bridge this gap, which they do with extensive orientation programs. Many nursing schools and service settings provide internships or opportunities to work as nursing assistants while completing basic programs. In addition to increasing competency, these opportunities provide wages while learning. Experience as a general staff nurse usually precedes assignment to a specialty area. Indeed, the changing image of nursing is well reflected in the growing number of areas for specialty practice and the many nontraditional career options.

Nurses who intend to advance significantly in *clinical nursing* (e.g., as midwives or nurse practitioners) are expected to receive advanced educational preparation in clinical nursing as opposed to some other functional specialty—for example, business administration. The purpose of master's education in nursing is to prepare nursing leaders for advanced clinical practice, teaching, and administrative positions. Nurses obtain degrees that are basically of two kinds: professional and academic. The professional degree, often the master of nursing (MN), may require fewer credits and tends not to have a research emphasis. Academic degrees are commonly the master of science (MS) or master of arts (MA). These graduate degrees usually take 1 to 2 years of full-time study (or the equivalent) and have a research emphasis, possibly requiring a formal project or thesis. Although full-time study may be educationally preferable, most nurses have multiple responsibilities and find part-time study necessary.

Nurses who expect to do independent research or teach in colleges offering graduate degrees should expect to be doctorally prepared. The doctor of philosophy (PhD) is the most common academic doctoral degree in nursing. Doctoral education emphasizes theory development and research skill. Doctoral programs in nursing have recently added postdoctoral fellowship programs that are comparable with those available in other sciences. A variety of educational opportunities are available at the doctoral level. Some common graduate professional degrees earned by nurses include the doctor of nursing science (DNS), doctor of nursing (DN), or, in other fields, such degrees as the juris doctor (JD), doctor of education (EdD), or doctor of public health (DPH). Perhaps the most exciting and significant development is that all major educational opportunities essential to professional nursing practice are available within nursing education.

The student body within all educational programs is becoming more diverse, e.g., many students are older, and more racial diversity is represented. More students are international, especially at the graduate level. Students at all levels are more globally aware as they travel personally or via the internet. Many students who grew up with computer technology are contributing to the diversity in technological skills among students.

Leadership

Leadership by nurses is needed for both nursing and health care. Nurses develop leadership abilities within educational programs and beyond. In addition to the formal and required educational activities that are aimed toward leadership development, individuals can initiate many other meaningful strategies.

A strategy is both a plan and action; it is the means to an end or goal. We are interested in the individual goal of self-actualization because we believe nurses, like their patients, have inherent self-actualization tendencies. We are interested in the professional goal of influencing health care policy because we believe nurses will move policy in the direction of helping clients of health care delivery to realize their inherent potential. How a profession is viewed by society is in large measure influenced by how the profession views itself and makes its worth known. The profession's view of itself arises from the self-image of individual practitioners. Each nurse needs to consider self-concept and its relationship to personal growth, the profession's image, and nursing's influence on health care policy.

In the lay view, all nurses tend to be the same. In the past, this view has sometimes considered nursing as a part of medicine. Public media have also tended to portray the nurse more often as a sweet young thing than as a mature practitioner.

For nursing to influence health care policy is a big order. You may have heard nursing scorned by feminists as traditional women's work done by unassertive workers. Sometimes, perhaps, this has been so. It is true that nurses have not always banded together to use their personal power as have feminists. Moreover, they have not regularly demonstrated the use of coalition strategies that politicians find so successful. These circumstances suggest that both individual and group strategies can and should be used by nurses of both genders to achieve personal self-actualization and to influence health care policy.

Individual Strategies

Selected individual strategies for increasing self-actualization and nursing influence are summarized in Table 12-1.

Most professionals are generally well-informed about society and the world. Professionals recognize that knowledge is power, whether in science, economics, or politics. Being well-informed is necessary for the strategy of effective planning. Membership in the American Nurses Association now provides a monthly copy of the American Journal of Nursing, an important source of information. Membership in the National Student Nurses' Association will provide a similar benefit. Familiarize yourself also with popular business classics that have been the basis of corporate restructuring, e.g., Hammer and Champy's *Reengineering the Corporation: A Manifesto for Business Revolution* (1994). All strategies suggested are intended to be points of departure for later professional growth and development.

Unless you know what you want personally, it is unlikely you will get it. To control both your personal and professional lives, you must be active rather than

TABLE 12-1 *Individual Strategies for Self-Growth and Nursing Influence*

Use information	Plan ahead	Participate	Be competent
Use person resources	Know yourself	Learn independently	Write and speak well
Gain access to professional literature through indexes and abstracts	Set goals	Interact with other health professionals	Project a professional image
Read widely	Share aspirations	Join health organizations	Assume accountability
		Mobilize support	Document practice
		Provide curriculum input	
		Support research	Commit yourself to lifelong learning
		Find a mentor	Strive for excellence
		Fight sex discrimination	

reactive. One reason for setting goals is to be able to identify obstacles in reaching them. With planning, it is possible to maintain a career focus even if you work part-time or anticipate time away from a career because of family or child-care responsibilities.

Not all persons who make long-term career commitments anticipate the potential personal conflicts that career decisions may provoke. A profession such as nursing, with expanding science and practice horizons, needs persons who are not reluctant to seize the available opportunities. When external barriers to independent behavior are removed, such as when laws and policies are changed, internal barriers such as lack of confidence and low self-esteem assume increased importance. Such unrecognized psychological barriers make some persons reluctant to plan and accept responsibility for their decisions. After all, hapless victims of circumstances are seldom held accountable for events beyond their control. Do you share your planning and aspirations with your significant others to gain their understanding, support, and encouragement?

Being informed and planning ahead are dead-end strategies unless they are accompanied by active participation. Several questions to ask yourself about participation follow:

Are you using your abilities and assets? To the fullest? To what end?
Do you give positive feedback and unsolicited support to peers for their accomplishments?
Do you recognize the urgency of research participation by all nurses?

Participation involves risk-taking behavior. It implies conviction about goals and willingness to be identified with them.

Competence is both an individual strategy and a goal. Nurses need to demonstrate competence in public ways to change the media image of nurses and nurs-

TABLE 12-2 *Group Strategies for Self-Growth and Nursing Influence*

Participate in politics	Build peer groups	Join formal organizations
Inform others and mobilize support	Form study groups	NSNA
Form coalitions	Interact with other health professionals	Sigma Theta Tau International
Vote	Create multidisciplinary teams	ANA when eligible
Work for candidates		NLN
Run for office		Health organizations

ing. Such change is critical to making nursing a potent force in shaping health care policy.

Sometimes we use the term *competent* to mean taking responsibility for your own actions and making appropriate decisions. You need to feel a certain fundamental personal competence to be personally powerful and to control your own life. In this sense, personal competence is basic to any professional competence. An extension of this competence is an ability to adapt to personal and professional stresses. Nurses need stress management skills to maintain the equilibrium necessary for their own adaptive living. Ideally, they also ought to be able to model the adaptive coping strategies they are advocating for their clients.

Professional certification as a validation of competency is an expression of commitment to caring that goes beyond the minimum to which society is entitled by basic licensure. Competent practitioners, managers, and leaders will be more effective change agents for improved health care delivery.

Group Strategies

Table 12-2 lists group strategies for self growth and nursing influence. Practitioners who have become competent through individual strategies for growth realize that change agents have power in groups.

Two powerful professional organizations of special significance for students are Sigma Theta Tau International and the autonomous National Student Nurses' Association. Sigma Theta Tau is open to both baccalaureate students and graduates and thereby enables students to identify early with a professional group of lasting professional importance. The NSNA, although comprised only of students, provides an important avenue for developing professional group skills. Another national organization that is concerned specifically with nursing is NLN. Membership in this organization is not limited to nurses, although the organization aims to influence nursing education and practice. An encouraging recent development is that nursing organizations have formed coalitions to advance the profession of nursing and to promote nursing's role in meeting the health care needs of society.

Professional Opportunities

The following selected opportunities are briefly described and only illustrate a few of the many available.

Develop a Significant Career

Nursing offers wide-ranging opportunities to develop a socially responsible and long-lasting career. Persons need nursing care from birth to death, so nurses have clients of all ages; also the geographic need for nursing is universal and timeless. Persons who have experienced professional nursing recognize and appreciate its social contribution. As health care reform continues, nursing, with its person-centered care focus, has an important role to play in advocating for person-centered care.

Nursing is nursing wherever it happens. Many health care settings need nurses around the clock, increasing both the number of jobs available and the compensation offered. Interstate relocation for nurses is facilitated by a national licensing examination. Licensure in a new state is usually expedited by endorsement of previous licensure.

Nursing, in contrast to most careers, offers professional status after baccalaureate education. Smaller initial investments of both money and education provide beginning entry into the occupational field, and this entry enables early gainful employment and relevant experience. The similarity of nursing across settings and specialties also enhances career security and the number of opportunities for movement and variety within nursing practice—especially if practitioners practice life-long learning. Additionally, persons entering nursing can become advanced specialty practitioners, scientists, administrators, teachers, and business entrepreneurs.

Practice Creative Nursing in Unlimited Settings

Creativity means different things to different people. To create is to evolve from one's own thoughts. Few answers exist about the specifics of creativity as a thought process. People have creative ideas, perceptions, and experiences. Creativity is both a process and a product of creative behavior. Because creativity is a uniquely human quality, creativity or creative potential undoubtedly exists to some degree within each of us. Nurses can be as creative as other professionals; they can be creative in the ways in which they both practice nursing and expand nursing practice. A recent graduate of a baccalaureate program felt inspired both to continue her education and to *create* a vision of a Family Nurse Practitioner clinic that was very real to her:

> As you walk into the clinic, on the left side there will be pictures of all the patients. How wonderful would you feel to walk into a clinic and have a picture of you on the wall? I believe that it would give each patient a feeling of home and warmth and comfort. There will be classical music playing and the smell inside will be that

of freshly cut flowers, not alcohol or antiseptics. The clinic will be warm enough to not leave you with goose bumps while in a gown. [*Monica Patel, R.N.*]

Whether or not this is the kind of a clinic you would *create*, you can imagine the ambience and uniquely personal nature of her creation. Nursing urgently needs creative leadership and creative practice: in a cost-conscious health care world, both nursing leaders and practitioners will create ways to demonstrate efficient and effective nursing care. That is, nursing care will produce the desired effect with a minimum of effort, expense, or waste. This demonstration will require creative problem solving and innovation. Innovation is the introduction of new methods; the National Institute of Nursing Research gave a top priority to funding research about both AIDS (human immunodeficiency virus [HIV]) and innovative nursing care delivery patterns.

Innovative professionals shape their practice arenas within the limits of law and policy, but creatively extend their control and influence. Creative ideas and behavior start with one person. No one can tell someone else how to be creative. Each individual's most immediate sphere of influence is over oneself, but sharing creative approaches may stimulate creativity in others, so influence can be far-reaching. Innovation in nursing will come from nurses.

Innovation is also uniqueness in the way of doing things. As Peters (1987) suggested, "[The] value of uniqueness as a source of empowerment is the basis for market value" (p. 142). This distinction suggests that creative nurses will convince the public about what creative nursing is worth. Nurses as professionals must assume responsibility for demonstrating their value to society and must say, "This is what we have to offer!" Even beginning nursing students will learn about nursing's unique service. Innovation in nursing care will come especially from new persons entering the field with new perspectives. How would you be creative in nursing? The opportunities for you are twofold: to strive to increase your creativity, and to bring innovation to nursing.

The authors assert that professional nursing is professional nursing wherever it is practiced, i.e., in unlimited settings. Kiplinger and Kiplinger (1996), citing statistics from the Bureau of Labor Statistics, claim that the assistive jobs in health care (including home-care aides, home health aides, and medical assistants) will be some of the fastest-growing jobs between now and 2005 (p. 3). They also note that care for the elderly will be provided by a variety of persons including the above and nurses.

No one knows exactly how the future healthcare system will evolve. We do know, however, that persons' needs for nursing care will increase. There are many reasons for this increase, including the following:

Health care is more cost effective than illness care.
The need for illness care will continue and increase for some populations.
Health and illness care is needed across the life span.

To capitalize on this situation, professional nurses must exercise creativity in their practice. That is how they will maintain control of nursing practice and assure that the public's needs for quality *professional* nursing care are met. We predict that location of practice will be less important for professional nurses than their ability to demonstrate their worth and effectiveness through creative practice. Why are we optimistic?

❏ Nurses are health care experts!
❏ Nurses are illness care experts!
❏ Health and illness care is needed by all persons from birth to death.

Extend Nursing Science Through Research and Theory Development

Few aspiring nurses are aware of the opportunities in nursing to be a research scientist or a theorist. Given that not many nurses may choose this role, perhaps this point seems minor. However, such a lack of awareness suggests that many practicing nurses do not recognize and publicize the scientific potential of nursing. Therefore, young persons who aspire to health science careers generally may not realize the particular opportunities in nursing for exciting scientific investigation. Furthermore, the loss to nursing of such scientific person-power is unfortunate at this stage in nursing's scientific development.

Nursing needs to increase its ability to predict what the outcomes of specific nursing interventions will be in actual practice. The research to support such prediction is known as clinical trials, intervention research, or experiments conducted in the real world of practice. Theory development is needed to both guide research and increase nursing's scientific credibility.

Nursing currently is evolving as a scientific community with national and international visibility and political influence. Health care reform has indeed created a window of opportunity for nursing as a science and profession, that is, to help solve many current and future health care dilemmas. National research funding is increasing rapidly for nursing science. Scholarly societies, research forums, and journals unite nurse–scientists. Nursing, as Meleis (1985) said, "is one of very few disciplines that isolates the components of research design and methodology and helps students develop necessary skills to undertake a research career" (p. 304). Yet, because not all nurses consider themselves scientists, nurse–scientists have unique opportunities within the professional nursing and health care communities. Also, because nursing is a new science, there is much uncharted territory. Opportunities to extend nursing science through research and theory development are particularly rich for interested professional nurses.

Manage or Administer Health Care Organizations

Health care encompasses medical and nursing care as well as a number of other clinical disciplines. Nurses represent the largest number of health care providers, and they have always been excellent and practical problem solvers. Increasingly, nurses are recognizing that complex health care organizations require contemporary nurses to have additional skills related to management, leadership, and fiscal responsibility. Long gone are the days when the "head nurse" on a hospital unit was concerned only with nursing care. With recent consolidation of middle management positions, even traditional titles such as "head nurse" are being changed. However, the need to "manage" and "administer" nursing and health care is more crucial than ever before.

Some corporate directors of health care might argue that nursing is best done by nurses and managing is best done by professional managers. However, management and administration are not foreign concepts for nurses. Baccalaureate nursing programs offer courses that focus on nursing management; social, political, and professional issues that affect nursing practice; and leadership. Students learn how to assess a health care setting, analyze nursing within the setting, and design planned change. Students learn individual and collective strategies to influence professional nursing practice and health care delivery. They also learn management theory and organizational principles. Increasingly, opportunities for beginning-level management positions in nursing are being filled by baccalaureate-prepared nurses; nurses with advanced nursing preparation fill such positions when these nurses are available.

Management and administrative positions at the corporate level require more sophisticated skills and knowledge related to budgeting and general business matters. This preparation is available in master's and doctoral programs in nursing, although many nurses have sought advanced degrees in business administration. Such preparation, from either source, opens the door to the corporate boardroom. Here, nursing has the potential to participate in senior management decisions. The unique perspective that nurses bring to the boardroom is the understanding of nursing care requirements.

In many health care settings—for example, nursing homes, home-care agencies, and community health agencies—nurses may be the only health professionals consistently on site or available in the agency. Clearly, it is in nursing's best interest to assume leadership in many of these situations, and it also may be in society's best interest for nursing to do so. As Meleis (1985) commented, "Nursing goals are generally congruent with those of the recipients of its care; nursing operates from a health and holistic approach and purports to enhance coping and harmony with one's environment" (p. 305). Kelly and Joel (1995) devote an entire chapter in *Dimensions of Professional Nursing* to "Leadership for an era of change."

Teach Consumers or Professionals

In addition to practicing, researching, and administering, nurses teach. In the past, the particulars of this teaching role were more often derived from physician prescription or doctor's orders than is currently the case. With the American Nurses Association (ANA) publication of its social policy statement in 1980, nursing was defined as "the diagnosis and treatment of human responses to actual or potential health problems" (p. 3).

As Mundinger (1980) wrote,

> Unhealthful responses, or the absence of some healthful responses, often can be the primary reason for nursing care. . . . Teaching and counseling for resolution and

self-care of disease or pathology are unique elements of professional nursing. Pathology resolution is the scope of medicine; resolution of responses to pathology is nursing. . . . Nursing is one of the only professions using primary physical and emotional data and intellectual and hands-on skill to identify and resolve unhealthful responses. . . . Only nurses have the full scope for identification and care to resolve health problems (p. 58).

The functional abilities that define health are in part those abilities needed to perform the activities of daily living. The necessary knowledge and skill-learning may be related to such basic activities as eating, sleeping, and exercising. Additionally, persons may need to learn basic information about body structure and function to promote and maintain health or to fully rehabilitate after medical intervention for disease.

In the future, many more opportunities will exist for nurses to teach clients outside the hospital setting. With hospital stays decreasing in length and increasing in the severity of illness and the level of care required, much health teaching by nurses will be done preadmission and postdischarge, and in alternative health care settings. Increasingly, nurses will be teaching family members how they can play a more active role in home health care for clients of all ages, but especially for the elderly. They will teach basic physical care as well as how to do treatments and dressings and manage pain, diets, and medications. The explosion of health education materials available via computer on-line is mind-boggling.

Many nurses find themselves drawn to the role of teacher as a way to greatly increase their influence on the improvement of nursing care. A heavy demand will remain for teachers of nurses in all levels of basic and continuing educational programs. In baccalaureate and higher degree programs, the role of teacher will be combined with that of researcher–scientist.

*B*e a Health Care Entrepreneur

Throughout this book, "health" has been consistently claimed as the domain of nursing. An *entrepreneur* is a contractor and also someone who undertakes projects requiring unconventional activity and some risk. Nurses are logical persons to be health care entrepreneurs. Private-duty nurses who provided nursing care at home during the early 20th century may have been the first health care entrepreneurs. Perhaps a difference between turn-of-the-century nurses and nurses today is that early entrepreneurs usually worked independently of institutions. Today's nurse–entrepreneurs work both independently of and within institutions and formal organizations. A new word has been coined: intrapreneur. *Intrapreneurs,* in the health care industry as in other businesses, offer nontraditional services within traditional organizations. These services not only provide opportunities for creative nurses but also enable large health care agencies to market health care competitively. Traditional acute-care centers are diversifying their "product lines" to offer services that meet nursing needs beyond hospitalization. Such services may include screening, counseling, and instruction before same-day surgery, home health care planning and coordination, extended skilled nursing care, and individualized home care. Additionally, the alternative birthing arrangements originally offered by enterprising nurse–midwives currently are being sponsored by hospitals eager to meet consumer demand and claim a market share.

Entrepreneurial practice activities made headlines in the 1970s as *independent nursing practice*. Since then, many nurses have set up entrepreneurial services to help clients manage chemical dependency and severe pain, for example. Orem set up a consulting firm based on her unique theoretical perspective. Nurses are also consultants to retirement communities and businesses such as organizational management and accounting firms, insurance companies, architects, and manufacturers of health care equipment. In 1991, the National Nurses in Business Association published *How I Became a Nurse Entrepreneur: Tales From 50 Nurses in Business*.

By their very nature, entrepreneurial opportunities arise over time through the originality of professionals entering the field. Who knows what opportunities your generation of practitioners will conceive?

Apply Computer Skills to Nursing

Although computers are not new to health care, their importance has escalated rapidly in recent years. It is now apparent that computerization throughout the health care industry affects nursing profoundly. To ignore this reality is to enter the next century walking backward. Just as the industrial revolution affected manufacturing, computerization has affected information processing. Computerized information processing is the key that enabled pricing of health care linked to medical diagnosis-related groups. Now, much client-related information is collected and processed by way of computers as the basis for important health care decisions.

Nursing was late to recognize the need to integrate nursing information with other client-related information. Also the complexity and nature of nursing information contributed to the lag in translating it to computer format. Attempts to standardize nursing diagnoses have been important advances toward nursing computerization. Identification of the Nursing Minimum Data Set (Werley & Lang, 1988) was an important effort to compile comparable uniform data across clinical settings. Nursing needs such integrated information to determine nursing costs per client, per medical diagnosis, per nursing diagnosis, per care delivery unit, and so forth. The computerized Nursing Intervention Classification (NIC) and Nursing Outcome Classification (NOC) extend original efforts to integrate nursing information into computerized health care data bases.

Nurses with computer skills will find varied opportunities to use these skills in the health care world of today and tomorrow. The full array of skills will be needed. These skills range from word processing to file management to accessing information. More advanced skills enable the computer to be a management tool using data base and spreadsheet strategies.

The most important computer skill is openness to learning the basics of a technology that will have applications in both professional and personal life. Computers can make many personal and professional tasks easier. The same word processing skills used to write personal letters and term papers help nurses create

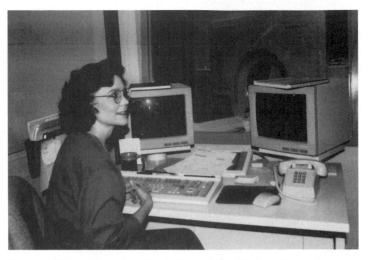

Computerization will profoundly affect nursing and the health care industry.

computerized care plans. Accessing information can include accessing college academic records, on-line personalized student evaluations from an instructor, professional literature, or client data bases. The American Nurses Association now publishes its Career Directory on line in addition to maintaining a NursingWorld website. Practicing nurses can apply computer skills to accessing the continuing education information that will keep practice current through lifelong learning. Technology available for entrepreneurial nurses (as well as other health professionals) to make services available on-line nationwide will force resolution of nursing licensure issues that were previously the business of states and are now being revisited.

Despite nursing's rather late interest in computing, there are many software programs that fit nursing's many clinical specialties and functional areas. These programs include general education in basic areas, for example, physiology, safety, medications, and case simulations. Software on general education in these areas helps nurses practice problem-solving skills in preparation for clinical activity or state board licensure exams; applying basic computer skills with user-friendly programs, students can review for state boards in either a tutorial or a practice test mode. Basic computer literacy also includes being able to read basic computer-generated reports.

Other applications of computer skills include engaging in data management for staffing and scheduling, accessing expert practice consultants, writing resumes, constructing tests, writing papers and presentations, and finding appropriate educational materials for client–patient use. Interactive computer instruction, which combines computer program basics with videotape examples, holds much promise for learning both manual skills (psychomotor) and feeling (affective) responses. Nurses can apply computer skills as both consumers and creators of such media.

Working collectively, nurses could advance nursing into profession-wide computer literacy that would do wonders for nurses' intelligence-gathering in the world of health care. User groups, message systems, and public domain software sponsored by nurses and for nurses would be helpful. Use of computers is less a technical skill problem and more a mental attitude opportunity. It is not the equipment per se but what it allows you to do that offers the great potential. In the past, nurses used mechanical lifts to augment their muscles in lifting and moving clients; now robots do such lifting, and also some hospital delivery tasks that nurses once did. Data management requires that nursing expand its collective brain power to work smarter by applying computer technology. Commitment to doing this will ensure that nursing as a profession is not left behind in this mind-boggling age of health care technology. Such technology will always require that nurses supplement the technology with human perception and analysis. As the futurist Naisbitt (1984) claimed, increased technology (hi-tech) will only increase the importance of human caring (hi-touch).

Promote Sports Health and Physical Fitness

Given the increasing interest in health and physical fitness, nursing has also been late to recognize the professional service opportunities in this area. Sports medicine and sports injuries have dominated the scene. There is even a well-established journal, *The Physician and Sports Medicine.* Interest in prevention usually follows rather than precedes interest in cure. Perhaps a journal titled *The Nurse and Sports Health* will be forthcoming. Much interest in this area is focused on amateur and professional competitive sports. However, health and fitness related to lifetime individual sports offer the potential involvement of an entire society. Consultancy to retirement communities suggests explorations in this area may be under way, and nurses will develop this window of opportunity.

The physical fitness of children has come under increasing scrutiny and criticism in recent years. When funds for public school education diminish, societal interest in nonacademic aspects of public education wanes. Art, music, and physical education programs are often at risk of cuts or closures. However, given the overall increased interest in sports, other segments of society may assume responsibility for children's health and physical fitness. As they do, nurses have much valuable information and many insights to share. It could be argued that the needs for physical fitness and sports health are important for all youths, even before formal public education begins. To accommodate this concern, nurses may increase their consultancy about physical fitness and health to the growing preschool childcare industry.

Fitness facilities in the workplace are also gaining increasing prominence. The traditional occupational health nurse's role is changing from focusing only on injury prevention and treatment in factory settings to health consultation in all kinds of business enterprises.

Pioneer in Space Health

The nurse is a uniquely appropriate health care specialist to staff either a traveling spacecraft or a permanently based space station: For the space nurse, the traditional nursing skills of expert care and sensitive communication will be basic to prolonged confinement. Nurses have the ability to assess and improvise solutions for novel problems of health maintenance and altered health. Carefully selected space travelers will need basic instruction about health maintenance and activities of daily living that a nurse is well-suited to provide. Of course, modifications will need to be made for the confined quarters and zero gravity of space flight.

The manned space activities have produced an enormous amount of new information, especially regarding physiology and communication. Humans' physiologic responses in space include parallels to the known changes after bedrest, for example, loss of skeletal calcium. New problems that accompany weightlessness include the pooling of blood in upper body parts rather than lower extremities. Sleep, nutrition, exercise, and mobility, common concerns for nurses, will become everyday concerns for space travelers. Human psychosocial responses in space will increase the need for purposeful interventions to decrease stress, counteract boredom and isolation from loved ones, and facilitate constructive interpersonal activity.

Space travel is a high-tech enterprise that includes health care equipment utilized for sampling and analyzing various body products and processes. Data from laboratory samples, imaging, and psychological testing will be beamed to Earth for interactive computer analysis, whereas computerized instruction and electronic stimulation can be beamed back to maximize the person's adaptive capabilities for biopsychosocial processes. Computer smart cards will contain complete individual health histories to assist space and Earth personnel. Computer literacy for health specialists will be a given and as important as for early pilot–astronauts. Because computer literacy will be increasingly required in Earth health care settings, it will seem commonplace to space travel. Just as computer science is now making its way into nursing curricula, space science and its attention to physics and bioengineering will not be far behind. Although little of nursing's present scientific literature speaks directly to space nursing today, that, too, will change. If aspiring nurses want to be health care providers in space, they will need to insist upon the necessary education and preparation. Other life scientists are already partners in planning for the activities and equipment that will support space travel and work stations; now nursing needs to assert its interest and expertise to be included. How exciting it will be to test Martha Rogers's theoretical principles about energy fields that transcend time and space in actual space travel!

The applications of early space travel, for example, Velcro (a nylon fabric that can be fastened to itself), dehydrated food, and so forth, are so overshadowed by new marvels of bionics, robotics, and artificial intelligence that it is difficult to imagine what new space-age marvels will soon dominate health care. These marvels will literally bring space nursing to Earth in your professional lifetime.

Arthur C. Clarke's (1986) *July 20, 2019: Life in the 21st Century* opens a window on astounding technologic predictions for space and Earth based on present science and futuristic speculation. If you are looking for a yet-to-be-publicized career option that blends concern for people with space-age technology, read his fantasy and dream, and then remember that some of these space-age technologies—for example, computer assisted self-medication, odorless human waste disposal, and muscle stimulators—already exist.

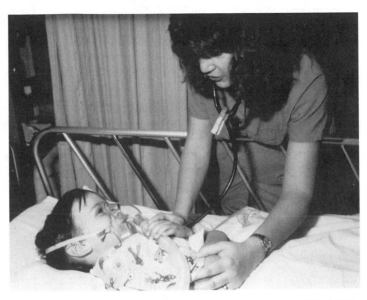

In this new age of modern technology, nurses have the opportunity of maintaining compassion in health care.

Gain Personal Understanding

Long before women generally made commitments to professional careers and work outside the home, nursing was considered a good preparation for living and family life. Although times have changed, nursing remains a scientific discipline and a clinical practice experience that contributes much to personal understanding. Through interactions with clients and their families, nurses expand their life experiences greatly. Many persons entering nursing have not experienced birth or death, poverty or wealth, fatal diagnoses or chronic disability, or pain or suffering. They probably have not observed a rescue from the brink of psychological despair by nurses, the wonder of surgical reconstruction by surgeons, or the togetherness of families in crisis. Although the potential of such experiences may seem frightening, fear of the unknown is perhaps the greatest fear of all. By thoughtful observation and guidance from others, nurses learn ways to help professionally without having lived through experiences personally. In doing so, they gain personal understanding that can, in turn, be used for increased understanding of and caring for others.

Understanding is a thinking function that combines knowledge with comprehension and application. It implies analysis and evaluation. Personal understanding brings together awareness of personal self, interpersonal interactions, but also the relationship between this awareness and these interactions. Nurses are privileged to witness life's most tender and intense moments. Doing so enables one to work through thoughts and feelings about how you would respond if it were your life being so affected; in this way it is possible to confront dilemmas you might otherwise not have anticipated. It is possible to gain personal understanding as a participant observer in the lives of other persons; doing so enriches your own life.

Create Dual Careers

There is an often unrecognized opportunity in nursing to blend nursing with unique personal abilities for a dual career.

Many unique abilities will combine with nursing knowledge and skill to find expression in nursing. Some of us are more artistic, whereas others are more analytic. For example, some practitioners use music, art, or drama regularly in their nursing (e.g., pediatric and psychiatric mental health nurses), whereas for other practitioners, verbal skills may predominate over their mathematical abilities. Furthermore, some of us write better than we speak and relate more comfortably one-on-one than in groups. Some nurses are fascinated with high-tech equipment and critical care; others are primarily people-persons and prefer interpersonal interaction in ambulatory care settings to high-tech drama in the operating room. Nursing needs all kinds of practitioners. All can find their special niche in direct care, management, teaching, research, and administration.

Nursing is also solid preparation for living and self-understanding. Nurses learn stress and time management, broad problem-solving techniques, communication techniques, strategies for dealing with ethical dilemmas, and teaching skills. With this educational foundation and self-understanding, nurses are qualified candidates for additional education in other fields. Two of the more common fields entered by nurses are law and business. The combination of nursing and law lends itself to careers mixing health care policy with legal defense. The combination of nursing and business lends itself to careers ranging from entrepreneurial endeavors to corporate health care management. The transition to professional person involves maximizing personal potential. Nursing education in combination with personal abilities or other education offers many opportunities to satisfy the individual and enrich nursing, health care, and society.

Challenges

Some of the following selected challenges have been stated explicitly or alluded to in previous discussions. All professions present challenges to their practitioners, and certainly nursing is no exception.

Humanize Health Care

Perhaps one of the greatest fears of both health care professionals and their clients is that modern technology will dehumanize health care. Health care professionals are apprehensive that some of their professional skills (e.g., diagnosing) may be replaced by automation. Clients fear the loss of human compassion. They worry that they will lie alone amidst whirring and ticking machines, attended to by robots and monitored by way of computers and television.

Two currently prominent health care problems may fuel these concerns. These problems are AIDS (HIV) and the increasing demand for health care services by the elderly. AIDS is frightening for its fatality, transmission to unsuspecting persons, and the continuing misunderstanding about how persons become infected. AIDS turns independent adults into physically wasted and dependent beings. Aging is frightening to some because it is a situation from which no one escapes. Aging is often accompanied by chronic disease and diminishing functional abilities. There is continuing misunderstanding about the usual abilities and deficits of healthy older persons. Additionally, the increasing priority given to youth, physical attractiveness, and stamina causes some older persons to question their worth and to fear that they have outlived their usefulness to society. Both AIDS clients and the elderly dread being unable to exercise their will and also becoming a burden on society and loved ones. They also worry that their diminishing physical beings will cause them to be devalued as persons.

Care of AIDS clients and elderly persons presents challenges for health professionals in general. However, because nursing's domain is both health and caring, nursing is the one health profession that has the most to contribute to the "care" of persons in both these circumstances.

Interestingly, "Proud to Care" was the theme of the 1988 Biennial Convention of the ANA. With this theme, nurses publicly reaffirmed their commitment to care. Aspiring nurses seem to respond to this theme also: a beginning nursing student wrote in an anonymous course evaluation, "Clinicals were always exciting and fun. I never realized how many people need care."

AIDS

In 1983 the first major article about AIDS for the general public appeared in *Science* magazine (Marx, 1983). In the mid-1980s, aspiring nurses and their loved ones voiced explicit concerns about nurses' contracting AIDS from clients.

AIDS challenges all caregivers, including aspiring nurses, to understand several facts:

- ❐ AIDS is a difficult disease to catch.
- ❐ The CDC Universal Precautions are easy-to-understand guidelines that will protect health care workers—including nurses—if followed. The highlights of these are handwashing, preventing needle sticks, and using gloves for all invasive procedures and for handling all body substances. Interestingly, similar precautions have been used for years for other infections.
- ❐ A government agency, the Occupational Safety and Health Administration, is enforcing the CDC guidelines in health care workplaces.
- ❐ The care required by AIDS clients is not unique.

Health Care of the Elderly

The elderly segment of our population is not well understood by society in general or by health care professionals in particular. Although the proportion of elderly persons is increasing in society, these persons are often isolated by early retire-

TABLE 12-3 *Myths and Realities*

Myth	Realities
Old age equals sickness	Although the probability of having chronic disease is higher in older people, most older people are adapting successfully in their homes and communities with the help of their families and health care professionals as needed
After 65, people age dramatically	Many body functions vary enormously throughout old age, depending on heredity, diet, occupation, environmental factors, lifestyle, and mental attitude
Older people form a homogeneous group	There is no such single entity as "the elderly"
Older years are tranquil, golden years of pleasure	Old age is a challenge of adaptation and some persons may be lonely, poor, and frustrated
Older persons are rigid, fixed, and unable to change	Many social, environmental, and personal factors affect adaptability

ment, the trend away from extended families, and the trend toward segregated retirement communities.

Myths about aging and elderly persons arise partly from fears of growing older and partly from generations of tales and jokes, but mostly from inexperience in dealing with elderly people (Table 12-3). Gerontologic research has produced a variety of perspectives about how persons age. Older persons are variously described as the vulnerable or fragile elderly, or more optimistically as the hale elderly. Diverse descriptors are undoubtedly appropriate in different circumstances.

There are both developmental tasks of aging (e.g., retirement) and adaptation tasks to biophysical changes of aging. The most pervasive security need among the elderly derives from a common fear of neglect, especially in crisis. Love and belonging needs are also important for older persons. The longer a person survives in this world, the greater the number of losses he or she will encounter in terms of family, friends, meaningful roles, and possessions. As meaningful roles are lost, so may self-esteem be lost. When an older person loses decision-making control over his or her life, he or she is also at risk for suffering lowered self-esteem and feelings of helplessness, hopelessness, and worthlessness. Self-actualization, the highest of Maslow's needs, is perhaps the most elusive for the elderly. One prerequisite of self-actualization, however, is the satisfaction of basic and preceding needs. For this satisfaction, many elderly persons depend on nursing services to keep them healthy and to help them adjust to change.

Elderly people worry about not staying healthy, and especially about the devastation of catastrophic illness. In 1988, both houses of Congress were finally able to agree on the largest expansion of Medicare in the program's 23-year history. This expansion was hailed as a landmark piece of legislation that would bring peace of mind to millions. Hospital coverage increased six-fold in length-of-stay provisions. Also included were doctors' bills, drug costs, hospice care, and skilled nursing care. Another major step forward was a change in Medicaid to prevent the impoverishment of a spouse caused by the nursing home care of a mate. These expansions also brought a variety of unanticipated problems.

Perhaps with the fear of devastating illness diminished, more attention can be focused on staying healthy. Additionally, perhaps elder abuse, an increasingly serious societal problem, may subside if some frustrations related to management of health care problems of the elderly are decreased.

Similarities of Care

Many similarities exist between the health care needs of persons with AIDS and the elderly. Both populations have been misunderstood and in many ways ostracized by society. Both will experience decreasing functional abilities and increasing dependency on others for assistance. To maintain independence will require maximizing remaining functional abilities. Susceptibility to infection is increased for both groups because of compromised immune systems (in AIDS clients) or decreased adaptability (in the elderly). Loneliness resulting from isolation is a potential threat to both populations. People in both groups are survivors and need care to continue to survive.

For both groups, nurses can be caregivers, respecters of personhood, advocates, and teachers to the affected as well as to their informal caregivers. AIDS clients and elderly persons represent a challenge to society, health care, and nursing. Nurses have the knowledge, caring skills, and compassion to make a difference in the care of these persons. Nursing as a health profession can use this window of opportunity: nurses can demonstrate both the essence of nursing and also the value of the care nurses provide. If nursing chooses to do so, it can make a powerful professional statement: nurses meet the challenge to humanize health care in a most significant way.

Responses to the Challenges

A FORM OF TREATMENT CALLED CARE

Care may be given to a person to ease discomfort, to aid and speed recovery, and most of all to enhance the quality of life despite a patient's condition or prognosis. Some conditions create irreversible and incurable symptoms. In the case of a patient suffering from such a condition, only care and comfort can be provided.

As medical technology advances, so does the life expectancy of humans. The older we get, the more help we need to function. As we age, our bodies become frail and weak. Part of the aging process involves the deterioration of the human body. In many instances, it will disable the patient's mobility, and it often involves the deterioration of the body's ability to fight off diseases, that is, a breakdown of the immune system. This will result in the person's need for personalized health and medical care as well as assistance with everyday needs. In many ways, old age is like an incurable ailment. The only thing that can be done is to recognize and treat the symptoms causing the person's discomfort. The results of this personalized care are the restoration and preservation of the person's human dignity and, most preferably, the stabilization of the person's health status. Provision of this care to the elderly will enhance the quality of life they deserve.

AIDS (HIV) is a disease that remains incurable, but it is not untreatable. Many of its symptoms are easily identified and effectively treated. All symptoms of AIDS (HIV) are just complications of the disease and are incurred due to the breakdown of the body's natural defenses. Many AIDS (HIV) patients suffer from pneumonia and anemia, both of which are more treatable, if not curable, in unaffected persons. When we talk about an incurable ailment such as AIDS or old age, here the key treatment is called care. AIDS victims as well as the elderly must be treated with care and compassion.

PERSONAL GLIMPSES

As another response to the challenges of humanizing health care, we offer personal glimpses from a person with AIDS and from a nursing student. Both illustrate the treatment called care.

Living with AIDS

Living with AIDS is not easy; in fact, it is a nuisance. It brings one all too abruptly to look squarely into the face of his or her mortality. Not an easy task, but one that can have rewards.

I want nurses to treat me in a compassionate manner. It is important to offer compassionate care without degrading the patient. Don't make me feel like a second-class citizen. I still look for respect. I've noticed how judgmental people's reactions are until AIDS becomes a personal issue. Like it's "those people and their disease," but AIDS is no longer a single minority's infection. We don't want pity either. We look for support to make very difficult decisions about organizing wills, arranging Power of Attorney, and that most difficult decision—when enough is enough!

To relieve the burden of AIDS patients on the medical system, the patient must be allowed to receive treatment in the comfort of one's home as long as deemed possible. The individual with AIDS must be given as much independence as possible. I want independence as long as I can have it and home care as long as it is wise. Allowing family to stay in the hospital to be near their loved one is important, as our family knows from personal experience.

I pray to always be accorded the utmost respect. As medical intervention progresses, I pray for no undue prolonging of life. Once the quality of life has ceased, there is no reason to continue and I hope I will be allowed to "cross over" with dignity—to have my family gathered about me, and I will transcend peacefully. When quality of life is gone, I want dignity to die peacefully and I want to be comfortable, even if in a medical state of coma. [*Michael G. Koteles*]

Note: As Mike's sister said in his presence, when it's time for us to let him go, it is important for us—his family—to be accorded that. Michael Koteles was the registrar for the University of Michigan School of Nursing for many years. After taking long-term disability leave, he offered to share his personal experiences with AIDS. It was his hope that doing so could help nursing students learn to care for persons with AIDS. Having lost both a brother and his own companion to AIDS, Mike faced his situation realistically and with courage, and taught those of us who knew him more than he will ever know. Mike Koteles died during the autumn of 1994.

BIRCH FAMILY CAMP

As a senior student in a baccalaureate nursing program, and having most of my clinical course-work at a major university medical center, I have seen that the stigma and dread of AIDS remain all too common among hospital staff. There are patients who are not only judged, but are feared—and as a result, their care may be compromised. In my own recent experience, an endearing little girl was hospitalized with full-blown AIDS that she had contracted perinatally from her mother. This woman became infected by a tainted blood transfusion. One day the patient's grandparents tearfully told me of the anguish they felt when nurses would not even touch the little girl to comfort her when she cried.

The Surgeon General of the United States and the Centers for Disease Control have made great strides in educating the public about the spread of HIV. In 1987, the CDC issued Universal Precautions for care providers to use as guidelines for infection control. Yet in spite of these efforts, the stigma of AIDS prevails in many health care settings.

This summer, however, my faith in human compassion and caring was restored. I had the opportunity to participate in a training program at a summer camp for families affected by AIDS. The experience was deeply meaningful and profoundly inspiring.

Located north of New York City, the Birch Family Camp is a superb example of holistic health care at its best! The camp is run mostly by dedicated volunteers—nurses, doctors, counselors, and staff. It provides a warm, accepting, non-judgmental environment that enhances the growth of the campers, young and old. Psychosocial and physiological aspects of these families' struggles are cared for with nurturing and empathy.

When I arrived at Birch Camp, I knew immediately it was a very special place. Warmth and support and joy infused the air. During the subsequent days, what I experienced was purely magical. I was witness to an amazing transformation: dozens of children moved from feeling shamed and burdened with stigma to being just plain happy kids, spirited and at peace. After a week of receiving unconditional acceptance, nonjudgmental friendship, and true heart-felt caring, the children were smiling and laughing. Even the very ill wheel-chair bound were empowered as they participated in all camp activities, including the hilarious evening talent shows.

Part of Birch Family Camp's philosophy is that if one family member is *infected* with AIDS, the whole family is *affected* by AIDS. At this camp, family needs and support are at the core of the environment. At Birch Camp, families are released, at least temporarily, from the pressures of both caretaking and keeping a shameful family secret. This respite allows them to experience playfulness and joy in a milieu of sensitivity, compassion, and unconditional acceptance.

As a nursing student, I was constantly inspired by the sense that this environment felt like the most caring place I had ever been. In an attempt to discover what it was about Birch Camp that created such an atmosphere, I sought insight from those who knew. As I talked with the children, I discovered that for them the magic was "having fun" and the freedom they felt in "having no secrets." The adult campers used the terms "understanding," "caring," "no secrets," and "warm feelings." They said, "It's the only place I can be myself and feel accepted." The counselors explained the magic with terms like "accepting," "fun," "wholesome," "emotional," "exhausting," "inspiring," "fulfilling," and "unconditional love."

Birch Camp's volunteer staff and counselors give two weeks of their summer for the simple reason that they are committed to easing the despair and turmoil which describe the lives of children and families with AIDS. This caring commitment begins with the founders and directors and has a ripple effect that spreads to all camp participants. This environment of unconditional acceptance, empathy, and heart-felt caring, enables maximum healing and coping for individuals and families. Today the nursing profession is in a unique position in the deeply complex AIDS health care phenomenon. It is we who can learn to bring more acceptance and human compassion—our special magic—into the lives of our patients. [*Nancy J. Bidlack, SN4*]

Nurses will certainly be challenged to provide person-centered care for increasing numbers of elderly patients and persons with AIDS. These challenges, although poignant and compelling in themselves, also illustrate the importance of the other challenges that follow.

Continue Professionalization of Nursing

Although professions arise from the needs of society, they flourish under the nurturance of the professionals themselves. On the one hand, such nurturance can obviously be viewed as self-serving to the profession. On the other hand, it should be obvious that the profession itself is best able to develop its services and make them known. Despite nursing's name and the nurturance of its clients, nurses have been remarkably slow to nurture their profession. To do so will require the concerted and collective efforts of both new and established professionals who are convinced of nursing's value, and these nurses must also be comfortable with their own self-worth so that they can be assertive with a purpose.

Society's need for nursing is not going to disappear, but whether this need can be fully met by organized nursing is a real question and challenge. Assistive personnel, not managed by nursing, may be a managed care solution to the increased "nursing" demand. However, that such a solution will not really meet the increased public demand for "nursing care" is clear. Nonetheless, nursing need not face this care challenge alone. The public is ready to be a partner and must be asked to help. Prospective nurses and the public might also be concerned about whether the extensive use of assistive personnel would adequately protect clients' health care interests.

Extend Practice Through Research

The National Center for Nursing Research has featured a phrase, "Nursing science: Serving health through research." The research programs of the National Institute of Nursing Research focus on both actual and potential health problems; these include health promotion and disease prevention—decreasing the vulnerability of persons to illness and disability throughout life; acute and chronic illness; and approaches to nursing care delivery that include quality, cost, and ethical issues. Even beginning nursing students recognize the importance of care as noted in the anonymous comment cited earlier: "I never realized how many people need care." But predicting and controlling the outcomes of care are other matters. These outcomes will require a sophisticated level of nursing research as well as a greatly increased quantity of research. In effect, this major challenge will require large numbers of well-qualified nurse–scientists. The challenge will await nurses entering the profession and established practitioners for decades to come.

The challenge to extend practice through research will be met in part by individual nurses believing in their own problem-solving skills and identifying problems from actual clinical practice. Some of the needed studies will be sophisticated, whereas others will be quite straightforward. The following example illustrates how one student discovered research as an undergraduate.

I entered the University of Michigan with the ultimate goal of graduating with a Bachelor's of Science in Nursing. I was an older student, and graduating from the university had been a life-long dream of mine. I certainly never even dreamed of pursuing graduate studies.

During my opening semester at the University of Michigan, however, I was inspired by my first research class. Being a 1963 high school graduate, I had not had many of the opportunities high school students have these days. Sure, we did research in high school, but it was different then. It was before computers and Xerox machines, making literature searches time-consuming and tedious. In those days, I would use one 3x5 index card for each reference, resulting in a stack of cards that I then transformed into a handwritten paper, that I then typed and retyped on a manual typewriter. There was no "Medline" or "Mirlyn" computerized library search or Internet—and certainly no white-out. There were no poster presentations. In high school, I thought the subjects assigned for our research papers were rather dull, and the process boring. Needless to say, I was not really looking forward to taking a required research class thirty-three years later. I decided to grab the bull by the horns, though, and take the class in my first semester to get it out of the way.

It was in that class, taught by Dr. Susan Boehm, that I discovered research was much different than I had remembered. As one of the requirements for this course, each student was to work on the research team of a School of Nursing faculty member. Since I was interested in the functioning of the brain, I joined Dr. Barbara Therrien's team studying disorientation and cognition, using an animal model. To my delight, there was an electricity throughout her lab as she gave me a tour and explained her study to me. The lab was buzzing with activity. A student was swimming rats in a large water maze for a behavioral investigation. In another room, a doctoral student was performing brain surgery on rats. In yet another room were doctoral students and post-docs who were slicing frozen rat brains and mounting them onto slides. In the next room, students were preparing impressive-looking professional posters for presentations at the Society for Neuroscience. It looked like fun, and a very hands-on type of experience—very different from the dry literature searches I had remembered. I was hooked! This was the place where I might find some answers to my own questions about the relationships of brain and behavior.

With the impetus of that research class, with the support and resources provided by Dr. Therrien, I wrote, designed, and prepared my first poster presentation. Since then, I have continued participating in Dr. Therrien's research, as well as taking advantage of other research opportunities as they have arisen. I have been involved with many aspects of research by now, and have seen first hand that by using a carefully controlled scientific method, nursing research can dramatically impact nursing practice.

A highlight of my undergraduate research opportunities was attending a spring conference of the Midwest Nursing Research Society. This enabled me to see all kinds of nursing research from around the country. Hundreds of poster and slide presentations—ranging from the role of preceptors in clinical settings, to the effectiveness of ear protection in noisy factories, to pain assessment of children, to the effects of stress on the immune system—were too many for one person to attend, but the exposure was phenomenal.

I may never have experienced these exciting and enriching opportunities had it not been a requirement to take that undergraduate research class. It hooked me on research, and now I don't want to stop! Graduation is soon, and I am hoping to make a contribution to the nursing profession, and subsequently to the relief of human affliction, by continuing my studies and making a career in nursing research.
[*Nancy J. Bidlack, SN4*]

*I*ncrease Public Awareness of Nursing's Contribution to Health Care

Nurses need to make the public aware of nursing's contribution to health care. This awareness is particularly important in an era of health care reform. Nurses could make more of a public impact in this regard if they would publish in newspapers for lay persons and in popular magazines. Such topics as women's health, sexuality, coping with life's stressors in healthy ways, dangers of substance abuse, sexually transmitted diseases, and care of the elderly and chronically ill in the home are all within nursing's expertise. For the public to see such topics widely and expertly discussed by nurses would increase nurse credibility and greatly expand the public's knowledge of nursing.

In their verbal presentations and everyday conversations, nurses can also increase public awareness of nursing's contribution to health care. In addition to dispensing information in community forums, they can make clear that well-educated nurses are prepared to offer care that is scientific and up to date, and they can differentiate between medical care and nursing care. Because the public often fails to differentiate, it may attribute to medicine efforts for which nursing deserves credit—for example, close, around-the-clock observation for untoward responses to surgery, or recognition of early deviations from health. Maraldo (1990) specifically noted nurses' abilities to decrease the length of hospital stay by preventing such conditions as phlebitis and pressure sores related to inadequate mobility and exercise (p. 44).

The public needs to know that nurses care for persons of all ages and in all levels of sickness and wellness, and that nurses do this in ways that maximize their clients' strengths so that they can maintain optimal independence in activities of daily living. The public also needs to know nursing's commitment to giving comforting care in those situations in which "cure" is currently impossible, as with AIDS clients and the elderly. In all settings, nurses advocate on the client's behalf for the fullest possible client control of health care decision making.

Increase Nursing Influence on Health Care Policy and Delivery

Several individual and group strategies for nurses to increase nursing influence were enumerated in some detail in Tables 12-1 and 12-2.

A high order of response to political pressure is action by organized government at the national level. The registered nurse shortage of the mid 1980s was identified not as a nursing issue but as a health care issue. Similarly, Felton (G. Felton, personal communication, April 7, 1988) likened nursing to a public utility that was a national necessity. Although the situation today is very different, the issue of whether persons have the kind of professional nursing care they need remains a *health care* issue.

The real challenge is for organized nursing as a single powerful voice, speaking for nursing and in the public interest, to lead the way in increasing nursing's influence on both health care policy and delivery. The challenge to increase nursing influence encompasses an important related challenge.

Control Nursing Activities Performed by Assistive Personnel

If assistive, ancillary personnel perform tasks labeled *nursing* by the profession, then nurses should supervise such individuals: nursing should have some say in the competence of such individuals, as well as which tasks they should perform. Nurses should also control matters related to staffing patterns and hiring practices. Only in this way can nursing claim accountability for that which is called *nursing care*.

Become More Globally Aware

In this day of global trade and travel, merely transforming national health care policy will be a partial, although important, victory. Global transformation of health care will be sorely needed, given economic and demographic predictions. Maraldo (1990) has suggested that

> the cornerstone of a nursing strategy for international health policy . . . will reside in the ability of nurses around the world to shape and advance policies that will reduce the inordinate and costly bias toward expensive inpatient care and costly technology, and to place a new and unprecedented emphasis, in industrialized and developing nations alike, on (1) prevention and primary services, (2) long-term care, and (3) the need to develop high-quality community-based systems of care (p. 215).

The wisdom of her words is reinforced by widespread natural disasters and famine, prolonged by tribal wars, that illustrate how *basic* care needs truly are. Although progress has been made toward recognizing the importance of primary care, much necessary work has yet to be done. Students who have global awareness will be better able to meet this challenge as licensed professionals. As one baccalaureate student wrote upon her return from spending two months in Nyamira, Kenya:

> After seeing the problems of their culture, I realized that the problems in this world are really social problems. . .There are so many things to learn about other cultures,

but in addition to learning the cultural ways, I was able to understand ideas on a more worldly level. By living in the village and working with residents, I saw that people are people wherever you are. They have the same problems we have with disciplining children, domestic violence, hunger, alcohol and drug abuse, uneven distribution of wealth, and social pressures. . .It is easy to look at another culture in a book and think of them as not human, but to live and work with them helps both cultures to see how similar we are. [*Mary Pohanka, SN4*]

An experienced nurse educator from New Zealand who has also observed nursing education in this country offers another international perspective called "Flying the Flag":

Flags are of many kinds, shapes, and colours but they all signify some special relationship to a people, a place, an event or a celebration. A number of flags could be flown for nurses and nursing, but there are only two I wish to unfurl in a brief moment of reflection on core issues for nurses in practice, nurses preparing to qualify for practice, and for those whose need for care bestows purpose and meaning on the practice of nursing.

Flag number one signifies, and celebrates, the purpose of nursing—which is simple, constant and unchanging. Within a wide variation of the 'world of nursing', common elements must exist to be consistent with the purpose of nursing. A most important common element I believe is related to a sincere, concernful regard for the well being of the person or 'being' of some other(s) with whom we interact in a nursing encounter. Underpinning all the principles that guide the concernful practices that nurses engage in is this one principle which speaks to the purpose of nursing, calls nursing into being, and has done so throughout time. *Nursing exists, always has and always will, through a deep sincere regard called forth by the expressed or observed need of individuals and communities for some assistance with their daily life practices; to be mediated with skill and understanding in ways appropriate to each person's needs and lifespace.*

Flag number two also celebrates the constancy of nursing's purpose but extends the celebration to the embracing of change as not the *disturber of the even tenor of our days* but as the companion to constancy of purpose. After all, everything changes, constantly! Change is a natural part of living-a-life that we adapt to, consciously and unconsciously. As Heraclitus, a Greek philosopher, pointed out, we cannot step into the same river twice for the river will be different and we will have changed. Hence flag number two offers a challenge to fly with, to transform our practices by developing research oriented practices, practices that are based on learning experiences that value and acknowledge the personhood, the 'being,' of students and beginning or advanced nurse practitioners. Research has us traveling a path that questions the relevancy and effectiveness of our daily practices in both educational and work settings. And not as an add-on activity, but as an integral part of the daily round of work. When we appreciate the community as the location of care, the user of care, and the provider of care, we will also appreciate the need to be alert that the context of care, like all else, is subject to two constancies. The constancy of the purpose of nursing is met, paradoxically, by nurses when they consistently adjust their practices to the constancy or unremitting regularity of change in the daily lifeworld of individuals and communities.

When self directed learning and self-organization approaches are core to the learning experiences planned for nursing students, research oriented practice will develop naturally. When that happens, nurses will mediate the purpose of nursing in ways that correspond to the context of need and the particularities of people. In contemporary socio-health contexts, and when a competitive spirit is confused with the health desire of an individual to excel and to actualize their potential, nurses/nursing need(s) special vision. They need to 'look along' the entire picture of what is desirable in creating communities of care that are inclusive of those who receive care and those who provide care. We have to contend with the world as we find it, but in partnership with all involved in the 'circle of care' we can transform, in affirmative ways, the challenges that contemporary communities present to us. Finding its place in the postmodern/industrial health care context compels nurses/nursing to look for new opportunities and new partnerships. The purpose of nursing may remain constant, but the practice of nursing must change as relevant to the context of need. Heidegger (1962) in "Being and Time" expressed this well when he wrote, "The passing of the past is something else than what has been, it is the gathering of what endures."

*I*ncrease the Number of Nurses in Health Care Leadership and Administrative Roles

Nurses have the appropriate problem-solving and interpersonal skills to represent the public interest in health care leadership and administrative roles. However, to date, nurses have been underrepresented in these roles. Two major reasons for this situation have been nurses' failure to assert themselves and others' failure to acknowledge nurses' abilities. Nurses themselves are largely responsible for both of these situations. As the most numerous of health care professionals, nurses should exert more influence just by sheer numbers alone.

The rationale for taking up this challenge is not merely to bring prestige to nursing. Rather, the public interest would be served by humanizing health care and bringing cost economies. Although it is clear nursing could provide leadership for the humanizing of health care, it is less clear to those outside nursing that nurses could bring about economies of cost. Unquestionably, the gauntlet has been thrown down, especially by the public; it remains to be seen whether nurses will rise to the challenge.

Some might interpret this challenge as confrontational to medicine, which is not the intent. Rather, it may be that nurses have not assumed their fair share of responsibility for collaborative action on the wide range of challenges facing health care. It is partly because cure has been so successful in prolonging life that many of the care problems now loom large. Care to stay healthy and care to comfort humanely are now assuming ever larger roles in health services delivery. As this happens, the potential for leadership by nurses will grow dramatically.

*A*chieve Cultural Diversity and Gender Balance in Nursing

In recent years, the nursing profession has become acutely aware of cultural variations and their impact on providing person-centered care. Official statements have been published recognizing nursing's contribution toward meeting the "health needs of a diverse and multicultural society" (National League for Nursing, 1977, p. 13) and toward considering "individual value systems and lifestyles" (ANA, 1976, p. 4).

As discussed in Chapter 5, ethnic origin and racial background greatly influence how a person reacts and is reacted to by others in the health care environment. *Ethnicity* is association based on common race, language, or religious or cultural heritage. Other cultural variables important in the health care setting include value orientation, family system, healing beliefs and practices, and nutritional behavior. As nursing comes of age as a science, nurses will grow in awareness of how biophysical variations among ethnic minority groups influence their own ability to carry out appropriate and accurate physical assessments, as well as other aspects of the nursing process, for clients different from themselves.

Nurses also need to be aware of both differences and similarities cross-culturally as a way of developing sensitivity to persons with varied cultural backgrounds, and as a way of avoiding stereotypical approaches in relieving psychological and physical stress. Especially in the past fifteen years, there has been an influx of culturally sensitive nursing education literature to enable the nurse to learn about cultural and ethnic differences. Yet, nursing exhibits relatively little cultural diversity within its ranks. Real-life diversity of professionals contributes a rich multicultural sensitivity to practice issues that cannot be duplicated in any other way.

A large number of ethnic minorities (i.e., African-Americans, Hispanics, and Native Americans) are part of low socioeconomic/poverty groups characterized by high unemployment, low income, poor housing and living conditions, and low educational standards. These socioeconomic conditions have a profound effect on the level of health among such groups. African-American and other minorities suffer proportionately greater rates of death and illness than the population as a whole. The 1985 report of the HHS Task Force on Black and Minority Health cited excess deaths from heart disease and stroke, homicide and accidents, cancer, infant mortality, chemical dependency, and diabetes. In addition, AIDS is disproportionately found among African-American populations.

Clearly, the current health care system is woefully inadequate for the health care of African-American and other ethnic minorities. To enrich its multicultural sensitivity and better serve the country's health care needs, nursing requires both ethnic and gender diversity.

Undoubtedly, some of the same socioeconomic conditions that are decreasing access to the health care system also decrease access to educational preparation for health care professions such as nursing. For example, African-Americans represent fewer than 4% of the total practicing RN population. Some capable minority scholars are unaware of career options in nursing, or are being recruited to other professions. Other minorities may not recognize their potential for nursing or realize the access available through community college programs.

The benefits of recruiting more minority persons to nursing are multiple: providing more sensitive nursing care to minorities, increasing health care access for minorities in the population, providing secure employment in an area of demand, and increasing sensitivity of all health care professionals to diverse population groups. Furthermore, because all minorities are underrepresented in nursing, minorities are an untapped pool for recruitment to fill critical nursing positions in all health care settings.

The number of men in nursing has changed relatively little despite social change and the entrance of women into traditionally male-dominated fields. The rationale for needing men in nursing is both different from and similar to that for needing ethnic minority persons. Unlike ethnic minorities, men are not generally disadvantaged as a group; however, like ethnic minorities, men are grossly under-represented in nursing proportionate to their health care needs.

In the past, men in nursing have been heavily concentrated in care populations that have been primarily male—for example, the military. Growing prison and substance abuse populations that are also primarily male will need increasing health care services; however, caring men would be an asset to all areas of nursing. Some men enter nursing from industry and bring valuable experience with them, as the following example illustrates:

> Dave began working for a large lumber mill in a small midwest community in 1982. There he learned much about leadership from his work with a large production team. The 100 production employees were divided into three teams. Two of the team leaders he described as follows: "Our team leader was firm, assertive, and well prepared. He expected a lot from us and made those expectations very clear. Quickly we evolved into a very efficient team, setting many production records and doing it safely. Their team leader was a pal and practiced a laissez-faire style of management whether she knew it or not. There was little leadership or discipline and attitudes were generally negative. They worked poorly together and it showed. They were lowest in productivity and highest in injuries. Eleven years later when I left the mill, they were still problematic and we were still productive. I remember years ago solving the evolutionary patterns of these two teams. They both bore traits consistent with the leadership they received."
>
> After graduation from an AD program at age 40, Dave had an opportunity to put some of his observations into practice as a team leader of a nursing team that included many CNA's (Certified Nursing Assistants). Although Dave initially lacked the *experience* he recognized in his industry team leader, he wrote me, "I'm constantly learning, and as my level of knowledge and experience grows, so does my level of confidence. I've a long way to go to become the leader I'm striving for, and chances are it will be a career-long process of continuous improvement." While one might have thought Dave an unlikely candidate for nursing, he clearly contributed much valuable experience and insight in addition to contributing to gender diversity. [*Dave Svenson, RN*]

Balancing the gender distribution of nurses would be likely to increase the sensitivity across the genders to nursing's goals and challenges. Such balance might also decrease the likelihood that the profession's problems would be viewed as women's problems. Also, it would seem that the expanding scientific and technologic opportunities available in nursing would be intriguing to men as well as to women.

Care Strategies for Self-Development

This section presents care strategies for self-development. The intent is to encourage the professional nurse to explore personal career development and management by focusing care strategies on his or her self. **Career development** is the purposeful advancement of skill level or professional experience involving greater depth and breadth.

Care Strategies for Self-Renewal

Caring for others demands commitment. It also demands self-renewal over time, because one cannot effectively care for others without also caring for oneself. Nurses encourage self-care and renewal strategies for their clients, but often are less attentive to their own self-renewal needs. Self-renewal needs are biopsychosocial and spiritual for nurses, just as they are for their clients. Nursing care is frequently physically demanding of its practitioners. Physical renewal may be achieved through a combination of rest and healthful exercise that is personally invigorating and individualistic. Hobbies and other interests outside the profession often combine several aspects of self-renewal. Psychic renewal comes from a variety of sources, including positive self-assessment, satisfying friendships, and the emotional support of significant others. Social support may come from a wider group of less intimate acquaintances and other persons of similar interests, culture, and perhaps religion. Spiritual renewal may come from shared religious experience or from solitary religious quest. Many and varying strategies and activities are needed over time to help even the most dedicated nurses maintain high energy levels and avoid burnout from professional demands.

In addition to the self-renewal activities that maintain personal well-being, nurses can initiate personal activities that will enhance their own professional well-being and facilitate career development. Such activities enable nurses to recognize and maximize opportunities and also to meet the challenges that face nurses and nursing. We believe that each nurse has unique individual strengths and career potential to focus on these opportunities and challenges, and also on individual career development.

Nurses who are interested in personal growth, professional success, and career development will use their individual strengths to maximize career potential. Such nurses will recognize that career development demands an initial investment and also a continuing reinvestment and shaping of a career over a lifetime. This reinvestment in career development can begin at any time.

Career Goals

Career development is goal directed. A **goal** is a specific end as a result of design, not chance. We assume, however, that career goals often change over time. The individual nurse is the single most informed person about his or her initial and changing career goals. That is, the individual knows his or her own personal interests, abilities, and also strengths and weaknesses. Although strengths are ready assets, remember that weaknesses signal challenges and growth opportunities. The individual professional nurse also knows his or her own personal values, energy level, and resources. Motivation and career commitment are needed both to capitalize on strengths and to transform weaknesses. Laura, a physical therapy student, wrote about learning to be good motivators. Her comments apply to motivating self as well as clients. She wrote,

> As future physical therapists, our job will be to get someone to do things differently (to gasp! CHANGE). . .Motivations change with our family and work responsibilities, our age, our economic circumstances, our personal experience. People may make the identical positive behavioral changes for vastly different reasons. Make it a habit to observe others—without being nosy!—whenever you can, attempting to discern why they do what they do. Read biographies and autobiographies. Seek out case studies. [*Laura Knight*]

Informed nurses not only recognize requirements for various positions and educational programs, but are able to evaluate past successes and failures in the context of these requirements. Remember also that the single most important predictor of future success is past success. Furthermore, many satisfying and dissatisfying aspects of your career are under your control. Initially, for example, you can decide to take a "career" approach rather than a "job" approach to your professional life. There are always options! Many options do not involve more than a baccalaureate education. Professional colleagues can provide guidance to enhance your career development. Such persons may be peers, supervisors, academic advisers, or mentors. A **mentor** is a person who assumes professional sponsorship for a less experienced colleague. To summarize, we assume the following:

- ❒ A career is different than a job.
- ❒ Just as persons grow and develop, careers develop over a lifetime.
- ❒ You are already at some unique point in your career development.
- ❒ You have choices.
- ❒ Career development is an active process with you in charge.
- ❒ You have valuable information about yourself that is pertinent to whatever career goals you may be considering.

At this point, you are having or have had unique experiences in nursing. You can probably place yourself quite accurately on a continuum between novice and expert. A **novice** is a person who is new to the practice of nursing, whereas an **expert** is a skilled and knowledgeable nurse. Even if you have given minimal consideration to your nursing career development previously, you have facts and perceptions that you can combine with your individual strengths and career potential. Assessing yourself to examine these assets assists goal setting and, hence, career development. Validating your assumptions and perceptions with others contributes to realistic assessment.

Career goals can be defined in many ways. A goal is both worth attaining and attainable. Therefore, a reasonable short-term goal is usually a significant achievement that might take 5 years to accomplish. An example of a short-term goal might be a step up a clinical ladder of recognition, in which one gains acknowledgment for growth and expertise in the field. Or a short-term goal may be a new position of increased responsibility, or the next educational degree. A long-term career goal, such as national recognition in a specialty area, the top managerial position within an organization, or academic tenure, might take considerably longer to achieve. In a career plan, attaining several short-term goals may be preliminary to reaching a long-term goal.

Once personal goals have been realistically set, informing others of your career goals is important. Do not assume that others know your career aspirations. Colleagues are often willing, however, to be supportive or give advice if you are explicit about your goals and needs. Colleagues can help identify strengths and also illuminate ways to reach career goals. Networking with colleagues and their contacts can increase the number of potential supporters geometrically. As Puetz (1991) stated, "Ultimately, all your networking efforts should assist you in meeting specific career goals . . . you should identify several career goals you'd like to achieve and put together a working list of personal and professional contacts who could help you achieve each goal" (p. 24). Support systems might also include professional colleagues' written works, in addition to peers, co-workers, managers, family members, personal friends, mentors, and former teachers. For example, Henderson and McGettigan (1994) have offered a full array of suggestions in *Managing Your Career in Nursing*. Today with computer access to the internet, the resources for career development are virtually unlimited. You can join interest groups online for moral support and information. Web pages for universities and nurse experts of all specialities are just a few keystrokes away.

Stress Management

Regardless of the goals or career options chosen, you will have periods of stress in your life. Therefore, learning strategies to reduce stress is necessary for successful career management. Stress reduction depends on a person's ability to either alter stressful situations or change his or her responses to them. Stress reduction strategies learned during student days can serve you well for years to come. Only some of the many individual strategies that you may already use or wish to explore are listed as follows:

- ❐ Exercising
- ❐ Deep breathing
- ❐ Learning self-hypnosis
- ❐ Imaging/visualizing
- ❐ Practicing progressive muscle relaxation
- ❐ Resetting goals
- ❐ Extending time lines
- ❐ Enjoying massage
- ❐ Relinquishing control by delegating responsibilities
- ❐ Improving basic skills (e.g., writing, speaking, computer skills)
- ❐ Improving time management
- ❐ Mobilizing social support systems
- ❐ Enjoying solitude
- ❐ Engaging in diversionary activities
- ❐ Contracting with self (e.g., rewarding self for achievement)

❐ Being satisfied with less than perfection

❐ Generating multiple solutions for any given problem

These activities provide ways for you to take care of yourself, which, after all, is the critical point. You will choose the activities and the methods that are best for you. Once you have considered goals and the educational preparation necessary, as well as your personal abilities and characteristics, evaluating your personal situation becomes important. For example, unavoidable demands on your time and energy may affect your career development options during particular periods. However, making such assessments and drawing conclusions purposefully can enable you to feel that your career decision has been right for you. You will know that you based your decision on a thoughtful data-gathering process and, after considering options, took responsibility for making those decisions within your control.

Career Paths

Today's and tomorrow's workers will change careers many times over a lifetime. That reality is good or bad news, depending on your occupation. Members of many other occupations will be forced to find career options outside of their field. Nurses, however, will continue to be in demand for the foreseeable future. The specialist of tomorrow may have a different name or title than the nurse of today. Other career development possibilities may extend practice to another client population, to another setting, or to another functional component of the nursing role. These components of nursing, such as teacher, manager, educator, and consultant, are often delineated in advanced practice but found at all levels. Many opportunities also exist in other fields such as business, law, and public health.

Sometimes self-development and career management may reflect a much less formal progression than implied here, especially if career is conceptualized as a process rather than a destination. James (1986) in her book *Success is the Quality of Your Journey* has suggested a more flexible career development view. In this view, career management is not planned in extreme detail, but rather remains open to adventure. Such a plan enables the nurse to find satisfaction in the unexpected, discover and use untapped talents, and seek the extraordinary opportunity—perhaps without ever changing position or setting.

Developing a career is a bit like solving a puzzle or crafting a collage: one piece creates the starting point for the complete picture. Certainly the old adage "nothing ventured, nothing gained" applies to the myriad of career management processes within career development. Career management and professional development both involve understanding yourself, assuming responsibility for the present, and taking control of the future. Self-assessment and growth pave the way for advancement and success. You can be in charge and use all available resources to shape your career path.

KEY CONCEPTS

✔A variety of opportunities and challenges await today's professional nurses.

✓Personal opportunities are enhanced by active career management.

✓Meeting professional challenges is the responsibility of nurses individually and collectively.

✓Care of the elderly and persons with ADIS illustrate but two of many opportunities for humanizing health care.

✓Personal care strategies enhance personal and professional quality of life and contribute to self-growth and growth of the profession.

CRITICAL THINKING QUESTIONS

1. How might your unique personal abilities find expression in nursing?

2. Which of the challenges presented do you think has the highest priority, and why? (Give a rationale for your answer.)

3. Identify a personal contribution you can make to AIDS education in your community.

4. Identify resources in your community to assist home care of chronically ill elderly persons.

5. Identify three career development actions that would be appropriate for you to take at this point in your education.

6. Familiarize yourself with two international in scope nursing journals. Compare and contrast the topics and issues with those found in U.S. nursing journals.

7. Familiarize yourself with a politically active nurse in your state.

8. Devise political strategies for a health care issue in your community.

9. Select an elected official in your state and pay attention to his or her activities and statements related to health care issues.

10. What are your creative thoughts for meeting the following challenges?
    a. Increasing the value of nursing to health care reform
    b. Preparing adequate and diverse numbers of advanced practitioners and scientists
    c. Preparing nurse professionals who are life-long learners

REFERENCES

American Nurses Association. (1980). *A social policy statement* (Publication No. NP-63 35M). Kansas City, MO: Author.

American Nurses Association. (1976). *Code for nurses with interpretive statements.* Kansas City, MO: Author.

Clarke, A.C. (1986). *July 20, 2019: Life in the 21st century.* New York: Macmillan.

Cody, W.K. (1994). Radical health care reform: The person as case manager. *Nursing Science Quarterly, 7*(4), 180–182.

Ellis, J.R. & Hartley, C.L. (1994). *Nursing in today's world: Challenges, issues and trends* (3rd ed.). Philadelphia: J.B. Lippincott.

Hammer, M. & Champy, J. (1994) *Reengineering the corporation: A manifesto for business revolution* (1st pbk ed.). New York: Harper Business.

Heidegger, M. (1962). Being and Time. NY: Harper.

Henderson, F.C. & McGettigan, B.O. (1994). *Managing your career in nursing* (2nd ed.). New York: National League for Nursing. (Pub. No. 14-2640)

James, J. (1986). *Success is the quality of your journey.* New York: Newmarket.

Joel, L.A. (1996). Map a new course for your career. AJN Career Guide for 1996. N.Y.: American Journal of Nursing Co., 8–9.

Kelly, L.Y. & Joel, L.A. (1995). *Dimensions of professional nursing* (7th ed.). New York: McGraw-Hill.

Kiplinger, K. & Kiplinger, A. (1996). *The Kiplinger Washington Letter 73*(52), p. 3.

McCloskey, J. (1994). *Current issues in nursing* (4th ed.). St. Louis: Mosby.

Maraldo, P. (1990). The case of nursing's preeminence in international health. In C.M. Fagin (Ed.), *Nursing leadership: Global strategies* (Publication No. 41-2349, pp. 209–220). New York: National League for Nursing.

Marx, J.L. (1983). Spread of AIDS sparks new health concern. *Science, 219*(4580), 42–43.

Meleis, A.I. (1985). *Theoretical nursing: Development and progress.* Philadelphia: J.B. Lippincott.

Mundinger, M. (1980). *Autonomy in nursing.* Germantown, MD: Aspen.

Naisbitt, J. (1984). *Megatrends: Ten new directions transforming our lives.* New York: Warner Books.

National League for Nursing, Department of Baccalaureate and Higher Degree Programs. (1977). *Criteria for the appraisal of baccalaureate and higher degree programs in nursing* (Publication No. 15-1251, 4th ed.). New York: Author.

National Nurses in Business Association. (1991). *How I became a nurse entrepreneur: Tales from 50 nurses in business.* Petaluma, CA: Author.

Perrin, M.M. (1985). Space nursing: A professional challenge. *Nursing Clinics of North America, 20*(3), 497–503.

Peters, T. (1987). *Thriving on chaos: Handbook for a management revolution.* New York: Knopf.

Puetz, B.E. (1991). Networking: Making it work for you. *Healthcare Trends and Transition, 3*(1), 21–28.

U.S. Department of Health and Human Services. (1985). *Report of the secretary's task force on black and minority health, Vol. 1—Executive summary* (HHS Publication No. O-487-637 [QL-3]). Washington, DC: Author.

Werley, H. & Lang, N. (1988). *Identification of the nursing minimum data set.* New York: Springer.

Glossary

Accommodation: The alteration of internal schemes to fit reality; reconciling new experiences or objects by revising the old plan to fit the new input (Piaget).

Accountability: Responsibility for the services one provides or makes available.

Accurate observation: Observation based on fact rather than conjecture.

Active listening: The cultivated skill of deriving meaning from the words and non-verbal vocalization of another.

Actual problem: A problem that can be identified clearly from the data at hand.

Adaptation: The dual process of assimilation and accommodation (which leads to adaptation) is a continuing process of learning from the environment and learning to adjust to alterations in the environment (per Piaget).

Adaptation: The process of changing throughout life by persons when faced with new, different, or threatening experiences without loss of health, sense of wholeness, or integrity of self.

Advance directives: ''Documents such as Durable Powers of Attorney and Living Wills that allow a person to plan for the management of health care and/or financial affairs in the event of incapacity.'' (Singleton et al., 1992, p. 42)

Affective learning or behavior: Reflects feelings, attitudes, and values.

Affirmative action: Positive steps to bring a deteriorating situation under control, for example, intervening to control unusual bleeding.

Aggregating: The process of collecting and summarizing many nursing interventions and their outcomes and determining relationships among the outcomes such that predictions can be made about the most effective interventions for a given age, sex, culture, health concern, life-style, and so forth.

AIDS: Acquired immune deficiency syndrome; a complex of infectous diseases caused by a severe infection with the human immunodeficiency virus (HIV).

Anxiety: A diffuse, unpleasant, vague feeling of apprehension, nervousness, or dread expressed both somatically and psychically.

Asepsis: Freedom from infectious agents.

Assertiveness: A verbal communication skill that states one's own rights positively without infringing upon the rights of others.

Assessing: The collection of information, data, or facts about the person so that the nurse may better understand his or her feelings, ideas, values, and biophysical responses.

Assimilation: The process of taking novel information and making it fit a preconceived notion about objects or the world.

Assistive personnel: Less expensive technical workers, minimally trained, doing activities formerly considered nursing.

Autonomous: Independent; self-governing.

Behavior: An emitted response (action or reaction); it is overt, observable, and measurable.

Behavioral objectives: Learning goals; statements of what a person will do or say as evidence of learning; expected outcomes.

Behaviorism: A theoretical approach that represents learning as a process of making connections through association; developed by J. B. Watson (1878–1958) and concerned primarily with objectively observable and measurable data rather than subjective phenomena such as ideas or emotions.

Bioethics: A subspecialty of the discipline of ethics; issues of an ethical nature that concern health professionals.

Biofeedback: That altered physiological or psychological state or response (and awareness of it) that can be measured objectively and/or subjectively.

Body image: How one views or thinks of the physical part of the self.

Boundaries: These separate the members of a social system from the environment.

Capitation: A system of reimbursement in which providers receive a fixed amount of income per enrollee regardless of the services they perform.

Career: One's major life work.

Career development: A purposeful advancement of skill level or professional experience.

Care maps: Similar to critical pathways, but broader, and including statements from all disciplines that address problems frequently related to specific diagnosis-related groups.

Case management: A collaborative process which assesses, plans, implements, coordinates, monitors, and evaluates the options and services to meet an individual's health needs, using communication and available resources to promote quality, cost-effective outcomes.

Certification: "Certification of specialists in nursing practice is a judgment made by the profession, upon review of an array of evidence examined by a selected panel of nurses who are themselves specialists and who represent the area of specialization." (American Nurses Association, *A Social Policy Statement*, 1980, p. 24).

Civil law: Law concerned with legal rights and duties of private persons.

Client: A person who engages the professional advice or services of another; a person served by or using the services of an agency; a person.

Climate: Average weather conditions at a place over a period of years, including factors such as average temperature, humidity, precipitation, and wind velocity.

Closed system: A system that cannot exchange matter, energy, or information with its environment.

Cognitive learning or behavior: Demonstrates results of the thinking process.

Cognitive learning theories: Those theoretical approaches that focus on the intellectual processes of thinking, language, and problem solving; term includes theories of Gestaltists (Wertheimer and Lewin) and developmental psychologists (Piaget).

Communication: A complex process in which two or more persons exchange messages and derive meanings; it is both verbal and nonverbal.

Community: A group of persons living in the same locality and under the same government; having common norms and cultures, health interests, and needs.

Conflict resolution: The effective management of conflict to produce positive change.

Consent: Voluntary granting of permission, for example, for treatment procedures or research.

Consumer: An individual, a group, or a community that uses a commodity or a service.

Continuity of care: An interdisciplinary process that includes clients and significant others in the development of a coordinated care plan. This process facilitates the client's transition between settings, based on changing needs and available resources.

Coordinator of care: One of the roles of the nurse; the act of helping the client use appropriately all resources available to him or her.

Coping: One's ability to deal with stressful situations or conditions.

Coping behavior: Adaptive or maladaptive responses consisting of cognitive function, motor activity, affect, and psychological defenses. Consists of actions or reactions in response to stress.

Criminal law: Law concerned with behavior detrimental to society as a whole.

Crisis: A turning point, a crucial period of increased vulnerability and heightened potential; may be biologic, psychological, or social; individual experiences disequilibrium when usual coping behaviors are not operating.

Critical pathways: Key events in the hospitalization of a particular care type that must occur for the client to reach the outcomes set by diagnosis-related group parameters.

Critical thinking: A professional skill that combines both framework thinking and flexible viewing.

Critique: Thoughtful and detailed responses to another's intent of presentation, ideas, or communication.

Cultural healing belief: Belief that reflects a specific cultural orientation toward health and illness.

Cultural variables: Characteristics that a person exhibits or with which he or she identifies from a particular cultural group.

Culture: A system of symbols shared by groups of humans and transmitted to new generations; a group's design for living.

Culture shock: Profound disorientation suffered by the person who has plunged without adequate preparation into an alien culture.*

Cyberspace: That abstract communication medium consisting of the internet and

---

* *Toffler, A. (1970). Future shock. New York: Random House, p. 308.*

world wide web within which information and persons can be accessed electronically. Created by linking computer networks globally through telecommunication.

Deductive reasoning: The process of applying general information or principles to specific situations.

Defining characteristics: Signs or symptoms that can be observed in the client.

Deontological: A classification of ethical theory; belief that the moral right or wrong of an act is considered separately from the goodness or badness of consequences.

Dependent nursing behavior: Those activities performed under delegated medical authority or supervision or according to a priori routines.

Development: The patterned, orderly, lifelong changes in structure, thought, or behavior that evolve as a result of the maturation of physical and mental capacity, experiences, and learning and that result in a new level of maturity and integration.

Developmental task: A growth responsibility that arises at a certain time in the course of development (Erikson).

Diagnosing: Investigator analysis of the cause or nature of a condition, situation, or problem; the act of reaching a conclusion about the nature or cause of some phenomenon; the phase of nursing process that involves analyzing assessment data and making a nursing diagnosis.

Diagnosis: A statement or conclusion concerning the nature or cause of some phenomenon.

Diagnosis-related groups: A system of classifying health care needs according to an accepted list of diagnosed illnesses and conditions of health deficits; used to determine Medicare payments for health care services, and thus affect the extent of services provided by many institutions.

Distance learning: Education in which the teacher and learner are separate during most of the instruction. Examples include correspondence courses, interactive television, and virtual reality (electronic simulation through interactive computer technology).

Distress: A state induced by unpleasant stimuli.

Documentation: The collection or provision of written information for reference.

Durable power of attorney: "A document that gives a surrogate decision maker called the attorney-in-fact the authority to make health care and/or property management decisions for the principal, who executes the document." (Singleton et al., 1992, p. 42).

Ecology: The study of the relationship between humans and the external environment.

Empathy: Ability to participate in the life of another individual and to perceive his or her thoughts and feelings.

Environment: An open system comprising social, cultural, physical, economic, and political subsystems.

Epidemiology: The study of the incidence, distribution, and control of disease in a human population.

Ethics: A discipline concerned with social, political, and legal philosophy and principles of good and bad, moral duty, obligation, and values; rules of conduct.

Ethnicity: A group's affiliation due to shared linguistic, racial, religious, or cultural background.

Eugenics: The science of improving human genes.

Eustress: A state induced by pleasant stimuli.

Evaluating: The act of determining the client's progress toward the outcomes established in the planning step of the nursing process.

Expert: A skilled and knowledgeable nurse.

Family: A group of persons who are emotionally joined, who live in close geographic proximity.

Function: The kind of action or activity proper to a person in a certain role, for example, functions of a professional nurse.

Geography: The physical features of an area; the physical components of land, sea, air and the plant and animal life that are supported by these physical features.

Goal: A specific end as a result of design, not chance.

Good Samaritan law: A state law intended to encourage health professionals to offer assistance in emergency situations.

Group: An assembly of persons who share specific functions or goals and who interact over time.

Growth: An actual biologic or quantitative increase in physical size, that is, the enlargement of any body component by an increase in the number of cells.

Health: A state of complete physical, mental, and social well-being, not merely the absence of disease or infirmity (World Health Organization, 1947, Ch. 6).

Health behavior: Actions by persons who believe they are well to avoid an encounter with illness.

Health care delivery: The methods of and approaches to health care, sometimes described as a system or as an industry.

Health education: Facilitating persons' learning to live and adapt in the healthiest possible style, a shared responsibility of health professionals.

Health maintenance organization: A group health care practice whose major distinguishing feature is prepayment.

Health promotion: Increasing the level of one's well-being and actualizing one's health potential.

Health promotion behavior: Behavior directed toward increasing the level of well-being and actualizing the health potential of individuals, families, communities, and society.

Health protection behavior: Preventive behavior that is directed toward decreasing the probability of illness, facilitating early diagnosis and treatment of disease, and rehabilitating following disease.

High-level wellness: An integrated method of functioning that is oriented toward maximizing the potential of which the individual is capable within the environment in which he is functioning (Dunn, 1959, Ch. 6).

Holism: A theory that the universe, and especially living nature, is correctly seen as interacting wholes that are more than the mere sum of elementary particles; a theory that describes the parts of a person as dependent on each other and coordinated in a systematic fashion (Smuts, 1926, Ch. 4).

Homeodynamics: A reciprocal interaction of living systems that maintains a balance within each system and a balance among them.

Hospice: An agency devoted to providing care to persons with life-limiting illnesses either in their own home or in a residence facility, with a focus on the entire family.

Humanistic approaches to learning: Those philosophical approaches to learning that emphasize affective or feeling responses to learning; growing out of humanistic or "third force" psychology, these approaches are also sometimes called "existential" or "phenomenologic."

Illness: A dynamic process, a disturbance in equilibrium between humans and their environments; illness is a reaction of the whole organism, a consequence of factors in a reaction, that is, internal and external stimuli as well as predisposition of the individual.

Illness behavior: The initial response of the person to psychological and somatic cues that are perceived as incapacitating, and therefore are signs of illness.

Implementing: The activation of the care plan.

Independent nursing behavior: Those activities initiated as a result of the nurse's own knowledge and skill rather than as a result of delegated authority from another, for example, a physician.

Inductive reasoning: The process of relating reality and past experience to principles or generalities.

Influence: The power of producing effects by invisible or insensible means.

Information superhighway: That channel of communication in cyberspace created by linking computer networks globally.

Interdependent nursing behavior: Those activities that overlap functions or activities of other health professionals; this type of nursing behavior recognizes the desirability of collegial relationships in which each profession contributes according to knowledge, skills, or focus.

Interview: An interaction with a purpose.

Intuition: The ability to obtain knowledge without the apparent use of rational processes; involves direct cognition and rapid insight.

Knowledge deficit: "The state in which the individual experiences a deficiency in cognitive knowledge or psychomotor skills that alters or may alter health." (Carpenito, 1984, p. 42).

Lateral thinking: A process of divergent thinking as contrasted with the vertical thinking processes of inductive and deductive reasoning; also called flexibility, or creative or innovative thinking.

Learning: Involves a change in behavior and implies adaptation to a behavioral situation; occurs in three domains: (1) cognitive or thinking, (2) affective or feeling, and (3) psychomotor (action or skills).

Legal right: A claim recognized and enforceable by law.

Liability: Responsibility or obligation because of position or particular circumstances; a legal responsibility for professional behavior.

Lifelong learning: Behavioral changes over time that contribute to personal empowerment and career advancement for professionals.

Litigation: A trial in court to settle legal issues; a lawsuit.

Maladaptation: The process of using inadequate ways of dealing with stress in an attempt to maintain equilibrium.

Malpractice: Negligence in carrying out professional services; improper professional action.

Managed care: The organization of unit-based care so that specific client outcomes can be achieved within fiscally responsible time frames.

Mandatory licensure: A kind of state law controlling nursing practice; requires all persons who nurse for compensation to be licensed.

Maturation: Development of cells until they can be completely used by the organism.

Maturational (normative, developmental) crisis: Expected life changes such as birth, puberty, marriage, pregnancy, and so forth.

Medicaid: Title XIX of the Social Security Act of 1966, which provides health care insurance for certain needy and low-income persons.

Medicare: Title XVIII of the Social Security Act of 1966, which provides health care insurance for persons older than age 65 years and for certain other persons.

Mentor: A person who assumes professional sponsorship for a less-experienced colleague.

Motivation: That which stimulates or moves someone to learn; whereas children are primarily motivated to learn by extrinsic rewards, adults are more likely to be motivated by intrinsic rewards.

NANDA: The North American Nursing Diagnoses Association, formerly known as the National Group for the Classification of Nursing Diagnoses.

National health insurance: A proposed insurance program that would provide guaranteed coverage so that health care could be obtained by everyone.

Negligence: Failure to exercise that degree of care required by law for the protection of others.

NIC: Nursing Interventions Classification: A classification of nursing interventions linked to the NANDA nursing diagnoses.

NOC: Nursing-Sensitive Outcomes Classification: An outcomes classification for patient care developed by a research team at the University of Iowa.

Noise: Unwanted sound.

Norms: Expected behavior that provides rules about standards of appropriate behavior in particular situations.

Nosocomial infection: Infection that originates in a hospital or medical facility.

Novice: A person who is new to the practice of nursing.

Nursing diagnosis: The conclusion drawn by the nurse, or the nurse and the person, from the data collected in the various functional areas; may represent a strength, a need, or a problem.

Nursing process: A series of five scientific steps that assist the nurse in using theoretical knowledge to diagnose the strengths and the nursing needs of persons and to implement therapeutic actions to attain, maintain, and promote optimal biopsychosocial functioning and to evaluate the client's progress.

Nursing research: Scientific study or investigation about nursing practice.

Nursing science: That body of unique knowledge derived from scientific thinking about the discipline or field of nursing and/or the profession of nursing.

Nursing theory: The systematic abstraction or formation of mental ideas about nursing practice reality.

Object permanence: Realization by a child that objects can exist apart from himself or herself; understanding that although he or she may not see the object, it still exists.

Open system: A system that can exchange matter, energy, and information with its environment.

Operation: An interiorized action, or an action performed in the mind (Piaget).

Paternalism: Fatherly interference with a person's autonomy or independence.

Pathogens: Microorganisms that are capable of causing disease.

Patient (adjective): To bear pains or trials calmly and without complaint; to be steadfast despite opposition or adversity; to be able or willing to bear.

Patient (noun): An individual awaiting or under medical care and treatment; the recipient of any of various person services.

Permissive licensure: A kind of state law controlling nursing practice; it permitted nurses to practice without a license if they did not claim licensure or use the RN (registered nurse) initials.

Person: A unique human who has some characteristics in common with others as well as his or her own individual thoughts, feelings, and ways of responding.

Person–environment fit: The match between needs and resources of the individual and demands and resources of the environment.

Planning: Decisions by the nurse and client about the outcomes to be achieved and the actions both need to take.

Policy: A purposefully chosen plan of action (or inaction) aimed toward some end.

Politics: Power and control; promotion of an interest using whatever resources are available to protect and advance it.

Position: Synthesis of related roles that represent the location of persons in a social system.

Possible problem: A problem for which some data have been obtained, but not enough to identify it as an actual problem.

Potential problem: A problem the person is at high risk of developing, given that person's particular situation.

Power: The ability to secure a particular outcome.

Preventive health care: Activities that promote health by reducing factors that contribute to illness and by reinforcing a person's strengths.

Primary nursing: A system of nursing care that renders the nurse responsible and accountable, although not necessarily present or available, on a 24-hour basis.

Primary preventive health care: Intervention with persons who have no symptoms but who are at risk for developing behaviors that could diminish their health.

Principle: An essential element or motivating force that serves as a basis for action.

Problem: A situation that requires specific action to be taken.

Professionalism: Professional character, spirit, or methods; also, activities found in various occupational groups whose members aspire to be professional.

Professionalization: The process of acquiring or changing characteristics in the direction of a profession.

Professions: Traditionally, the occupations of medicine, law, and the ministry.

Psychological competence: Ability to function adequately cognitively, emotionally, and behaviorally.

Psychomotor learning or behavior: Involves actions or skills.

Quality assurance: The establishment of professional standards and the monitoring of performance by colleagues.

Quality of life: The subjective experience of well-being that includes physical, mental, and social dimensions.

Reasonable care: That degree of skill and knowledge customarily used by a competent health practitioner of similar education and experience in treating and caring for the sick and injured in the community in which the individual is practicing or learning his or her profession.

Responsible consumerism: The act of controlling and providing input into those things that affect one as an individual; it is an obligation as well as a right.

Role: Set of expected behaviors, normatively defined, that serves to make behavior predictable.

Schema: A more complex mental image, an action organization that a person uses to explain what he or she sees and hears (Piaget).

Science: Knowledge gained by systematic study.

Scientific method: The most advanced approach to acquiring knowledge and solving scientific problems. Comprised of four steps: 1) define the problem 2) collect data from observation and experimentation 3) devise and execute a solution 4) evaluate the solution.

Secondary preventive health care: Education, counseling, and treatment that assist persons to minimize factors that are a part of their lifestyles and that could affect their health.

Self-care: Activities that individuals personally initiate on their own behalf in maintaining or enhancing life, health, and well-being (Orem).

Self-concept: A collection of notions, feelings, and beliefs about the self with which one identifies and through which one relates and communicates with others and interacts with the environment.

Self-esteem: One's personal judgment of one's own worth.

Self-ideal: How one believes he or she ought to function and behave given his or her personal value system and set of personal standards.

Sensory overload and sensory deprivation: Syndromes caused by too much or too little sensory stimulation, characterized by altered perception and disorientation.

Situational (accidental) crisis: Unexpected or hazardous events such as illness, catastrophic circumstances, and natural disasters.

Social support: Interpersonal transactions that include expression of positive affect. Affirmation of another's behaviors or perceptions and giving aid to another.

Societies: Groups of people sufficiently organized to carry out the conditions necessary to live together.

Standard: Something set up and established by authority as a rule for the measure of quantity, weight, extent, value, or quality.

Strength: An internal resource; a biologic, psychological, social, or spiritual quality that contributes to a person's character, integrity, and uniqueness and that can be mobilized to cope with a problem or to attain a goal.

Stress: The nonspecific response of the body to any demand made on it (Selye); everyday wear and tear of living.

Stressor: Anything that induces stress; the stimulus that places demands on persons to prepare for change (e.g., pain, cold, or a test).

Structure: The way in which information is organized within the person to make a simple mental image or pattern of action (Piaget).

Subculture: A system of patterns and meanings that has shared characteristics of a larger culture but also has characteristics that are unqiue.

System: "An organized unit with a set of components that mutually react" (Abbey, 1978, pp. 20–21).

Teachable moment: A circumstance in which a learner is uniquely motivated or susceptible to motivation.

Teaching: A special type of communication that is carefully structured and sequenced to produce learning; a direct or indirect communication intended to facilitate learning.

Teleological: A classification of ethical theory; belief that ends justify the means.

Tertiary care: That care that occurs in highly specialized institutions that provide sophisticated diagnosis and treatment.

Tertiary preventive health care: Care that focuses on persons who have encountered a specific stressor that has already compromised their health.

Torts: Civil wrongs that may be intentional or unintentional; violations of reasonable behavior.

23-hour admission: An admission less than a full 24-hour day, making reimbursement different and to the advantage of both the agency and the insurer.

Universal Precautions: Special techniques for handling and coming into contact with blood and body fluids.

Utilitarianism: An approach to ethics that advocates the greatest good for the greatest number.

Value: A belief or a custom that frequently arises from cultural or ethnic backgrounds, family tradition, peer group ideas and practices, political philosophies in one's country, and educational and religious philosophies with which one identifies.

Value judgment: A personal decision about whether something is right or wrong.

Variable: "A characteristic or attribute of a person or object that varies (i.e., takes on different values) within the population under study (e.g., body temperature, age, heart rate)" (Polit & Hungler, 1991, p. 657).

Violence: Any nonaccidental act that results in physical or psychological injury including homicide, assault, rape, sexual abuse, emotional abuse, and physical abuse.

Virtual reality: Interactive audiovisual presentations via computer that enable a viewer to participate in realistic simulations of actual or imagined situations for entertainment or educational experience.

Wellness: A dynamic process, a condition of change in which the person moves toward a higher potential of functioning.

Work redesign: A restructuring of the system of a particular type of work; a changing of the actual structure of the job performed.

Index

Page numbers followed by *f* indicate illustrations; those followed by *t* indicate tabular material.